MCQs in Radiology for Residents & Technologists

MCQs in Radiology for Residents & Technologists

Second Edition

Dr. SUMEET BHARGAVA
MBBS, DNB (Radiodiagnosis); MNAMS; FCGP; FIAMS; FICRI
Assistant Professor, Deptt. of Radiology and Imaging,
Rama Medical College & Superspeciality Hospital,
Delhi-Hapur Road, Hapur

and

Prof. (Dr.) SATISH K. BHARGAVA
Head, Department of Radiology and Imaging,
Rama Medical College & Superspeciality Hospital,
Delhi-Hapur Road, Hapur
Formerly: Head, Deptt. of Radiology & Imaging,
University College of Medical Sciences (Delhi University) and
associated G.T.B. Hospital,
Dilshad Garden, Delhi-110095

CBSPD

CBS Publishers & Distributors Pvt Ltd

New Delhi • Bengaluru • Chennai • Kochi • Kolkata • Lucknow • Mumbai
Hyderabad • Jharkhand • Nagpur • Patna • Pune • Uttarakhand

MCQs in
Radiology for
Residents and Technologists
Second Edition

ISBN: 978-93-86217-63-9

Second Edition: 2017
Reprint: 2017, 2018, 2019, 2020, 2021, 2022, 2023, 2024, 2025
2026
First Edition: 2012
Reprint: 2015

Published by **Satish Kumar** Jain and Produced by **Varun Jain** for
CBS Publishers & Distributors Pvt Ltd
4819/XI Prahlad Street, 24 Ansari Road, Daryaganj, New Delhi 110 002, India.
Ph: 011-23289259, 23266861, 23266867 Fax: 011-23243014 Website: www.cbspd.com
e-mail: delhi@cbspd.com; cbspubs@airtelmail.in.

Corporate Office: 204 FIE, Industrial Area, Patparganj, Delhi 110 092, India
Ph: 011-4934 4934 Fax: 011-4934 4935 e-mail: publishing@cbspd.com; publicity@cbspd.com

Branches

- **Bengaluru:** Seema House 2975, 17th Cross, KR Road, Banasankari 2nd Stage, Bengaluru 560 070, Karnataka, India
  Ph: +91-80-26771678/79 Fax: +91-80-26771680 e-mail: bangalore@cbspd.com
- **Chennai:** 18/8B, Subbaraya Street, Shenoy Nagar, Chennai 600 030, Tamil Nadu, India
  Ph: +91-044-42032115, 044-26681266 e-mail: chennai@cbspd.com
- **Kochi:** 42/1325, 1326, Power House Road, Opp KSEB, Power House, Ernakulam Kochi 682 018, Kerala, India
  Ph: +91-484-4059061-65,67 Fax: +91-484-4059065 e-mail: kochi@cbspd.com
- **Kolkata:** 147, Hind Ceramics Compound, 1st Floor, Nilgunj Road, Belghoria, Kolkata-700056, West Bengal, India
  Ph: +033-25633055, 033-25633056 e-mail: kolkata@cbspd.com
- **Lucknow:** Basement, Khushnuma Complex, 7 Meerabai Marg (Behind Jawahar Bhawan), Lucknow-226001, UP, India
  Ph: +0522-4000032 e-mail: tiwari.lucknow@cbspd.com
- **Mumbai:** PWD Shed, Gala no 25/26, Ramchandra Bhatt Marg, Next to JJ Hospital Gate no. 2, Opp. Union Bank of India, Noorbaug, Mumbai-400009, Maharashtra, India
  Ph: 022-66661880/89 e-mail: mumbai@cbspd.com

Representatives

- Gujarat • Hyderabad • Jharkhand • Nagpur • Patna • Pune • Uttarakhand

For trade terms please contact customercare@cbspd.com
For general enquiries please contact info@cbspd.com

Printed at Glorious Printers, Jhilmil Industrial Area, Delhi, India

Preface to the Second Edition

With the process of digitization in the country progressing and to keep more transparency, more and more institutions and examining bodies are opting for MCQs as mode of recruitment.

Keeping in view the above and more demand of MCQs by the readers, it was decided to update the book with large number of important MCQs so as to benefit the students. I am sure our sincere efforts will be helpful to the aspirants.

Sumeet Bhargava
Satish K. Bhargava

Preface to the First Edition

It is an overwhelming situation/occasion when our young students want to take up as a career in the professional institution to do M.B.B.S. or technologist course in Radiology like B.Sc. Medical Imaging technologist or M.Sc. Medical Imaging Technologist course. There are a lot of mixed moments of joy, euphoria and depression during this period of preparation because of change of the perception from theoretical knowledge to a competition. The popularity of the Radiology in this imaging era and the pivotal role played by the technologists, the book has been prepared with most expected MCQs covering almost all from basic to the latest in the imaging including artifacts. The pattern of the questions vary from simple, straight forward to tough ones, which offer a good mental exercise to all. The standard Textbook of Radiology has been used to prepare these MCQs and the answer appeared are standard and universally accepted. The book is one of its kind as it offers complete preparation of the subject aiming to get entrance examination for technologist, M.B.B.S. and F.R.C.R. examination.

Sumeet Bhargava
Satish K. Bhargava

List of Contributors

1. **Prof. Satish K. Bhargava**
   Head, Department of Radiology & Imaging,
   Rama Medical College & Superspeciality Hospital,
   Delhi-Hapur Road, Hapur

2. **Dr. Sumeet Bhargava**
   Assistant Professor, Department of Radiology & Imaging,
   Rama Medical College & Superspeciality Hospital,
   Delhi-Hapur Road, Hapur

3. **Dr. Anurag Agarwal**
   Additional Director, National Board of Examination,
   Ansari Nagar, New Delhi

4. **Ms. Rachna Khera Murdeshwar**
   R.S.O. & Ex Lecturer,
   Symbiosis Institute of Health Science, Pune

5. **Dr. Swati Gupta**
   Ex Resident, Department of Radiology & Imaging,
   University College of Medical Sciences (Delhi University)
   and G.T.B. Hospital, Dilshad Garden, Delhi-110095

6. **Packia Agnes Vimalan**
   Ex Resident, Department of Radiology & Imaging,
   University College of Medical Sciences (Delhi University)
   and G.T.B. Hospital, Dilshad Garden, Delhi-110095

7. **Niranjan Baghel**
   Radiological Technologist, Deptt. of Radiology & Imaging, Vardhman Mahavir Medical College (VMMC) and associated Safdarjung Hospital, New Delhi

8. **Ms. Usha**
   Technologist, Department of Radiodiagnosis & Imaging, Postgraduate Institute of Medical Sciences & Research, Chandigarh.

9. **Dinesh K. Baghel**
   Medical Physicist,
   Department of Medical Physics & Radiation Oncology, Delhi State Cancer Institute, (DSCI), New Delhi

10. **Ms. Bushra Khan**
    Sr. Lecturer, SAHS Sharda University,
    Greater Noida

11. **Ms. Ankita Deshmana**
    Lecturer, SAHS Sharda University,
    Greater Noida

Contents

CHAPTER

1

Anatomy and Physiology

1. Posterior communicating artery is the branch of

(a) External carotid
(b) Internal carotid
(c) Ophthalmic
(d) Middle cerebral

Ans. (b). *Textbook of Radiology for Residents & Technicians, 5th ed., S.K. Bhargava & Sumeet Bhargava, p. 48-96.*

2. The vertebral artery traverses all of the following except

(a) Foramen magnum
(b) Subarachnoid space
(c) Intervertebral foramen
(d) Foramen transversarium

Ans. (c). *Textbook of Radiology for Residents & Technicians, 5th ed., S.K. Bhargava & Sumeet Bhargava, p. 48-96.*

3. All of the following are the branches of the external carotid artery except

(a) Superior thyroid artery
(b) Anterior ethmoidal artery
(c) Occipital artery
(d) Posterior auricular artery

Ans. (b). *Textbook of Radiology for Residents & Technicians, 5th ed., S.K. Bhargava & Sumeet Bhargava, p. 48-96.*

4. Which one of the following found in the mandibular canal

(a) Lingual artery
(b) Mental artery
(c) Myelohyoid nerve
(d) Inferior alveolar nerve

Ans. (d). *Textbook of Radiology for Residents & Technicians, 5th ed., S.K. Bhargava & Sumeet Bhargava, p. 48-96.*

5. Skull consists of _______ bones.

(a) 20
(b) 22
(c) 24
(d) 28

Ans. (b). *Textbook of Radiology for Residents & Technicians, 5th ed., S.K. Bhargava & Sumeet Bhargava, p. 1-20.*

6. Following foramen are found in greater wing of the sphenoid except

(a) Rotundum (b) Ovale
(c) Spinosum (d) Optic canal

Ans. (d). *Textbook of Radiology for Residents & Technicians, 5th ed., S.K. Bhargava & Sumeet Bhargava, p. 1-20.*

7. Isthmus of the tracheal gland is across _______ tracheal ring.

(a) 2nd to 4th (b) 3rd to 5th
(c) 5th and 6th (d) 4th only

Ans. (a). *Textbook of Radiology for Residents & Technicians, 5th ed., S.K. Bhargava & Sumeet Bhargava, p. 1-20.*

8. The length of the external acoustic meatus is approximately

(a) 16 mm (b) 20 mm
(c) 24 mm (d) 30 mm

Ans. (c). *Textbook of Radiology for Residents & Technicians, 5th ed., S.K. Bhargava & Sumeet Bhargava, p. 1-20.*

9. Common carotid artery usually bifurcates at the level of _______ cervical vertebrae.

(a) 4th (b) 5th
(c) 3rd (d) 2nd

Ans. (a). *Textbook of Radiology for Residents & Technicians, 5th ed., S.K. Bhargava & Sumeet Bhargava, p. 48-96.*

10. Which of the following does not pass through jugular foramen?

(a) Internal jugular vein (b) Internal carotid artery
(c) Inferior petrosal sinus (d) ix, x, xi cranial nerves

Ans. (b). *Textbook of Radiology for Residents & Technicians, 5th ed., S.K. Bhargava & Sumeet Bhargava, p. 48-96.*

11. Crista galli is a crest on _______ bone.

(a) Sphenoid (b) Frontal
(c) Ethmoid (d) Occipital

Ans. (c). *Textbook of Radiology for Residents & Technicians, 5th ed., S.K. Bhargava & Sumeet Bhargava, p. 1-20.*

12. Bifurcation of the trachea is at the level of

(a) Upper border of third thoracic vertebrae
(b) Lower border of third thoracic vertebrae

(c) Upper border of second thoracic vertebrae
(d) Lower border of fourth thoracic vertebrae

Ans. (d). Textbook of Radiology for Residents & Technicians, 5th ed., S.K. Bhargava & Sumeet Bhargava, p. 48-96.

13. Dentate nucleus is a part of

(a) Mid brain (b) Pons
(c) Medulla (d) Cerebellum

Ans. (d). Textbook of Radiology for Residents & Technicians, 5th ed., S.K. Bhargava & Sumeet Bhargava, p. 48-96.

14. True about orbit is

(a) Medial wall formed by frontal, lacrimal and maxillary bone
(b) Infra-orbital foramen opens at the junction of medial 1/3rd and lateral 1/3rd
(c) Lateral wall is formed by lesser wing of sphenoid, zygomatic, temporal bones
(d) Nasal aperture is formed by frontal, temporal bone

Ans. (a). Textbook of Radiology for Residents & Technicians, 5th ed., S.K. Bhargava & Sumeet Bhargava, p. 48-96.

15. C.S.F. is principally secreted by

(a) Arachnoid granulation (b) Choroid plexus
(c) Floor of IV ventricle (d) Peri aqueduct gray matter

Ans. (b). Textbook of Radiology for Residents & Technicians, 5th ed., S.K. Bhargava & Sumeet Bhargava, p. 48-96.

16. Filum terminale is formed by

(a) Pia mater (b) Arachnoid
(c) Dura mater (d) Spinal cord

Ans. (a). Textbook of Radiology for Residents & Technicians, 5th ed., S.K. Bhargava & Sumeet Bhargava, p. 48-96.

17. Complete sulcus is

(a) Calcrine sulcus (b) Central sulcus
(c) Temporal sulcus (d) Frontal sulcus

Ans. (a). Textbook of Radiology for Residents & Technicians, 5th ed., S.K. Bhargava & Sumeet Bhargava, p. 48-96.

18. In brain, there is maximum representation of

(a) Thumb (b) Face
(c) Trunk (d) Leg

Ans. (a). Textbook of Radiology for Residents & Technicians, 5th ed., S.K. Bhargava & Sumeet Bhargava, p. 1-20.

19. The weight of the pituitary gland is

(a) 2.0 gm (b) 1.0 gm
(c) 1.5 gm (d) 0.5 gm

Ans. (d). *Textbook of Radiology for Residents & Technicians, 5th ed., S.K. Bhargava & Sumeet Bhargava, p. 48-96.*

20. The oldest part of cerebellum is

(a) Paleocerebellum (b) Archicerebellum
(c) Neocerebellum (d) Lingula

Ans. (b). *Textbook of Radiology for Residents & Technicians, 5th ed., S.K. Bhargava & Sumeet Bhargava, p. 48-96.*

21. The circle of the Willis is formed by the following arteries except

(a) The anterior cerebral artery
(b) Anterior communicating artery
(c) Posterior cerebral arteries and Posterior communicating artery
(d) Middle cerebral artery

Ans. (d). *Textbook of Radiology for Residents & Technicians, 5th ed., S.K. Bhargava & Sumeet Bhargava, p. 48-96.*

22. The filum terminale is composed of

(a) Pia mater (b) Dura mater
(c) Ganglion cell (d) White matter

Ans. (a). *Textbook of Radiology for Residents & Technicians, 5th ed., S.K. Bhargava & Sumeet Bhargava, p. 48-96.*

23. Cerebellopontine angle contains all except

(a) Styloglossus (b) Stylopharyngeus
(c) Palatoglossus (d) Hypoglossus

Ans. (d). *Textbook of Radiology for Residents & Technicians, 5th ed., S.K. Bhargava & Sumeet Bhargava, p. 48-96.*

24. Hilum of the right lung is arched by

(a) Recurrent laryngeal nerve (b) Azygous vein
(c) Thoracic duct (d) Superior vena cava

Ans. (b). *Textbook of Radiology for Residents & Technicians, 5th ed., S.K. Bhargava & Sumeet Bhargava, p. 48-96.*

25. Bronchopulmonary segment contains all of the followings, except

(a) Independent pulmonary artery
(b) Independent pulmonary vein
(c) Tertiary bronchiole
(d) Conical segment

Ans. (b). Textbook of Radiology for Residents & Technicians, 5th ed., S.K. Bhargava & Sumeet Bhargava, p. 48-96.

26. Right middle lobe consists of which broncho-pulmonary segment

(a) Superior and inferior (b) Medial and lateral
(c) Anterior and posterior (d) Apical and lateral

Ans. (b). Textbook of Radiology for Residents & Technicians, 5th ed., S.K. Bhargava & Sumeet Bhargava, p. 1-20.

27. Broncho-pulmonary segment is a unit in the architecture of the lung. The best guide to the intersegment planes would be the

(a) Segmental bronchi
(b) Branches of the segmental artery
(c) Veins draining the segment
(d) Connective tissue septa

Ans. (c). Textbook of Radiology for Residents & Technicians, 5th ed., S.K. Bhargava & Sumeet Bhargava, p. 1-20.

28. The functional tissue of lung is

(a) Alveoli (b) Bronchi
(c) Respiratory bronchiole (d) Terminal bronchiole

Ans. (a). Textbook of Radiology for Residents & Technicians, 5th ed., S.K. Bhargava & Sumeet Bhargava, p. 1-20.

29. The blood supply of the lung tissue is

(a) Pulmonary veins (b) Pulmonary arteries
(c) Bronchial arteries (d) Lower thoracic aorta

Ans. (c). Textbook of Radiology for Residents & Technicians, 5th ed., S.K. Bhargava & Sumeet Bhargava, p. 48-96.

30. Lingula is a part of

(a) Left upper lobe (b) Left lower lobe
(c) Right upper lobe (d) Right middle lobe

Ans. (a). Textbook of Radiology for Residents & Technicians, 5th ed., S.K. Bhargava & Sumeet Bhargava, p. 48-96.

31. The most dependant part of the lung in the supine position is

(a) Upper atria (b) Lower apical
(c) Basal (d) Upper anterior

Ans. (b). Textbook of Radiology for Residents & Technicians, 5th ed., S.K. Bhargava & Sumeet Bhargava, p. 1-20.

32. Base of the heart is formed by

(a) Left apical (b) Both atria

(c) Right atria
(d) Left ventricle

Ans. (b). Textbook of Radiology for Residents & Technicians, 5th ed., S.K. Bhargava & Sumeet Bhargava, p. 48-96.

33. Inferior surface of the heart is formed by

(a) Right and left ventricles
(b) Separated from base by right ventricle
(c) Posterior AV groove
(d) Right and left atria

Ans. (a). Textbook of Radiology for Residents & Technicians, 5th ed., S.K. Bhargava & Sumeet Bhargava, p. 48-96.

34. Superior vena cava is formed at the level of

(a) First costal cartilage
(b) First intercostal space
(c) Second intercostal space
(d) Second costal cartilage

Ans. (a). Textbook of Radiology for Residents & Technicians, 5th ed., S.K. Bhargava & Sumeet Bhargava, p. 48-96.

35. Which is true regarding the membranous part of the septum?

(a) Situated at the anterosuperior part of the septum
(b) Separates right ventricle from left atrium
(c) Separates left ventricle from right atrium
(d) All of the above

Ans. (a). Textbook of Radiology for Residents & Technicians, 5th ed., S.K. Bhargava & Sumeet Bhargava, p. 48-96.

36. Erb's point is

(a) C4, C5
(b) C5, C6
(c) C6, C7
(d) C7, C8, T1

Ans. (d). Textbook of Radiology for Residents & Technicians, 5th ed., S.K. Bhargava & Sumeet Bhargava, p. 21-47.

37. The medial wall of the axilla is formed by

(a) Serratus
(b) Subcapsularis muscle
(c) Pectoralis major muscle
(d) Teres major muscle

Ans. (a). Textbook of Radiology for Residents & Technicians, 5th ed., S.K. Bhargava & Sumeet Bhargava, p. 48-96.

38. Clavicular part of the deltoid is associated with

(a) Lateral rotation
(b) Medial
(c) Abduction
(d) Adduction

Ans. (b). Textbook of Radiology for Residents & Technicians, 5th ed., S.K. Bhargava & Sumeet Bhargava, p. 48-96.

39. Nerve supply of the nail blade of the thumb is

(a) Median (b) Ulnar
(c) Radial (d) All of the above

Ans. (a). *Textbook of Radiology for Residents & Technicians, 5th ed., S.K. Bhargava & Sumeet Bhargava, p. 48-96.*

40. Elevation of the scapula is caused by except

(a) Trapezius (b) Levator scapulae
(c) Lattismus dorsi (d) Rhomboid major

Ans. (c). *Textbook of Radiology for Residents & Technicians, 5th ed., S.K. Bhargava & Sumeet Bhargava, p. 48-96.*

41. The following structure pass through the carpal tunnel except

(a) Flexure digitorum profundus (b) Flexure pollucis longus
(c) Median nerve (d) Ulnar nerve

Ans. (d). *Textbook of Radiology for Residents & Technicians, 5th ed., S.K. Bhargava & Sumeet Bhargava, p. 48-96.*

42. Winging of the scapula is due to injury to

(a) Nerve supplying serratus anterior
(b) Pectoralis nerve
(c) Subscapular nerve
(d) Ulnar nerve

Ans. (a). *Textbook of Radiology for Residents & Technicians, 5th ed., S.K. Bhargava & Sumeet Bhargava, p. 48-96.*

43. "Dropped shoulder" occurs due to paralysis of

(a) Deltoid (b) Trapezius
(c) Deltoid and teres minor (d) Serratus anterior

Ans. (b). *Textbook of Radiology for Residents & Technicians, 5th ed., S.K. Bhargava & Sumeet Bhargava, p. 48-96.*

44. The floor of the Femoral triangle is formed by all, except

(a) Adductor longus (b) Psoas major
(c) Pectineus (d) Sartorius

Ans. (d). *Textbook of Radiology for Residents & Technicians, 5th ed., S.K. Bhargava & Sumeet Bhargava, p. 1-20.*

45. Artery in anatomical snuff box

(a) Radial (b) Brachial
(c) Ulnar (d) Interosseous

Ans. (a). *Textbook of Radiology for Residents & Technicians, 5th ed., S.K. Bhargava & Sumeet Bhargava, p. 1-20.*

46. Femoral ring is bounded by the following structures except

(a) Femoral vein
(b) Inguinal ligament
(c) Femoral artery
(d) Lacunar ligament

Ans. (c). *Textbook of Radiology for Residents & Technicians, 5th ed., S.K. Bhargava & Sumeet Bhargava, p. 1-20.*

47. Deep palmar arch

(a) Formed by the continuation of the radial artery
(b) Gives 3 digital branches
(c) Lies behind lumbricals
(d) Lies at proximal palmar crease

Ans. (a). *Textbook of Radiology for Residents & Technicians, 5th ed., S.K. Bhargava & Sumeet Bhargava, p. 1-20.*

48. Longest ligament around the hip joint is

(a) Iliofemoral
(b) Ischiofemoral
(c) Pubofemoral
(d) Ligamentous teres

Ans. (a). *Textbook of Radiology for Residents & Technicians, 5th ed., S.K. Bhargava & Sumeet Bhargava, p. 48-90.*

49. Short saphenous vein is a tributary of

(a) Medial marginal vein
(b) Popliteal vein
(c) Posterior tibial vein
(d) Dorsal venous arch

Ans. (b). *Textbook of Radiology for Residents & Technicians, 5th ed., S.K. Bhargava & Sumeet Bhargava, p. 1-20.*

50. Foot drop is caused by damage to

(a) Interrosseous nerve
(b) Superficial peroneal nerve
(c) Deep peroneal nerve
(d) Deltoid ligament of the ankle joint

Ans. (c). *Textbook of Radiology for Residents & Technicians, 5th ed., S.K. Bhargava & Sumeet Bhargava, p. 48-96.*

51. Femoral nerve does not supply to

(a) Sartorius
(b) Rectus femoris
(c) Tensor fasciae latae
(d) Articularis genu

Ans. (c). *Textbook of Radiology for Residents & Technicians, 5th ed., S.K. Bhargava & Sumeet Bhargava, p. 1-20.*

52. Which of the following muscles are flexors of the thigh?

(a) Psoas
(b) Pectineus
(c) Rectus femoris
(d) Vastus lateralis

Ans. (a). Textbook of Radiology for Residents & Technicians, 5th ed., S.K. Bhargava & Sumeet Bhargava, p. 1-20.

53. The following structures pass through the sub-sartorial canal, except the

(a) Posterior division of the obturator nerve
(b) Saphenous nerve
(c) Femoral artery
(d) Nerve to vastus intermedius

Ans. (d). Textbook of Radiology for Residents & Technicians, 5th ed., S.K. Bhargava & Sumeet Bhargava, p. 1-20.

54. Saphenous opening is situated

(a) Just above the pubic tubercle
(b) Just below the pubic tubercle
(c) Above and medial to pubic tubercle
(d) Below and lateral to pubic tubercle

Ans. (d). Textbook of Radiology for Residents & Technicians, 5th ed., S.K. Bhargava & Sumeet Bhargava, p. 1-20.

55. All of the following are abductors of hip joint except

(a) Gluteus maximus
(b) Gluteus minimus
(c) Gluteus medius
(d) Tensor fascia latae

Ans. (a). Textbook of Radiology for Residents & Technicians, 5th ed., S.K. Bhargava & Sumeet Bhargava, p. 1-20.

56. Ascending part of duodenum is _______ cm long.

(a) 5
(b) 6
(c) 7.5
(d) 10.0

Ans. (a). Textbook of Radiology for Residents & Technicians, 5th ed., S.K. Bhargava & Sumeet Bhargava, p. 48-96.

57. The narrowest part of the ureter is at the

(a) Ureteropelvic junction
(b) Iliac vessel crossing
(c) Pelvic ureter
(d) Ureterovesical junction

Ans. (d). Textbook of Radiology for Residents & Technicians, 5th ed., S.K. Bhargava & Sumeet Bhargava, p. 48-96.

58. The gastroduodenal artery is derived from

(a) Celiac artery
(b) Hepatic artery
(c) Splenic artery
(d) It initiates cardiac conduction

Ans. (b). Textbook of Radiology for Residents & Technicians, 5th ed., S.K. Bhargava & Sumeet Bhargava, p. 48-96.

59. The neck of the pancreas is related on its posterior surface to

(a) Gastroduodenal artery
(b) Superior mesenteric vein
(c) Inferior vena cava
(d) Bile duct

Ans. (b). *Textbook of Radiology for Residents & Technicians, 5th ed., S.K. Bhargava & Sumeet Bhargava, p. 48-96.*

60. The right lobe of the liver consists of which of the following segments

(a) V, VI, VII & VIII
(b) IV, V, VI, VII & VIII
(c) I, V, VI, VII & VIII
(d) I, IV, V, VI, VII & VIII

Ans. (a). *Textbook of Radiology for Residents & Technicians, 5th ed., S.K. Bhargava & Sumeet Bhargava, p. 48-96.*

61. The prostatic urethrae is characterized by all of the following features, except that it

(a) Is the widest and most dilatable part
(b) Presents a concavity posteriorly
(c) Lies closer to anterior surface of prostate
(d) Receives prostatic ductules along its posterior wall

Ans. (b). *Textbook of Radiology for Residents & Technicians, 5th ed., S.K. Bhargava & Sumeet Bhargava, p. 48-96.*

62. Which of the following structures is not present within the lesser omentum?

(a) Portal vein
(b) Bile duct
(c) Inferior vena cava
(d) Hepatic artery

Ans. (c). *Textbook of Radiology for Residents & Technicians, 5th ed., S.K. Bhargava & Sumeet Bhargava, p. 48-96.*

63. The abdominal organ most frequently injured is

(a) Spleen
(b) Liver
(c) Kidney
(d) Pancreas

Ans. (a). *Textbook of Radiology for Residents & Technicians, 5th ed., S.K. Bhargava & Sumeet Bhargava, p. 48-96.*

64. False about mesentery is

(a) Sigmoid mesentery develops from apex
(b) Breadth of the mesentery is in central part (about 8 inches lower part)
(c) Intestinal border is 6 m long
(d) Fat is most abundant in lower part

Ans. (a). *Textbook of Radiology for Residents & Technicians, 5th ed., S.K. Bhargava & Sumeet Bhargava, p. 48-96.*

65. One of the branches of the celiac artery is the

(a) Right gastric (b) Common hepatic
(c) Gastroduodenal (d) Left gastroepiploic

Ans. (b). *Textbook of Radiology for Residents & Technicians, 5th ed., S.K. Bhargava & Sumeet Bhargava, p. 48-96.*

66. The Appendix may be found most often in the _______ space.

(a) Retrocaecal (b) Paracolic
(c) Subcaecal (d) Pelvic

Ans. (a). *Textbook of Radiology for Residents & Technicians, 5th ed., S.K. Bhargava & Sumeet Bhargava, p. 48-96.*

67. Which of the following is most posterior part of the stomach?

(a) Fundus (b) Body
(c) Cardiac orifice (d) Pylorus

Ans. (a). *Textbook of Radiology for Residents & Technicians, 5th ed., S.K. Bhargava & Sumeet Bhargava, p. 48-96.*

68. Meckel's diverticulum

(a) Contains all layers of the gut
(b) Represents the remains of the urachus
(c) Receives the blood supply from inferior mesenteric artery
(d) Represents the functional point of the mid and hind gut

Ans. (a). *Textbook of Radiology for Residents & Technicians, 5th ed., S.K. Bhargava & Sumeet Bhargava, p. 48-96.*

69. The shortest part of the colon is

(a) Ascending (b) Transverse
(c) Descending (d) Sigmoid

Ans. (a). *Textbook of Radiology for Residents & Technicians, 5th ed., S.K. Bhargava & Sumeet Bhargava, p. 48-96.*

70. The bloodless fold of Traves is

(a) Colocolic fold
(b) Jejunoileal fold
(c) Ileocaecal fold
(d) Is found in descending colon

Ans. (c). *Textbook of Radiology for Residents & Technicians, 5th ed., S.K. Bhargava & Sumeet Bhargava, p. 48-96.*

71. Superior mesenteric artery arises behind _______ and _______.

(a) Liver, T-12 (b) Pancreas, L-1
(c) Pancreas, L-2 (d) Spleen, L-2

Ans. ***(b).*** *Textbook of Radiology for Residents & Technicians, 5th ed., S.K. Bhargava & Sumeet Bhargava, p. 48-96.*

72. Following are the features of the ileum in contrast to jejunum except

(a) Thinner and less vascular
(b) Windows in mesentery
(c) Smaller and sparse circular mucosal folds
(d) Peyers patches are present

Ans. ***(b).*** *Textbook of Radiology for Residents & Technicians, 5th ed., S.K. Bhargava & Sumeet Bhargava, p. 48-96.*

73. Which is true regarding tail of pancreas?

(a) Lies in gastro splenic ligament
(b) Related to upper part of the spleen
(c) Has more islets of Langerhans
(d) Carcinoma is more common

Ans. ***(c).*** *Textbook of Radiology for Residents & Technicians, 5th ed., S.K. Bhargava & Sumeet Bhargava, p. 48-96.*

74. The pancreatic bed does not include

(a) Left kidney
(b) Splenic artery
(c) Left renal vein
(d) Left crus of the diaphragm

Ans. ***(b).*** *Textbook of Radiology for Residents & Technicians, 5th ed., S.K. Bhargava & Sumeet Bhargava, p. 48-96.*

75. Accessory pancreatic duct is also called _______ duct.

(a) Wirsung
(b) Bernard
(c) Hoffmann's
(d) Hensen's

Ans. ***(b).*** *Textbook of Radiology for Residents & Technicians, 5th ed., S.K. Bhargava & Sumeet Bhargava, p. 48-96.*

76. Pancreas is about _______ cm broad.

(a) 2
(b) 3
(c) 4
(d) 5

Ans. ***(b).*** *Textbook of Radiology for Residents & Technicians, 5th ed., S.K. Bhargava & Sumeet Bhargava, p. 48-96.*

77. The head of the pancreas is most likely related to which of the following?

(a) Second part of duodenum
(b) Spleen
(c) Left lobe of liver
(d) Ascending colon

Ans. ***(a).*** *Textbook of Radiology for Residents & Technicians, 5th ed., S.K. Bhargava & Sumeet Bhargava, p. 48-96.*

78. The length of ureter is

(a) 60 cm (b) 30 cm
(c) 25 cm (d) 45 cm

Ans. (c). *Textbook of Radiology for Residents & Technicians, 5th ed., S.K. Bhargava & Sumeet Bhargava, p. 48-96.*

79. The normal urethrovesical angle in female is

(a) 90 degree (b) 100 degree
(c) 110 degree (d) 129 degree

Ans. (b). *Textbook of Radiology for Residents & Technicians, 5th ed., S.K. Bhargava & Sumeet Bhargava, p. 48-96.*

80. Gartner duct is present in

(a) Vaginal wall (b) Broad ligament of uterus
(c) Transverse cervical ligament (d) Pouch of Dougles

Ans. (b). *Textbook of Radiology for Residents & Technicians, 5th ed., S.K. Bhargava & Sumeet Bhargava, p. 48-96.*

81. Seminal vesicles are present between

(a) Prostate and anus (b) Prostate and rectum
(c) Bladder and rectum (d) Prostate and bladder

Ans. (c). *Textbook of Radiology for Residents & Technicians, 5th ed., S.K. Bhargava & Sumeet Bhargava, p. 48-96.*

82. The percentage of the sensory fibers in a motor nerve is

(a) 0% (b) 10%
(c) 20% (d) 40%

Ans. (d). *Textbook of Radiology for Residents & Technicians, 5th ed., S.K. Bhargava & Sumeet Bhargava, p. 48-96.*

83. Vomiting center is located in

(a) Cervical spinal cord (b) Thalamus
(c) Hypothalamus (d) Medulla oblongata

Ans. (d). *Textbook of Radiology for Residents & Technicians, 5th ed., S.K. Bhargava & Sumeet Bhargava, p. 48-96.*

84. The normal amount of CSF in man is about

(a) 50 CC (b) 100 CC
(c) 150 CC (d) 200 CC

Ans. (c). *Textbook of Radiology for Residents & Technicians, 5th ed., S.K. Bhargava & Sumeet Bhargava, p. 48-96.*

85. The cerebellum

(a) Has a totally inhibitory output from its cortex

(b) Has only excitatory signal output from its deep nuclear fibers
(c) Has a conscience interpretation of motor activity
(d) Has inhibitory influence on muscle tone in humans

Ans. (d). *Textbook of Radiology for Residents & Technicians, 5th ed., S.K. Bhargava & Sumeet Bhargava, p. 48-96.*

86. First relay station of pain is

(a) Spinal cord (b) Medulla
(c) Pons (d) Thalamus

Ans. (a). *Textbook of Radiology for Residents & Technicians, 5th ed., S.K. Bhargava & Sumeet Bhargava, p. 48-96.*

87. Vessels not under sympathetic control are

(a) Cerebral (b) Splanchnic
(c) Cardiac (d) Cutaneous

Ans. (a). *Textbook of Radiology for Residents & Technicians, 5th ed., S.K. Bhargava & Sumeet Bhargava, p. 48-96.*

88. Relation between nerve thickness and conduction velocity is

(a) Linear (b) Parabolic
(c) Hyperbolic (d) No relation

Ans. (a). *Textbook of Radiology for Residents & Technicians, 5th ed., S.K. Bhargava & Sumeet Bhargava, p. 48-96.*

89. Genu of internal capsule has

(a) Sensory fibers from thalamus to brain
(b) Motor fibers from lower limb
(c) Motor fibers from upper limb
(d) Motor fibers from trunk

Ans. (a). *Textbook of Radiology for Residents & Technicians, 5th ed., S.K. Bhargava & Sumeet Bhargava, p. 48-96.*

90. Broca's area of speech lies at

(a) Superior border of the frontal lobe
(b) Inferior border of the frontal lobe
(c) Posterior border of the frontal lobe
(d) Superior temporal gyrus

Ans. (b). *Textbook of Radiology for Residents & Technicians, 5th ed., S.K. Bhargava & Sumeet Bhargava, p. 48-96.*

91. Gag reflux is mediated by cranial nerve

(a) VII (b) IX
(c) X (d) XII

Ans. (b). *Textbook of Radiology for Residents & Technicians, 5th ed., S.K. Bhargava & Sumeet Bhargava, p. 48-96.*

92. Vestibular fibers relay in

(a) Vermis
(b) Lateral genicular body
(c) Flocculonodular lobe of cerebellum
(d) Auditory cortex

Ans. (c). *Textbook of Radiology for Residents & Technicians, 5th ed., S.K. Bhargava & Sumeet Bhargava, p. 48-96.*

93. In children the cerebral blood flow is approximately _______ of the adult.

(a) Half
(b) Same
(c) 2 times
(d) 3 times

Ans. (c). *Textbook of Radiology for Residents & Technicians, 5th ed., S.K. Bhargava & Sumeet Bhargava, p. 48-96.*

94. Blood brain barrier is not present in

(a) Area postrema
(b) Corpus striatum
(c) Corpus callosum
(d) Cerebral cortex

Ans. (a). *Textbook of Radiology for Residents & Technicians, 5th ed., S.K. Bhargava & Sumeet Bhargava, p. 48-96.*

95. Endolymph drains into

(a) Extradural space
(b) Subdural space
(c) Subarachnoid space
(d) Virchow-Robin space

Ans. (b). *Textbook of Radiology for Residents & Technicians, 5th ed., S.K. Bhargava & Sumeet Bhargava, p. 48-96.*

96. Which ion is more in CSF?

(a) Cl^-
(b) HCO_3^-
(c) Na^+
(d) K^+

Ans. (a). *Textbook of Radiology for Residents & Technicians, 5th ed., S.K. Bhargava & Sumeet Bhargava, p. 48-96.*

97. SA node acts as a pacemaker of the heart because of the fact that it

(a) Is capable of generating impulses spontaneously
(b) Has rich sympathetic innervations
(c) Has poor cholinergic innervations
(d) Generates impulses at the higher rate

Ans. (d). *Textbook of Radiology for Residents & Technicians, 5th ed., S.K. Bhargava & Sumeet Bhargava, p. 48-96.*

98. During the cardiac cycle, the opening of the aortic valve take place at the
(a) Beginning of systole
(b) End of isovolumetric contraction
(c) End of diastole
(d) End of systole

Ans. (b). *Textbook of Radiology for Residents & Technicians, 5th ed., S.K. Bhargava & Sumeet Bhargava, p. 48-96.*

99. The main inhibitory center of heart is
(a) Nucleus tractus solitaris (b) Nucleus ambiguous
(c) Nucleus parabrachialis (d) Dorsal nucleus of vagus

Ans. (b). *Textbook of Radiology for Residents & Technicians, 5th ed., S.K. Bhargava & Sumeet Bhargava, p. 48-96.*

100. Normal systolic pressure (mmHg) in pulmonary artery is
(a) 0–10 (b) 10–20
(c) 25–32 (d) 90–120

Ans. (c). *Textbook of Radiology for Residents & Technicians, 5th ed., S.K. Bhargava & Sumeet Bhargava, p. 48-96.*

101. O_2 content of arterial blood (ml/100 ml) is
(a) 11.2 (b) 14.5
(c) 19.4 (d) 21.3

Ans. (c). *Textbook of Radiology for Residents & Technicians, 5th ed., S.K. Bhargava & Sumeet Bhargava, p. 48-96.*

102. In an average adult the stroke volume per minute is
(a) 20–40 cc (b) 40–50 cc
(c) 60–70 cc (d) 80–100 cc

Ans. (c). *Textbook of Radiology for Residents & Technicians, 5th ed., S.K. Bhargava & Sumeet Bhargava, p. 48-96.*

103. Platue phase of action potential is seen in
(a) SA node (b) AV node
(c) Atrial fibers (d) Ventricular fibers

Ans. (d). *Textbook of Radiology for Residents & Technicians, 5th ed., S.K. Bhargava & Sumeet Bhargava, p. 48-96.*

104. During BP measurement if the muffled sound does not disappear with return of mercury to '0', the conclusion is
(a) Aortic stenosis (b) Low haematocrit
(c) Zero diastolic pressure (d) Patent ductus arteriosis

Ans. (b). Textbook of Radiology for Residents & Technicians, 5th ed., S.K. Bhargava & Sumeet Bhargava, p. 48-96.

105. Pulmonary embolism is a complication of all except

(a) Vitamin K deficiency
(b) Oral contraception
(c) Atrial muscle
(d) Ventricular muscle

Ans. (a). Textbook of Radiology for Residents & Technicians, 5th ed., S.K. Bhargava & Sumeet Bhargava, p. 48-96.

106. The first Aortic sound (S1) occurs due to closure of AV valves during

(a) Isotonic relaxation
(b) Isotonic contraction.
(c) Iso volumetric contraction
(d) Iso volumetric relaxation

Ans. (c). Textbook of Radiology for Residents & Technicians, 5th ed., S.K. Bhargava & Sumeet Bhargava, p. 48-96.

107. Cardiac Index is the ratio of

(a) Cardiac output and body weight
(b) Cardiac output and surface area
(c) Cardiac output and work of heart
(d) Stroke volume and surface area

Ans. (b). Textbook of Radiology for Residents & Technicians, 5th ed., S.K. Bhargava & Sumeet Bhargava, p. 48-96.

108. Parasympathetic stimulation of the heart causes

(a) Decreased rate of SA node.
(b) Increased excitability of A-V junctional fibres.
(c) Prevent ventricular contraction
(d) None of the above

Ans. (a). Textbook of Radiology for Residents & Technicians, 5th ed., S.K. Bhargava & Sumeet Bhargava, p. 48-96.

109. Fibres of the A-V junction

(a) Modified muscle fibres
(b) Modified nerve fibres
(c) Highly contractible
(d) Conduct impulse rapidly

Ans. (a). Textbook of Radiology for Residents & Technicians, 5th ed., S.K. Bhargava & Sumeet Bhargava, p. 48-96.

110. Conduction velocity is least in

(a) SA node
(b) AV node
(c) His bundle
(d) Purkinje bundle

Ans. (b). Textbook of Radiology for Residents & Technicians, 5th ed., S.K. Bhargava & Sumeet Bhargava, p. 48-96.

111. When pace maker is another area of heart, it denotes

(a) Wrong with conducting tissue
(b) Wrong with S-A node
(c) Wrong with neural controlling system
(d) None of the above

Ans. (b). *Textbook of Radiology for Residents & Technicians, 5th ed., S.K. Bhargava & Sumeet Bhargava, p. 48-96.*

112. Carotid sinus on pressure causes

(a) Reflex bradycardia (b) Increased RR
(c) Increased HR (d) Decreased RR

Ans. (a). *Textbook of Radiology for Residents & Technicians, 5th ed., S.K. Bhargava & Sumeet Bhargava, p. 48-96.*

113. SA node is a pace maker because of its

(a) Neural control (b) Location of atrium
(c) Strength of impulse formation (d) Rate of impulse formation

Ans. (d). *Textbook of Radiology for Residents & Technicians, 5th ed., S.K. Bhargava & Sumeet Bhargava, p. 48-96.*

114. Heart rate is maximum in a normal

(a) Fetus (b) Newborn
(c) Adults (d) Old age

Ans. (a). *Textbook of Radiology for Residents & Technicians, 5th ed., S.K. Bhargava & Sumeet Bhargava, p. 48-96.*

115. A sign of nodal rhythm is

(a) Prolonged PR interval
(b) Prolonged QRS complex
(c) Increased sympathetic tone to SA node
(d) Increased parasympathetic tone to SA node

Ans. (d). *Textbook of Radiology for Residents & Technicians, 5th ed., S.K. Bhargava & Sumeet Bhargava, p. 48-96.*

116. Principal source of energy to heart in healthy individual is

(a) Glucose (b) Amino acid
(c) Free fatty acid (d) Lactase and pyruvate

Ans. (c). *Textbook of Radiology for Residents & Technicians, 5th ed., S.K. Bhargava & Sumeet Bhargava, p. 48-96.*

117. The ECG waves produced by ventricular repolarization is

(a) P (b) Q
(c) R (d) T

Ans. (d). *Textbook of Radiology for Residents & Technicians, 5th ed., S.K. Bhargava & Sumeet Bhargava, p. 48-96.*

118. U-waves are produced in ECG
(a) Just after Q-waves (b) Just after R-waves
(c) Just after S-waves (d) Just after T-waves

Ans. (d). *Textbook of Radiology for Residents & Technicians, 5th ed., S.K. Bhargava & Sumeet Bhargava, p. 48-96.*

119. Cardiac output is maximally increased in
(a) Anxiety (b) Eating
(c) Exercise (d) Pregnancy

Ans. (c). *Textbook of Radiology for Residents & Technicians, 5th ed., S.K. Bhargava & Sumeet Bhargava, p. 48-96.*

120. Heart rate is accelerated by the following, except
(a) Inspiration (b) Grief
(c) Exercise (d) Anger

Ans. (b). *Textbook of Radiology for Residents & Technicians, 5th ed., S.K. Bhargava & Sumeet Bhargava, p. 48-96.*

121. Heart rate is slowed by the following, except
(a) Inspiration
(b) Fear
(c) Increased intracranial pressure
(d) Hypoxia

Ans. (d). *Textbook of Radiology for Residents & Technicians, 5th ed., S.K. Bhargava & Sumeet Bhargava, p. 48-96.*

122. PR interval is
(a) From the beginning of P to the end of R
(b) Time taken for the conduction of impulse through the atria and SV node
(c) Time taken for the impulse to travel through the AV node
(d) None

Ans. (c). *Textbook of Radiology for Residents & Technicians, 5th ed., S.K. Bhargava & Sumeet Bhargava, p. 48-96.*

123. Heart pumps out blood to
(a) Provide nutrition to cell
(b) Remove waste product from the body
(c) Maintain temperature of the body
(d) All of the above

Ans. (d). *Textbook of Radiology for Residents & Technicians, 5th ed., S.K. Bhargava & Sumeet Bhargava, p. 48-96.*

124. Sudden drop in systemic BP occurs at

(a) Arteries (b) Arteriole
(c) Capillaries (d) Veins

Ans. (b). *Textbook of Radiology for Residents & Technicians, 5th ed., S.K. Bhargava & Sumeet Bhargava, p. 48-96.*

125. Which of the following regulates the fine control of blood pressure

(a) Medulla (b) Hypothalamus
(c) Midbrain (d) Median eminence

Ans. (a). *Textbook of Radiology for Residents & Technicians, 5th ed., S.K. Bhargava & Sumeet Bhargava, p. 48-96.*

126. Velocity of the blood flow is inversely proportional to

(a) Viscosity (b) Flow
(c) Cross-sectional area (d) Length

Ans. (c). *Textbook of Radiology for Residents & Technicians, 5th ed., S.K. Bhargava & Sumeet Bhargava, p. 48-96.*

127. Heart muscle, true are all except

(a) Acts as syncitium (b) Has multiple nuclei
(c) Has ap junction (d) Has branching

Ans. (b). *Textbook of Radiology for Residents & Technicians, 5th ed., S.K. Bhargava & Sumeet Bhargava, p. 48-96.*

128. CO_2 is primarily transported in the arterial blood as

(a) Dissolved CO_2 (b) Carbonic acid
(c) Carbamino-hemoglobin (d) Bicarbonate

Ans. (d). *Textbook of Radiology for Residents & Technicians, 5th ed., S.K. Bhargava & Sumeet Bhargava, p. 48-96.*

129. Carbon dioxide affects respiratory centre via

(a) Aortic bodies
(b) Carotid bodies
(c) Inflation and deflation receptors
(d) CSF H^+ concentration

Ans. (d). *Textbook of Radiology for Residents & Technicians, 5th ed., S.K. Bhargava & Sumeet Bhargava, p. 48-96.*

130. Hyperbaric oxygenation is useful in all, except

(a) Congenital heart disease (b) Gas gangrene
(c) Carbon monoxide poisoning (d) Nitrogen toxicity

Ans. (d). *Textbook of Radiology for Residents & Technicians, 5th ed., S.K. Bhargava & Sumeet Bhargava, p. 48-96.*

131. Total vital capacity is decreased but timed vital capacity is normal in

(a) Bronchial asthma (b) Scoliosis
(c) Chronic bronchitis (d) All of the above

Ans. (b). *Textbook of Radiology for Residents & Technicians, 5th ed., S.K. Bhargava & Sumeet Bhargava, p. 48-96.*

132. Arterial pO_2 is reduced in

(a) Anemia (b) KCN poisoning
(c) Pulmonary hypoventilation (d) CO poisoning

Ans. (c). *Textbook of Radiology for Residents & Technicians, 5th ed., S.K. Bhargava & Sumeet Bhargava, p. 48-96.*

133. Carbon monoxide is released in lungs from

(a) Iron of hema molecule (b) Plasma
(c) Transferrin (d) Serum

Ans. (c). *Textbook of Radiology for Residents & Technicians, 5th ed., S.K. Bhargava & Sumeet Bhargava, p. 48-96.*

134. CO_2 influences respiration by acting at

(a) 90–120 (b) 125–170
(c) 170–210 (d) 210–250

Ans. (d). *Textbook of Radiology for Residents & Technicians, 5th ed., S.K. Bhargava & Sumeet Bhargava, p. 48-96.*

135. Air in the pleural cavity causes all, except

(a) Reduction in the residual volume
(b) Abnormal dullness to percussion on the affected side
(c) Less obvious rib contours on the affected side
(d) Reduced vital capacity

Ans. (b). *Textbook of Radiology for Residents & Technicians, 5th ed., S.K. Bhargava & Sumeet Bhargava, p. 48-96.*

136. Diffusion capacity of lung for O_2 at rest in M/L min/mmHg is

(a) 5 (b) 10
(c) 20 (d) 30

Ans. (c). *Textbook of Radiology for Residents & Technicians, 5th ed., S.K. Bhargava & Sumeet Bhargava, p. 48-96.*

137. Vital capacity (litres) in man is

(a) 4.2 (b) 4.8
(c) 6.0 (d) 6.8

Ans. (b). *Textbook of Radiology for Residents & Technicians, 5th ed., S.K. Bhargava & Sumeet Bhargava, p. 48-96.*

138. CO_2 which is excreted per minute (ml) is

(a) 50
(b) 100
(c) 200
(d) 400

Ans. (c). Textbook of Radiology for Residents & Technicians, 5th ed., S.K. Bhargava & Sumeet Bhargava, p. 48-96.

139. Diffusion capacity (ml/min/mmHg) of lungs for carbon monoxide is

(a) 0–5
(b) 5–10
(c) 10–30
(d) 40–80

Ans. (c). Textbook of Radiology for Residents & Technicians, 5th ed., S.K. Bhargava & Sumeet Bhargava, p. 48-96.

140. Respiratory center controlled by pons is

(a) Gasping
(b) Pneumotoxic
(c) Inspiratory
(d) Expiratory

Ans. (b). Textbook of Radiology for Residents & Technicians, 5th ed., S.K. Bhargava & Sumeet Bhargava, p. 48-96.

141. Hyperpnea in exercise is because of

(a) Hypercapnia
(b) Hypoxaemia
(c) Reflex
(d) Stimulation of cortex and proprioceptors

Ans. (b). Textbook of Radiology for Residents & Technicians, 5th ed., S.K. Bhargava & Sumeet Bhargava, p. 48-96.

142. Most potent respiratory stimulant is

(a) Oxygen
(b) Carbon dioxide
(c) H^+
(d) K^+

Ans. (b). Textbook of Radiology for Residents & Technicians, 5th ed., S.K. Bhargava & Sumeet Bhargava, p. 48-96.

143. About 90% of the CO_2 entering the blood is carried as

(a) Dissolved CO_2
(b) Carbon anhydrase
(c) Carbamino CO_2
(d) Carbonic acid
(e) Bicarbonate

Ans. (e), Textbook of Radiology for Residents & Technicians, 5th ed., S.K. Bhargava & Sumeet Bhargava, p. 48-96.

144. Normal Adult lung weights is

(a) 100–200 gm
(b) 200–300 gm
(c) 300–400 gm
(d) 500–600 gm

Ans. (c). Textbook of Radiology for Residents & Technicians, 5th ed., S.K. Bhargava & Sumeet Bhargava, p. 48-96.

145. The difference between amount of O_2 entering body (ml/per min) and CO_2 excreted (ml/min) is _______ ml/min.

(a) 20 (b) 50
(c) 0 (d) –10

Ans. (b). Textbook of Radiology for Residents & Technicians, 5th ed., S.K. Bhargava & Sumeet Bhargava, p. 48-96.

146. Ventilation/perfusion ratio is maximum in

(a) Apical region (b) Middle region
(c) Base (d) Same all over

Ans. (a). Textbook of Radiology for Residents & Technicians, 5th ed., S.K. Bhargava & Sumeet Bhargava, p. 48-96.

147. From lung to tissue O_2 transported by

(a) 70% (b) 86%
(c) 91% (d) 97%

Ans. (d). Textbook of Radiology for Residents & Technicians, 5th ed., S.K. Bhargava & Sumeet Bhargava, p. 48-96.

148. Hypoxemia does not depend on

(a) FiO_2 (b) Altitude
(c) Hb (d) CO_2

Ans. (c). Textbook of Radiology for Residents & Technicians, 5th ed., S.K. Bhargava & Sumeet Bhargava, p. 48-96.

149. Renal blood flow is (L/min)

(a) 0.8–1.2 (b) 1.2–1.3
(c) 1.5–2.0 (d) 2.0–2.5

Ans. (b). Textbook of Radiology for Residents & Technicians, 5th ed., S.K. Bhargava & Sumeet Bhargava, p. 48-96.

150. The length of nephrons including the collecting ducts ranges from

(a) 5–10 mm (b) 25–45 mm
(c) 45–65 mm (d) 65–100 mm

Ans. (c). Textbook of Radiology for Residents & Technicians, 5th ed., S.K. Bhargava & Sumeet Bhargava, p. 48-96.

151. The length of distal convoluted tubule is

(a) 2 mm (b) 5 mm
(c) 8 mm (d) 12 mm

Ans. (b). Textbook of Radiology for Residents & Technicians, 5th ed., S.K. Bhargava & Sumeet Bhargava, p. 48-96.

152. Each kidney contains about _______ nephrons.

(a) One million (b) Two million
(c) Four million (d) Half million

Ans. (a). Textbook of Radiology for Residents & Technicians, 5th ed., S.K. Bhargava & Sumeet Bhargava, p. 48-96.

153. Which of the following is minimally excreted in urine

(a) Urea (b) Creatinine
(c) Uric acid (d) Chloride

Ans. (c). Textbook of Radiology for Residents & Technicians, 5th ed., S.K. Bhargava & Sumeet Bhargava, p. 48-96.

154. GFR is increased when

(a) Plasma osmotic pressure is increased
(b) Glomerular hydrostatic pressure is decreased
(c) Tubular hydrostatic pressure is increased
(d) Increased renal blood flow

Ans. (d). Textbook of Radiology for Residents & Technicians, 5th ed., S.K. Bhargava & Sumeet Bhargava, p. 48-96.

155. What is the glomerular filtration rate (ml/min)?

(a) 100 (b) 125
(c) 150 (d) 175

Ans. (b). Textbook of Radiology for Residents & Technicians, 5th ed., S.K. Bhargava & Sumeet Bhargava, p. 48-96.

156. All of the following are actively reabsorbed from the proximal tubules, except

(a) Sodium (b) Urea
(c) Amino acid (d) Urea and water

Ans. (d). Textbook of Radiology for Residents & Technicians, 5th ed., S.K. Bhargava & Sumeet Bhargava, p. 48-96.

157. Juxtamedullary nephrons in kidney are what percentage of total nephrons

(a) 15 (b) 50
(c) 70 (d) 90

Ans. (d). Textbook of Radiology for Residents & Technicians, 5th ed., S.K. Bhargava & Sumeet Bhargava, p. 48-96.

158. Following is least absorbable in tubules

(a) Creatinine (b) Glucose
(c) Urea (d) Sucrose

Ans. ***(a).*** *Textbook of Radiology for Residents & Technicians, 5th ed., S.K. Bhargava & Sumeet Bhargava, p. 48-96.*

159. In the nephron, reabsorption of the kidney consists of

(a) Proximal convoluted tubule (b) Loop of Henle
(c) Distal convoluted tubule (d) Collecting duct

Ans. ***(a).*** *Textbook of Radiology for Residents & Technicians, 5th ed., S.K. Bhargava & Sumeet Bhargava, p. 48-96.*

160. Maximum absorption of glucose is

(a) 370 (b) 150
(c) 180 (d) 120

Ans. ***(a).*** *Textbook of Radiology for Residents & Technicians, 5th ed., S.K. Bhargava & Sumeet Bhargava, p. 48-96.*

161. Following cells are responsible for acid secretion in kidney

(a) T-cell (b) P-cell
(c) Mesangial cell (d) Pericytes

Ans. ***(a).*** *Textbook of Radiology for Residents & Technicians, 5th ed., S.K. Bhargava & Sumeet Bhargava, p. 48-96.*

162. About renal physiology all are true, except

(a) DCT always receives hypo-osmotic solution
(b) Afferent artery supplies glomerulus
(c) GFR is controlled by afferent and efferent arteriole
(d) 5% cardiac output is received by kidney

Ans. ***(d).*** *Textbook of Radiology for Residents & Technicians, 5th ed., S.K. Bhargava & Sumeet Bhargava, p. 48-96.*

163. Vitamin B_{12} is absorbed from

(a) Jejunum (b) Proximal ileum
(c) Terminal ileum (d) Stomach

Ans. ***(c).*** *Textbook of Radiology for Residents & Technicians, 5th ed., S.K. Bhargava & Sumeet Bhargava, p. 48-96.*

164. Gastric secretion is not influenced by

(a) Diet (b) Gastrin
(c) Cholecystokinin (d) None of the above

Ans. ***(d).*** *Textbook of Radiology for Residents & Technicians, 5th ed., S.K. Bhargava & Sumeet Bhargava, p. 48-96.*

165. Sphincter of oddi is located in

(a) Gastrium (b) Urinary bladder
(c) Biliary system (d) Central nervous system

Ans. ***(c).*** *Textbook of Radiology for Residents & Technicians, 5th ed., S.K. Bhargava & Sumeet Bhargava, p. 48-96.*

166. Process of normal swallowing involves all, except

(a) Vocal cord approximation (b) Soft palate elevation
(c) Palatopharyngeal folds (d) Tracheal valves

Ans. ***(d).*** *Textbook of Radiology for Residents & Technicians, 5th ed., S.K. Bhargava & Sumeet Bhargava, p. 48-96.*

167. What hormone causes contraction of the gall bladder?

(a) Secretin (b) Gastrin
(c) Villikinen (d) Cholecystokinin

Ans. ***(d).*** *Textbook of Radiology for Residents & Technicians, 5th ed., S.K. Bhargava & Sumeet Bhargava, p. 48-96.*

168. Duodenal mucosa is protected from the action of acid and pepsin by

(a) Reduced secretion of bicarbonate
(b) Secretion of the Brunners gland
(c) Hyperplasia of the duodenal mucosa
(d) Stimulation of sympathetics

Ans. ***(b).*** *Textbook of Radiology for Residents & Technicians, 5th ed., S.K. Bhargava & Sumeet Bhargava, p. 48-96.*

169. Which of the following is the fastest to be absorbed from stomach

(a) Carbohydrate (b) Proteins
(c) Fats (d) Water

Ans. ***(d).*** *Textbook of Radiology for Residents & Technicians, 5th ed., S.K. Bhargava & Sumeet Bhargava, p. 48-96.*

170. After absorption, iron in blood is

(a) Apoferritin (b) Ferritin
(c) Transferrin (d) Ceruloplasmin

Ans. ***(c).*** *Textbook of Radiology for Residents & Technicians, 5th ed., S.K. Bhargava & Sumeet Bhargava, p. 48-96.*

171. Iron is absorbed almost entirely in

(a) Stomach (b) Duodenum
(c) Jejunum (d) Ileum

Ans. ***(b).*** *Textbook of Radiology for Residents & Technicians, 5th ed., S.K. Bhargava & Sumeet Bhargava, p. 48-96.*

172. Lipase is not present in

(a) Saliva (b) Pancreatic juice

(c) Succus entericus (d) Gastric juice

Ans. (d). *Textbook of Radiology for Residents & Technicians, 5th ed., S.K. Bhargava & Sumeet Bhargava, p. 48-96.*

173. Salivary amylase digests starch in

(a) Mouth (b) Stomach
(c) Duodenum (d) Jejunum

Ans. (d). *Textbook of Radiology for Residents & Technicians, 5th ed., S.K. Bhargava & Sumeet Bhargava, p. 48-96.*

174. The principal function of the gastro-esophageal sphincter is

(a) To allow stomach acid into esophagus
(b) To maintain food in the esophagus for digestion
(c) To prevent reflux of the stomach contents
(d) Non-existent

Ans. (c). *Textbook of Radiology for Residents & Technicians, 5th ed., S.K. Bhargava & Sumeet Bhargava, p. 48-96.*

175. Saliva differs from plasma in

(a) Hypo-tonicity (b) HCO_3^- concentration
(c) Protease enzyme (d) Aldosterone decreases

Ans. (d). *Textbook of Radiology for Residents & Technicians, 5th ed., S.K. Bhargava & Sumeet Bhargava, p. 48-96.*

176. When excess amounts of carbohydrates or proteins are consumed, they are stored in the body as

(a) Glucose (b) Glucogen
(c) Protein (d) Triglyceride

Ans. (d). *Textbook of Radiology for Residents & Technicians, 5th ed., S.K. Bhargava & Sumeet Bhargava, p. 48-96.*

177. The gas present in the fundus of the stomach is mostly due to

(a) Fermentation (b) Putrefaction
(c) Swallowing (d) Diffusion

Ans. (c). *Textbook of Radiology for Residents & Technicians, 5th ed., S.K. Bhargava & Sumeet Bhargava, p. 48-96.*

178. Which enzyme is secreted by intestine?

(a) Phospholipase (b) Dipeptidase
(c) Trypsin (d) Elastage

Ans. (b). *Textbook of Radiology for Residents & Technicians, 5th ed., S.K. Bhargava & Sumeet Bhargava, p. 48-96.*

179. Which of the following has the highest pH

(a) Gastric juice
(b) Pancreatic juice
(c) Bile
(d) Saliva

Ans. (c). Textbook of Radiology for Residents & Technicians, 5th ed., S.K. Bhargava & Sumeet Bhargava, p. 48-96.

180. Fat in duodenum

(a) Contracts gall bladder
(b) Inhibits CCK
(c) Increases gastric emptying
(d) Inhibits gastrin

Ans. (a). Textbook of Radiology for Residents & Technicians, 5th ed., S.K. Bhargava & Sumeet Bhargava, p. 48-96.

181. Axillary means

(a) Breast
(b) Armpit
(c) Cheek
(d) Hair

Ans. (b). Textbook of Radiology for Residents & Technicians, 5th ed., S.K. Bhargava & Sumeet Bhargava, p. 1-20.

182. Babies are born with how many bones?

(a) 300
(b) 289
(c) 256
(d) 206

Ans. (a). Textbook of Radiology for Residents & Technicians, 5th ed., S.K. Bhargava & Sumeet Bhargava, p. 1-20.

183. Human brain has how many percent of water in it?

(a) 70
(b) 80
(c) 85
(d) 95

Ans. (c). Textbook of Radiology for Residents & Technicians, 5th ed., S.K. Bhargava & Sumeet Bhargava, p. 1-20.

184. The full length of small intestine is

(a) 11 feet
(b) 16 feet
(c) 19 feet
(d) 22 feet

Ans. (d). Textbook of Radiology for Residents & Technicians, 5th ed., S.K. Bhargava & Sumeet Bhargava, p. 1-20.

185. Basic structural units

(a) Cell
(b) Chemical
(c) Tissue
(d) Organism

Ans. (a). Textbook of Radiology for Residents & Technicians, 5th ed., S.K. Bhargava & Sumeet Bhargava, p. 48-96.

186. Contributes to the formation of cilia and flagella

(a) Centrosome
(b) Endoplasmic reticulum
(c) Ribosomes
(d) Organelles

Ans. (a). Textbook of Radiology for Residents & Technicians, 5th ed., S.K. Bhargava & Sumeet Bhargava, p. 48-96.

187. Found on bone joints surfaces

(a) Fibrocartilage
(b) Hyaline
(c) Elastic cartilage
(d) All of the above

Ans. (b). Textbook of Radiology for Residents & Technicians, 5th ed., S.K. Bhargava & Sumeet Bhargava, p. 1-20.

188. No epithelial layer, line joint cavities and secrete synovial fluid

(a) Cutaneous
(b) Mucous
(c) Synovial
(d) All of the above

Ans. (c). Textbook of Radiology for Residents & Technicians, 5th ed., S.K. Bhargava & Sumeet Bhargava, p. 1-20.

189. Secrete antibodies

(a) Plasma
(b) Adipocytes
(c) Fibroblasts
(d) Cell

Ans. (a). Textbook of Radiology for Residents & Technicians, 5th ed., S.K. Bhargava & Sumeet Bhargava, p. 46-90.

190. Specialized for transmitting and converting stimuli and information

(a) Nervous tissue
(b) Muscle tissue
(c) Connective tissue
(d) Cartilage

Ans. (a). Textbook of Radiology for Residents & Technicians, 5th ed., S.K. Bhargava & Sumeet Bhargava, p. 46-90.

191. This type of plane is when the body is cut down the middle separating left from right

(a) Frontal
(b) Sagittal
(c) Transverse
(d) Oblique

Ans. (b). Textbook of Radiology for Residents & Technicians, 5th ed., S.K. Bhargava & Sumeet Bhargava, p. 21-47.

192. The mid-clavicular line passes through the

(a) Armpit
(b) Umbilicus
(c) Nipple
(d) Palm

Ans. (c). Textbook of Radiology for Residents & Technicians, 5th ed., S.K. Bhargava & Sumeet Bhargava, p. 48-96.

193. The trachea bifurcates into two at the level of

(a) D-4
(b) D-6
(c) D-1
(d) D-8

Ans. ***(a).*** *Textbook of Radiology for Residents & Technicians, 5th ed., S.K. Bhargava & Sumeet Bhargava, p. 48-96.*

194. Which of the following is not a valve in the heart?

(a) Aortic
(b) Pulmonic
(c) Tricuspid
(d) Ventral

Ans. ***(d).*** *Textbook of Radiology for Residents & Technicians, 5th ed., S.K. Bhargava & Sumeet Bhargava, p. 46-96.*

195. The left lung has _______ lobe(s).

(a) One
(b) Two
(c) Three
(d) Four

Ans. ***(b).*** *Textbook of Radiology for Residents & Technicians, 5th ed., S.K. Bhargava & Sumeet Bhargava, p. 46-96.*

196. The cervical vertebrae consist of _______ vertebrae.

(a) 5
(b) 12
(c) 7
(d) 3

Ans. ***(c).*** *Textbook of Radiology for Residents & Technicians, 5th ed., S.K. Bhargava & Sumeet Bhargava, p. 1-20.*

197. The organ in the form of a sac on the underside of the liver that stores bile produced by the liver is the

(a) Appendix
(b) Pancreas
(c) Colon
(d) Gallbladder

Ans. ***(d).*** *Textbook of Radiology for Residents & Technicians, 5th ed., S.K. Bhargava & Sumeet Bhargava, p. 46-96.*

198. Which of the primary germ layers of the embryo does the epidermis of the skin develop from?

(a) Endoderm
(b) Ectoderm
(c) Mesoderm
(d) All of these choices are correct.

Ans. ***(b).*** *Textbook of Radiology for Residents & Technicians, 5th ed., S.K. Bhargava & Sumeet Bhargava, p. 48-96.*

199. About 25% of all stress fractures involve which bone?

(a) Rib
(b) Clavicle
(c) Humerus
(d) Tibia

Ans. ***(d).*** *Textbook of Radiology for Residents & Technicians, 5th ed., S.K. Bhargava & Sumeet Bhargava, p. 1-20.*

200. These are considered bone-building cells

(a) Fibroblasts (b) Osteoclasts
(c) Osteocytes (d) Osteoblasts

Ans. (d). *Textbook of Radiology for Residents & Technicians, 5th ed., S.K. Bhargava & Sumeet Bhargava, p. 1-20.*

201. Which of the following two minerals are needed in large quantities when bones are growing?

(a) Calcium and chlorine (b) Magnesium and sulfur
(c) Calcium and phosphorous (d) Potassium and phosphorous

Ans. (c). *Textbook of Radiology for Residents & Technicians, 5th ed., S.K. Bhargava & Sumeet Bhargava, p. 48-96.*

202. Name the artery that carries blood from the left ventricle to the body.

(a) Pulmonary vein (b) Aorta
(c) Semilunar valve (d) Atria

Ans. (b). *Textbook of Radiology for Residents & Technicians, 5th ed., S.K. Bhargava & Sumeet Bhargava, p. 48-96.*

203. Aorta has

(a) 2 parts (b) 3 parts
(c) 4 parts (d) 8 parts

Ans. (a). *Textbook of Radiology for Residents & Technicians, 5th ed., S.K. Bhargava & Sumeet Bhargava, p. 48-96.*

204. Which of the following bones is found unpaired?

(a) Maxilla (b) Palatine
(c) Nasal (d) Vomer

Ans. (d). *Textbook of Radiology for Residents & Technicians, 5th ed., S.K. Bhargava & Sumeet Bhargava. p. 1-20.*

205. Protein synthesis within the cell is regulated by

(a) Cytoplasm (b) Organelles
(c) Genes (d) Cell membrane

Ans. (c). *Textbook of Radiology for Residents & Technicians, 5th ed., S.K. Bhargava & Sumeet Bhargava, p. 48-96.*

206. In order to continue to contract, muscle cells must have

(a) Carbohydrates (b) Oxygen
(c) ATP (d) All of the above

Ans. (c). *Textbook of Radiology for Residents & Technicians, 5th ed., S.K. Bhargava & Sumeet Bhargava, p. 48-96.*

207. The speed of chemical reactions that occur within the body is regulated by

(a) Exogenic reactions
(b) Endogenic reactions
(c) Entropy
(d) Enzymes

Ans. (d). Textbook of Radiology for Residents & Technicians, 5th ed., S.K. Bhargava & Sumeet Bhargava, p. 48-96.

208. What is the biggest organ in body?

(a) Liver
(b) Brain
(c) Muscle
(d) Penis

Ans. (a). Textbook of Radiology for Residents & Technicians, 5th ed., S.K. Bhargava & Sumeet Bhargava, p. 48-96.

209. Where does fertilization happen?

(a) In distal first of uterine tube
(b) In distal second of uterine tube
(c) In distal third of uterine tube
(d) In distal fourth of uterine tube

Ans. (c). Textbook of Radiology for Residents & Technicians, 5th ed., S.K. Bhargava & Sumeet Bhargava, p. 48-96.

210. What is corpus luteum?

(a) It secretes progesterone and estradiol.
(b) It secretes only estradiol.
(c) It secretes only progesterone.
(d) It secretes only luteal hormone.

Ans. (a). Textbook of Radiology for Residents & Technicians, 5th ed., S.K. Bhargava & Sumeet Bhargava, p. 48-96.

211. What are the routes in systemic circulation?

(a) Aorta to left ventricle to systemic arteries to systemic capillaries to systemic veins to right atrium.
(b) Left ventricle to aorta to systemic arteries to systemic capillaries to systemic veins to right atrium.
(c) Left ventricle to aorta to systemic arteries to systemic veins to right atrium.
(d) Systemic arteries to left ventricle to aorta to systemic capillaries systemic veins to right atrium.

Ans. (b). Textbook of Radiology for Residents & Technicians, 5th ed., S.K. Bhargava & Sumeet Bhargava, p. 48-96.

212. In the endometrial cycle, what happens in the uterus?

(a) Follicular phase begins on day 5

(b) Ovarian phase begins on day 5
(c) Luteal phase begins on day 5
(d) Proliferative phase begins on day 5

Ans. (d). *Textbook of Radiology for Residents & Technicians, 5th ed., S.K. Bhargava & Sumeet Bhargava, p. 48-96.*

213. Secrete mucus into urethra, below prostate

(a) Bulbourethral glands
(b) Accessory glands
(c) Prostate glands
(d) Pituitary gland

Ans. (a). *Textbook of Radiology for Residents & Technicians, 5th ed., S.K. Bhargava & Sumeet Bhargava, p. 48-96.*

214. A word for not enough oxygen in lungs is

(a) Hypoxic hypoxia
(b) Anemic hypoxia
(c) Oxyhemoglobin
(d) Maximum expiration

Ans. (a). *Textbook of Radiology for Residents & Technicians, 5th ed., S.K. Bhargava & Sumeet Bhargava, p. 48-96.*

215. What happens in the ovaries in luteal phase?

(a) On day 13, a burst of LH from anterior pituitary triggers ovulation; on day 14, causes remnant of folicle to form corpus luteum in ovary.
(b) On day 13, causes remnant of folicle to form corpus luteum in ovary; on day 14, a burst of LH from anterior pituitary triggers ovulation.
(c) On day 13, causes follicle to grow maturely; on day 14, a burst of LH from anterior pituitary triggers ovulation.
(d) On day 13, causes remnant of folicle to form corpus luteum in ovary; on day 14, causes a follicle to grow maturely.

Ans. (a). *Textbook of Radiology for Residents & Technicians, 5th ed., S.K. Bhargava & Sumeet Bhargava, p. 48-96.*

216. A word for not enough Hb in blood to transport oxygen

(a) Hypoxic hypoxia
(b) Anemic hypoxia
(c) Oxyhemoglobin
(d) Maximum expiration

Ans. (b). *Textbook of Radiology for Residents & Technicians, 5th ed., S.K. Bhargava & Sumeet Bhargava, p. 48-96.*

217. Causes follicle to grow to maturity in females

(a) FSH
(b) LH
(c) Oestrogen
(d) GH

Ans. (a). *Textbook of Radiology for Residents & Technicians, 5th ed., S.K. Bhargava & Sumeet Bhargava, p. 48-96.*

218. How many litres are pumped into the aorta per minute?

(a) 2 litres per minute at rest (b) 3 litres per minute at rest
(c) 4 litres per minute at rest (d) 5 litres per minute at rest

Ans. (d). *Textbook of Radiology for Residents & Technicians, 5th ed., S.K. Bhargava & Sumeet Bhargava, p. 48-96.*

219. What happens when arterial pressure decreases?

(a) Decreased arterial pressure (b) Increased arterial pressure
(c) Increased cardiac output (d) Decreased cardiac output

Ans. (d). *Textbook of Radiology for Residents & Technicians, 5th ed., S.K. Bhargava & Sumeet Bhargava, p. 48-96.*

220. Ovulation occurs on what day of a 28-day cycle?

(a) Day 30 (b) Day 7
(c) Day 14 (d) Day 28

Ans. (c). *Textbook of Radiology for Residents & Technicians, 5th ed., S.K. Bhargava & Sumeet Bhargava, p. 48-96.*

221. What happens after 6-8 days of fertilization?

(a) Formation gastrocyte (b) Mitosis-I
(c) Mitosis-II (d) Formation blastocyst

Ans. (d). *Textbook of Radiology for Residents & Technicians, 5th ed., S.K. Bhargava & Sumeet Bhargava, p. 48-96.*

222. What is follicle?

(a) Follicle is a progesterone plus surrounding cells.
(b) Follicle is a corpus luteum plus surrounding cells.
(c) Follicle is a spermocyte plus surrounding cells.
(d) Follicle is an oocyte plus surrounding cells.

Ans. (d). *Textbook of Radiology for Residents & Technicians, 5th ed., S.K. Bhargava & Sumeet Bhargava, p. 48-96.*

223. How long does it take for embryo to travel through uterine tube?

(a) Only 1 day (b) 3-4 days
(c) 4-5 days (d) 5-6 days

Ans. (b). *Textbook of Radiology for Residents & Technicians, 5th ed., S.K. Bhargava & Sumeet Bhargava, p. 48-96.*

224. Where is the site of gas exchange?

(a) Alveoli (b) Pharynx
(c) Larynx (d) Bronchi

Ans. (a). *Textbook of Radiology for Residents & Technicians, 5th ed., S.K. Bhargava & Sumeet Bhargava, p. 48-96.*

225. What is a soma?

(a) 80% lipid and 20% protein; helps insulate the axon; facilitates action potential; prevents signals from getting crossed between neurons.
(b) Cell body; contains the nucleus.
(c) Facilitates communication between neurons by releasing neuro-transmitters after they receive the electrical message sent down the axon.
(d) Space between terminal buttons of the cell sending the message (presynaptic cell) and the membrane of the cell receiving the message (postsynaptic cell).

Ans. (b). *Textbook of Radiology for Residents & Technicians, 5th ed., S.K. Bhargava & Sumeet Bhargava, p. 48-96.*

226. What is the terminal button?

(a) 80% lipid and 20% protein; helps insulate the axon; facilitates action potential; prevents signals from getting crossed between neurons.
(b) Cell body; contains the nucleus.
(c) Facilitates communication between neurons by releasing neuro-transmitters after they receive the electrical message sent down the axon.
(d) Space between terminal buttons of the cell sending the message (presynaptic cell) and the membrane of the cell receiving the message (postsynaptic cell).

Ans. (c). *Textbook of Radiology for Residents & Technicians, 5th ed., S.K. Bhargava & Sumeet Bhargava, p. 48-96.*

227. What is the synapse?

(a) 80% lipid and 20% protein; helps insulate the axon; facilitates action potential; prevents signals from getting crossed between neurons.
(b) Cell body; contains the nucleus.
(c) Facilitates communication between neurons by releasing neuro-transmitters after they receive the electrical message sent down the axon.
(d) Space between terminal buttons of the cell sending the message (presynaptic cell) and the membrane of the cell receiving the message (postsynaptic cell).

Ans. (d). *Textbook of Radiology for Residents & Technicians, 5th ed., S.K. Bhargava & Sumeet Bhargava, p. 48-96.*

228. The teeth break-up food into small parts by a process called

(a) Absorption (b) Deglutition

(c) Mastication (d) Ingestion

Ans. (c). *Textbook of Radiology for Residents & Technicians, 5th ed., S.K. Bhargava & Sumeet Bhargava, p. 48-96.*

229. Hydrochloric acid and pepsin are secreted by the

(a) Salivary glands (b) Stomach
(c) Pancreas (d) Liver

Ans. (b). *Textbook of Radiology for Residents & Technicians, 5th ed., S.K. Bhargava & Sumeet Bhargava, p. 48-96.*

230. Which of the following cell types is not a supporting cell or glial cell of the central nervous system?

(a) Schwann cell (b) Astrocyte
(c) Oligodendrocyte (d) Ependymal cell

Ans. (a). *Textbook of Radiology for Residents & Technicians, 5th ed., S.K. Bhargava & Sumeet Bhargava, p. 48-96.*

231. A stimulus that is just strong enough to initiate an impulse in a neuron is called a ________ stimulus.

(a) base line (b) synaptic
(c) threshold (d) differential

Ans. (c). *Textbook of Radiology for Residents & Technicians, 5th ed., S.K. Bhargava & Sumeet Bhargava, p. 48-96.*

232. Impulses are conducted to the soma by the

(a) Axon (b) Axon hillock
(c) Dendrites (d) All of the above

Ans. (c). *Textbook of Radiology for Residents & Technicians, 5th ed., S.K. Bhargava & Sumeet Bhargava, p. 48-96.*

233. An important structure in both learning and memory is the __________.

(a) hippocampus (b) pons
(c) medulla (d) cerebellum

Ans. (a). *Textbook of Radiology for Residents & Technicians, 5th ed., S.K. Bhargava & Sumeet Bhargava, p. 48-96.*

234. An individual who has an eating disorder along with intense thirst and wildly varying body temperatures may have a dysfunction of the __________.

(a) pons (b) medulla
(c) thalamus (d) hypothalamus

Ans. (d). *Textbook of Radiology for Residents & Technicians, 5th ed., S.K. Bhargava & Sumeet Bhargava, p. 48-96.*

235. Which of the following is not a lobe of the cerebral cortex?

(a) Occipital
(b) Parietal
(c) Cerebellar
(d) Temporal

Ans. (c). *Textbook of Radiology for Residents & Technicians, 5th ed., S.K. Bhargava & Sumeet Bhargava, p. 48-96.*

236. There are _____ pairs of cranial nerves and ____ pairs of spinal nerves.

(a) 10; 30
(b) 31; 12
(c) 12; 31
(d) 30; 10

Ans. (c). *Textbook of Radiology for Residents & Technicians, 5th ed., S.K. Bhargava & Sumeet Bhargava, p. 48-96.*

237. The 'knee jerk' reflex is an example of

(a) Axon reflex
(b) Extensor thrust reflex
(c) Cross-extensor reflex
(d) Stretch reflex

Ans. (d). *Textbook of Radiology for Residents & Technicians, 5th ed., S.K. Bhargava & Sumeet Bhargava, p. 48-96.*

238. Muscle stretch (monosynaptic) reflexes

(a) are dependent on descending activation from higher motor neurons.
(b) involve sensory neurons, spinal cord interneurons and motor neurons only.
(c) are not present in all skeletal muscles.
(d) include the knee jerk reflex response to striking the patellar tendon.

Ans. (d). *Textbook of Radiology for Residents & Technicians, 5th ed., S.K. Bhargava & Sumeet Bhargava, p. 48-96.*

239. Which statement regarding autonomic sympathetic neurons is false?

(a) They are usually activated as a single unit (mass activation).
(b) They emerge from the brain and sacral regions.
(c) They form white and grey rami communicantes fibres.
(d) They may have ganglia located along the spinal cord.

Ans. (b). *Textbook of Radiology for Residents & Technicians, 5th ed., S.K. Bhargava & Sumeet Bhargava, p. 48-96.*

240. Which neuron releases noradrenaline as a neurotransmitter?

(a) Preganglionic sympathetic fibres
(b) Postganglionic sympathetic fibres
(c) Preganglionic parasympathetic fibres
(d) Postganglionic parasympathetic fibres

Ans. ***(b).*** *Textbook of Radiology for Residents & Technicians, 5th ed., S.K. Bhargava & Sumeet Bhargava, p. 48-96.*

241. Accommodation, the ability of the eyes to keep the image focused on the retina as distance is changed, results from contraction of the

(a) Circular muscles
(b) Ciliary muscles
(c) Radial muscles
(d) Pupil

Ans. ***(b).*** *Textbook of Radiology for Residents & Technicians, 5th ed., S.K. Bhargava & Sumeet Bhargava, p. 48-96.*

242. Four refractory media of the eye, listed in the sequence in which they refract light, are

(a) Vitreous humour, lens, aqueous humour, cornea
(b) Cornea, aqueous humour, lens, vitreous humour
(c) Cornea, vitreous humour, lens, aqueous humour
(d) Lens, aqueous humour, cornea, vitreous humour

Ans. ***(b).*** *Textbook of Radiology for Residents & Technicians, 5th ed., S.K. Bhargava & Sumeet Bhargava, p. 48-96.*

243. Among the cells involved in inflammation that are part of the nonspecific immune system, the most numerous and first to be mobilized and arrive at the site of inflammation are the

(a) Macrophages
(b) Basophils
(c) Neutrophils
(d) Lymphocytes

Ans. ***(c).*** *Textbook of Radiology for Residents & Technicians, 5th ed., S.K. Bhargava & Sumeet Bhargava, p. 48-96.*

244. The role of the thymus is to

(a) monitor for specificity and potency of lymphocytes
(b) monitor for airborne pathogens
(c) monitor for pathogens in the blood
(d) monitor pathogens in the lymph

Ans. ***(a).*** *Textbook of Radiology for Residents & Technicians, 5th ed., S.K. Bhargava & Sumeet Bhargava, p. 48-96.*

245. Oxygen most likely binds to ____ in the hemoglobin in the ____.

(a) iron, lungs
(b) amino acids, lungs
(c) iron and amino acids, lungs
(d) amino acids, tissues

Ans. ***(a).*** *Textbook of Radiology for Residents & Technicians, 5th ed., S.K. Bhargava & Sumeet Bhargava, p. 48-96.*

246. The soft, fleshy V-shaped mass of tissue that hangs from the soft palate is the _______.

(a) epiglottis (b) esophageal hiatus
(c) uvula (d) gingival

Ans. (c). *Textbook of Radiology for Residents & Technicians, 5th ed., S.K. Bhargava & Sumeet Bhargava, p. 48-96.*

247. Thickened white patches on the oral mucous membranes characterize the disorder called

(a) Cholelithiasis (b) Peridontitis
(c) Pancreatitis (d) Leukoplakia

Ans. (d). *Textbook of Radiology for Residents & Technicians, 5th ed., S.K. Bhargava & Sumeet Bhargava, p. 48-96.*

248. ECG

(a) records the electrical activity of the heart.
(b) records the mechanical activity of the heart.
(c) records both electrical and mechanical activity of heart.
(d) None of the above

Ans. (a). *Textbook of Radiology for Residents & Technicians, 5th ed., S.K. Bhargava & Sumeet Bhargava, p. 48-96.*

249. In ECG, P-wave represents

(a) atria to ventricular conduction time
(b) duration of activation and recovery of the ventricular muscle
(c) ventricular repolarization
(d) depolarization of both atria

Ans. (d). *Textbook of Radiology for Residents & Technicians, 5th ed., S.K. Bhargava & Sumeet Bhargava, p. 48-96.*

250. Normal duration of ECG is

(a) 0.12 sec (b) 0.8 sec
(c) 1.6 sec (d) 2.0 sec

Ans. (b). *Textbook of Radiology for Residents & Technicians, 5th ed., S.K. Bhargava & Sumeet Bhargava, p. 48-96.*

251. The presence of U waves may indicate

(a) Ischemia (b) Hyperkalemia
(c) Hypokalemia (d) Bradycardia

Ans. (c). *Textbook of Radiology for Residents & Technicians, 5th ed., S.K. Bhargava & Sumeet Bhargava, p. 48-96.*

252. Each lung is covered by a closed sac of serous membrane called

(a) Peritonium (b) Pericardium

(c) Pleura (d) Facia

Ans. (c). *Textbook of Radiology for Residents & Technicians, 5th ed., S.K. Bhargava & Sumeet Bhargava, p. 48-96.*

253. Pulmonary artery carries

(a) Oxygenated blood (b) Deoxygenated blood
(c) Mix blood (d) All of the above

Ans. (b). *Textbook of Radiology for Residents & Technicians, 5th ed., S.K. Bhargava & Sumeet Bhargava, p. 48-96.*

CHAPTER

2

Basic Physics and Radiation Physics

1. Ultrasound waves require to travel

(a) Medium (jelly or oil etc.) (b) Air
(c) Vacuum (d) Gas

Ans. (a). *Textbook of Radiology for Residents & Technicians, 5th ed., S.K. Bhargava & Sumeet Bhargava, p. 97-114.*

2. For X-rays to travel, it require

(a) No medium required (b) Presence of water
(c) Presence of oxygen (d) None

Ans. (a). *Textbook of Radiology for Residents & Technicians, 5th ed., S.K. Bhargava & Sumeet Bhargava, p. 97-114.*

3. The particle of discrete bundles of energy released from electromagnetic spectrum is known as

(a) Quantum (b) Radiation
(c) Angstrom (d) Frequency

Ans. (a). *Textbook of Radiology for Residents & Technicians, 5th ed., S.K. Bhargava & Sumeet Bhargava, p. 97-114.*

4. The Protons are _______ charged particles.

(a) positive (b) negative
(c) neutral (d) None

Ans. (a). *Textbook of Radiology for Residents & Technicians, 5th ed., S.K. Bhargava & Sumeet Bhargava, p. 98.*

5. Electrons are _______ charged particles.

(a) positive (b) negative
(c) neutral (d) None

Ans. (b). Textbook of Radiology for Residents & Technicians, 5th ed., S.K. Bhargava & Sumeet Bhargava, p. 98.

6. A unit of measurement of the electron energy is

(a) Electron volt (b) Kilovoltage
(c) Milliampere (d) None of the above

Ans. (a). Textbook of Radiology for Residents & Technicians, 5th ed., S.K. Bhargava & Sumeet Bhargava, p. 99.

7. Isotopes are those elements which has

(a) Same atomic number but different mass number
(b) Different atomic number but same mass number
(c) Equal number of protons and electrons
(d) None of the above

Ans. (a). Textbook of Radiology for Residents & Technicians, 5th ed., S.K. Bhargava & Sumeet Bhargava, p. 98.

8. Isobars are those elements which have

(a) Different atomic number but same mass number
(b) Same atomic number but different mass number
(c) Equal number of protons and electron
(d) None of the above

Ans. (a). Textbook of Radiology for Residents & Technicians, 5th ed., S.K. Bhargava & Sumeet Bhargava, p. 98.

9. X-ray beam when fall on the body, act as

(a) Reflected (b) Absorbed
(c) Transmitted (d) All above

Ans. (d). Textbook of Radiology for Residents & Technicians, 5th ed., S.K. Bhargava & Sumeet Bhargava, p. 97-114.

10. X-ray being invisible, the presence can be detected by their

(a) Effect on radiographic film (b) Effect on fluorescent screen
(c) Ability to ionize the air (d) Any of the above

Ans. (d). Textbook of Radiology for Residents & Technicians, 5th ed., S.K. Bhargava & Sumeet Bhargava, p. 97-114.

11. Electric current is measured in

(a) Watt (b) Erg
(c) Volt (d) Ampere

Ans. (d). Textbook of Radiology for Residents & Technicians, 5th ed., S.K. Bhargava & Sumeet Bhargava, p. 97-114.

12. Electric pressure is measured in

(a) Watt (b) Volts

(c) Ohm (d) Farad

Ans. ***(b).*** *Textbook of Radiology for Residents & Technicians, 5th ed., S.K. Bhargava & Sumeet Bhargava, p. 97-114.*

13. Electric resistance is measured in

(a) Ohm (b) Ampere
(c) Ergs (d) Farad

Ans. ***(a).*** *Textbook of Radiology for Residents & Technicians, 5th ed., S.K. Bhargava & Sumeet Bhargava, p. 98.*

14. The matter which convert one energy to another

(a) Pb. zirconate titanate (b) Calcium tungstate
(c) Zd cadmium sulphide (d) Barium sulphate

Ans. ***(a).*** *Textbook of Radiology for Residents & Technicians, 5th ed., S.K. Bhargava & Sumeet Bhargava, p. 347-348.*

15. The device which converts one value of alternating current to another is known as

(a) Rectifier (b) X-ray tube
(c) Transformer (d) Kenotron

Ans. ***(c).*** *Textbook of Radiology for Residents & Technicians, 5th ed., S.K. Bhargava & Sumeet Bhargava, p. 106-107.*

16. The types of the transformers used in basic X-ray units are

(a) Autotransformer (b) Step up transformer
(c) Step down transformer (d) All above

Ans. ***(d).*** *Textbook of Radiology for Residents & Technicians, 5th ed., S.K. Bhargava & Sumeet Bhargava, p. 106-108.*

17. A transformer which has more turns in the secondary coil than in the primary is said to be

(a) Step up (b) Step down
(c) Auto (d) None of the above

Ans. ***(a).*** *Textbook of Radiology for Residents & Technicians, 5th ed., S.K. Bhargava & Sumeet Bhargava, p. 106.*

18. The process by which AC is converted to DC is known as

(a) Rectification (b) Generator
(c) Thermionic emission (d) Transformation

Ans. ***(a).*** *Textbook of Radiology for Residents & Technicians, 5th ed., S.K. Bhargava & Sumeet Bhargava, p. 106.*

19. With the filament current, temperature of filament increases resulting in liberation of electrons by a process known as

(a) Fluorescent (b) Photoemission
(c) Thermionic emission (d) Light emission

***Ans.* (c).** *Textbook of Radiology for Residents & Technicians, 5th ed., S.K. Bhargava & Sumeet Bhargava, p. 116.*

20. The direction and the magnitude is changed repeatedly in
(a) Direct current (b) Alternating current
(c) Induced current (d) Pulsating current

***Ans.* (b).** *Textbook of Radiology for Residents & Technicians, 5th ed., S.K. Bhargava & Sumeet Bhargava, p. 98.*

21. The power loss in the transformer is due to
(a) Cable loss (b) Hysteresis
(c) Eddy current (d) All above

***Ans.* (d).** *Textbook of Radiology for Residents & Technicians, 5th ed., S.K. Bhargava & Sumeet Bhargava, p. 107.*

22. The power loss in a transformer caused through the cycles of magnetization and demagnetization is called
(a) Cable loss (b) Hysteresis
(c) Eddy current (d) None of the above

***Ans.* (b).** *Textbook of Radiology for Residents & Technicians, 5th ed., S.K. Bhargava & Sumeet Bhargava, p. 107.*

23. Rectification means
(a) Change AC to DC (b) Increasing the voltage
(c) Decrease the current (d) All of the above

***Ans.* (a).** *Textbook of Radiology for Residents & Technicians, 5th ed., S.K. Bhargava & Sumeet Bhargava, p. 125.*

24. Full wave rectifier consists of
(a) 4 diode valve in bridge form
(b) 2 diode valve in bridge form
(c) 2 diode valve with X-ray tube
(d) None of the above

***Ans.* (a).** *Textbook of Radiology for Residents & Technicians, 5th ed., S.K. Bhargava & Sumeet Bhargava, p. 129.*

25. Reduction of the exposure time, utilization of X-ray in both half cycles and high tube rating are the features of
(a) Full wave rectification (b) Half wave rectification
(c) Self wave rectification (d) None of the above

***Ans.* (a).** *Textbook of Radiology for Residents & Technicians, 5th ed., S.K. Bhargava & Sumeet Bhargava, p. 129.*

26. High frequency generator has

(a) High tube current with short exposure
(b) More efficient
(c) Ripple factor is minimum
(d) All of the above

Ans. (d). *Textbook of Radiology for Residents & Technicians, 5th ed., S.K. Bhargava & Sumeet Bhargava, p. 132.*

27. In step-up transformer, the voltage in secondary coil is more than primary, hence the

(a) Current in secondary is more
(b) Current in the secondary is less
(c) Current in the secondary is not effected
(d) None of the above

Ans. (b). *Textbook of Radiology for Residents & Technicians, 5th ed., S.K. Bhargava & Sumeet Bhargava, p. 124.*

28. The tendency to limit the emission of more electrons from the filament of the X-ray tube during heating is called as

(a) Thermionic emission (b) Space charge effect
(c) Voltage fluctuation (d) None of the above

Ans. (b). *Textbook of Radiology for Residents & Technicians, 5th ed., S.K. Bhargava & Sumeet Bhargava, p. 121.*

29. In Transformer, the laminated cores are used to reduce the power losses by

(a) Eddy current (b) Hysteresis
(c) Make the transformer light (d) None

Ans. (a). *Textbook of Radiology for Residents & Technicians, 5th ed., S.K. Bhargava & Sumeet Bhargava, p. 107.*

30. In modern X-ray tube, a vacuum is maintained equal to

(a) 10^{-3} mm/Hg (b) 10^{-2} mm/Hg
(c) 10 mm/Hg (d) None

Ans. (a). *Textbook of Radiology for Residents & Technicians, 5th ed., S.K. Bhargava & Sumeet Bhargava, p. 120.*

31. Soft X-ray have the tube voltage of

(a) 0–10 kV (b) 20–60 kV
(c) 150–400 kV (d) 400–3000 kV

Ans. (b). *Textbook of Radiology for Residents & Technicians, 5th ed., S.K. Bhargava & Sumeet Bhargava, p. 115.*

32. Hard X-rays have tube voltage of

(a) 0–10 kV (b) 20–60 kV
(c) 150–400 kV (d) 400–3000 kV

Ans. (c). *Textbook of Radiology for Residents & Technicians, 5th ed., S.K. Bhargava & Sumeet Bhargava, p. 115.*

33. Very Hard X-rays have the tube voltage

(a) 0–10 kV (b) 20–60 kV
(c) 150–400 kV (d) 400–3000 kV

Ans. (d). *Textbook of Radiology for Residents & Technicians, 5th ed., S.K. Bhargava. p. 115.*

34. Gas filled tubes has the following advantages

(a) KV and MAs are difficult to control independently.
(b) Produce blackening thus shortening its life
(c) Speed of the electron will be reduced thus energy of the X-rays would be lesser.
(d) All above

Ans. (d). *Textbook of Radiology for Residents & Technicians, 5th ed., S.K. Bhargava & Sumeet Bhargava, p. 119.*

35. Edison effect termed to the electron cloud surrounding the filament produced by

(a) Thermionic emission (b) Photoelectric effect
(c) Chemical effect (d) None of the above

Ans. (a). *Textbook of Radiology for Residents & Technicians, 5th ed., S.K. Bhargava & Sumeet Bhargava, p. 121.*

36. The filament of the X-ray tube is made-up of Tungsten due to

(a) High melting point
(b) Stable electron emission at high temperature
(c) Good mechanical strength and long life
(d) All above

Ans. (d). *Textbook of Radiology for Residents & Technicians, 5th ed., S.K. Bhargava & Sumeet Bhargava, p. 121.*

37. X-rays are produced when anode of high atomic number (tungsten) is bombarded by

(a) Accelerated light photons (b) High speed electrons
(c) Low speed electrons (d) None of the above

Ans. (b). *Textbook of Radiology for Residents & Technicians, 5th ed., S.K. Bhargava & Sumeet Bhargava, p. 120.*

38. In modern X-ray tubes line focus principle is used in focal spot to get

(a) Good radiographic detail
(b) Sharper anatomical detail
(c) Withstand larger tube current, thus less danger of destroying the X-ray tube
(d) All above

Ans. (d). *Textbook of Radiology for Residents & Technicians, 5th ed., S.K. Bhargava & Sumeet Bhargava, p. 120.*

39. Advantages of rotating anode X-ray tubes are

(a) Quick dissipation of heat
(b) High output of X-ray tube
(c) Short exposure time
(d) All above

Ans. (d). *Textbook of Radiology for Residents & Technicians, 5th ed., S.K. Bhargava & Sumeet Bhargava, p. 122.*

40. Ideal material for construction of anode should have

(a) High atomic number, hence high conversion efficiency for electrons into X-rays
(b) High melting point
(c) High specific heat
(d) All above

Ans. (d). *Textbook of Radiology for Residents & Technicians, 5th ed., S.K. Bhargava & Sumeet Bhargava, p. 122.*

41. Ideal material for construction of anode should have

(a) High thermal conductivity
(b) Low vapour pressure even at high temperature
(c) Suitable mechanical properties for construction purposes
(d) All above

Ans. (d). *Textbook of Radiology for Residents & Technicians, 5th ed., S.K. Bhargava & Sumeet Bhargava, p. 122.*

42. Anode is made up of

(a) Tungsten with rhenium
(b) Pure tungsten
(c) Molybdenum
(d) None of the above

Ans. (a). *Textbook of Radiology for Residents & Technicians, 5th ed., S.K. Bhargava & Sumeet Bhargava, p. 122.*

43. Heat is dissipated in most of the X-ray tubes by

(a) Conduction, convection and radiation
(b) Conduction and convection
(c) Conduction and radiation
(d) Convection and radiation

Ans. (a). *Textbook of Radiology for Residents & Technicians, 5th ed., S.K. Bhargava. p. 136.*

44. The glass envelope of diagnostic X-ray tube is made up of
(a) Borosilicate (b) Ordinary glass
(c) Steel (d) None of the above

Ans. (a). *Textbook of Radiology for Residents & Technicians, 5th ed., S.K. Bhargava & Sumeet Bhargava, p. 123.*

45. The leakage radiation is that radiation which comes out
(a) Through glass window (b) Through tube housing
(c) Both above (d) None above

Ans. (a). *Textbook of Radiology for Residents & Technicians, 5th ed., S.K. Bhargava & Sumeet Bhargava, p. 124.*

46. Most of the time the speed of the modern X-ray tubes is
(a) 3000 rpm (b) 1600 rpm
(c) 3500 rpm (d) 4000 rpm

Ans. (a). *Textbook of Radiology for Residents & Technicians, 5th ed., S.K. Bhargava & Sumeet Bhargava, p. 121.*

47. Penetration of the tube is directly related to
(a) KVP (b) MA
(c) Exposure time (d) Focus film distance

Ans. (a). *Textbook of Radiology for Residents & Technicians, 5th ed., S.K. Bhargava & Sumeet Bhargava, p. 121.*

48. The quantity of X-ray received at given point is dependant on
(a) KVP (b) MA
(c) MAs (d) Size of the focal spot

Ans. (c). *Textbook of Radiology for Residents & Technicians, 5th ed., S.K. Bhargava & Sumeet Bhargava, p. 122.*

49. In Goodge's principle, the X-ray tube is so designed that it have the following
(a) Angled target
(b) Line focus principle to have small effective target area
(c) Dual focus
(d) All above

Ans. (d). *Radiological Science for Technologists by Stewart Carlyce Bushang, 9th Ed., Mosby Elsevier, 2008, p. 198.*

50. The heat generated in the anode of the X-ray tube is
(a) Less than 1% (b) Less than 30%
(c) Less than 75% (d) More than 99%

Ans. (d). *Textbook of Radiology for Residents & Technicians, 5th ed., S.K. Bhargava & Sumeet Bhargava, p. 122.*

51. The amount of the kinetic energy utilized in the production of X-rays are

(a) Less than 1%
(b) Less than 40%
(c) Less than 90%
(d) More than 99%

Ans. (a). *Textbook of Radiology for Residents & Technicians, 5th ed., S.K. Bhargava & Sumeet Bhargava, p. 122.*

52. There are 5 types of the interaction that occur between the X-rays and atoms of the absorbing material, of which two occur in the range of the diagnostic radiology

(a) Coherent scattering
(b) Photoelectric absorption and compton scattering
(c) Pair production
(d) Photodisintegration

Ans. (b). *Textbook of Radiology for Residents & Technicians, 5th ed., S.K. Bhargava & Sumeet Bhargava, p. 159.*

53. In coherent scattering, the single electron is involved in interaction in

(a) Thompson scattering
(b) Rayleigh scattering
(c) Both above
(d) None above

Ans. (a). *Textbook of Radiology for Residents & Technicians, 5th ed., S.K. Bhargava & Sumeet Bhargava, p. 159.*

54. The photoelectric absorption involves

(a) Incident X-ray photons has more energy than binding energy of K-shell electron
(b) Involve tightly bound electron
(c) K-shell
(d) All above

Ans. (d). *Textbook of Radiology for Residents & Technicians, 5th ed., S.K. Bhargava & Sumeet Bhargava, p. 160.*

55. The SI unit for measurement of quantity of radiation is (are)

(a) Gray
(b) Gray, Sievert, Bequerrel
(c) Gray, Sievert
(d) Roentgen, Sievert

Ans. (b). *Textbook of Radiology for Residents & Technicians, 5th ed., S.K. Bhargava & Sumeet Bhargava, p. 98.*

56. Photoelectric interaction results in excellent quality image due to

(a) P.E. absorption does not produce scattered radiation
(b) Enhances natural tissue contrast

(c) Both
(d) None

Ans. ***(c).*** *Textbook of Radiology for Residents & Technicians, 5th ed., S.K. Bhargava & Sumeet Bhargava, p. 160.*

57. In photoelectric emission, patient dose is

(a) High (b) Low
(c) Medium (d) No effect

Ans. ***(a).*** *Textbook of Radiology for Residents & Technicians, 5th ed., S.K. Bhargava & Sumeet Bhargava, p. 160.*

58. Compton scattering involve

(a) Moderate energy strikes outer shell electron (loosely bound and eject an electron from its orbit)
(b) Energy of scattered photon is increased
(c) The incident photon is scattered in new direction
(d) All above

Ans. ***(d).*** *Textbook of Radiology for Residents & Technicians, 5th ed., S.K. Bhargava & Sumeet Bhargava, p. 161.*

59. Pair production occur, if energy is of

(a) 0.08 MeV (b) 0.02 MeV
(c) 0.10 MeV (d) 1.02 MeV

Ans. ***(d).*** *Textbook of Radiology for Residents & Technicians, 5th ed., S.K. Bhargava & Sumeet Bhargava, p. 162.*

60. Mass density of the lung is

(a) 320 kg/m (b) 100 kg/m
(c) 200 kg/m (d) 1000 kg/m

Ans. ***(a).*** *Textbook of Radiology for Residents & Technicians, 5th ed., S.K. Bhargava & Sumeet Bhargava, p. 164.*

61. Mass density of bone is

(a) 1850 kg/m (b) 320 kg/m
(c) 910 kg/m (d) 1000 kg/m

Ans. ***(a).*** *Textbook of Radiology for Residents & Technicians, 5th ed., S.K. Bhargava & Sumeet Bhargava, p. 164.*

62. Lead is used as a shielding material and has a K-edge of

(a) 29 keV (b) 88 keV
(c) 120 keV (d) 10 keV

Ans. ***(b).*** *Textbook of Radiology for Residents & Technicians, 5th ed., S.K. Bhargava & Sumeet Bhargava, p. 168.*

63. The glass envelope of an X-ray tube also filters the emerging X-ray beam and is called as

(a) Inherent filtration (b) Filters
(c) Leakage filtration (d) None above

Ans. (a). *Textbook of Radiology for Residents & Technicians, 5th ed., S.K. Bhargava & Sumeet Bhargava, p. 123.*

64. Collimator used in X-ray tube is for

(a) To reduce size and shape of the beam
(b) Decrease the patient dose
(c) Improve the quality of Image
(d) All above

Ans. (d). *Radiological Science for Technologists by Stewart Carlyce Bushang, 9th Ed., Mosby Elsevier, 2008, p. 187-194.*

65. The scattered radiation can be reduced by

(a) Collimation (b) Correct voltage
(c) Compression (d) All above

Ans. (d). *Radiological Science for Technologists by Stewart Carlyce Bushang, p. 187.*

66. The minimum base and fog density of X-ray film is about

(a) 0.02 (b) 0.05
(c) 0.12 (d) 1.0

Ans. (c). *Textbook of Radiology for Residents & Technicians, 5th ed., S.K. Bhargava & Sumeet Bhargava, p. 206.*

67. The average range of measuring density on the radiograph is

(a) 0.25–2.0 above and fog level (b) 1–3
(c) 0.02–0.12 (d) 0.5–1.5

Ans. (a). *Textbook of Radiology for Residents & Technicians, 5th ed., S.K. Bhargava & Sumeet Bhargava, p. 206.*

68. The radiation unit to record the radiation received by radiation worker

(a) Roentgen (b) Rad
(c) Curie (d) Milli-Sievert

Ans. (d). *Radiological Science for Technologists by Stewart Carlyce Bushang, 9th Ed., Mosby Elsevier, 2008, p. 571.*

69. The principle of radiation protection involves

(a) Time (b) Time and distance
(c) Time, distance and shielding (d) None above

Ans. (c). *Textbook of Radiology for Residents & Technicians, 5th ed., S.K. Bhargava & Sumeet Bhargava, p. 151.*

70. The filters used in diagnostic X-ray tubes are made up of

(a) Aluminium
(b) Copper
(c) Tin
(d) Lead

Ans. (a). *Textbook of Radiology for Residents & Technicians, 5th ed., S.K. Bhargava & Sumeet Bhargava, p. 123.*

71. Late causes of the X-ray tube failure are

(a) Gassy tube
(b) Failure due to filament, due to constant heating, progressive thinning of the filament.
(c) Progressive pitting of the anode area
(d) All above

Ans. (d). *Textbook of Radiology for Residents & Technicians, 5th ed., S.K. Bhargava & Sumeet Bhargava, p. 138-139.*

72. Early causes of X-ray tube failure are

(a) Overheating
(b) Mechanical damage of filament/glass envelope
(c) Electric failure
(d) Any of the above

Ans. (d). *Textbook of Radiology for Residents & Technicians, 5th ed., S.K. Bhargava & Sumeet Bhargava, p. 138.*

73. The X-ray tube said to be "gassy" when

(a) Filament has burnt out
(b) Presence of the gas molecule
(c) Pitting of the anode
(d) None of the above

Ans. (b). *Radiological Science for Technologists by Stewart Carlyce Bushang, 9th Ed., Mosby Elsevier, 2008, p. 134.*

74. "Gassy tube" is diagnosed by any one of the following

(a) No exposure
(b) MA meter does not move
(c) MA meter shows fluctuation
(d) MA meter shows full deflection during exposure

Ans. (d). *Radiological Science for Technologists by Stewart Carlyce Bushang, 9th Ed., Mosby Elsevier, 2008, p. 134-35.*

75. The tube which acts as secondary switch as well as production of X-rays (grid controlled X-ray tubes) used in

(a) Conventional radiology units
(b) Mobile X-rays
(c) Fluoroscopic X-rays
(d) Cine-angiography units

Ans. (d). Textbook of Radiology for Residents & Technicians, 5th ed., S.K. Bhargava & Sumeet Bhargava, p. 142.

76. The Aluminium filter used in the diagnostic X-ray tube is

(a) For absorption of the low energy photons
(b) For absorption of scattered photons
(c) For absorption of high energy photons
(d) None of the above

Ans. (a). Textbook of Radiology for Residents & Technicians, 5th ed., S.K. Bhargava & Sumeet Bhargava, p. 166.

77. When energic electron passes by the nucleus, it is decelerated, resulting in loss of kinetic energy of the electron which is then converted into X-rays and is known as

(a) Bremsstrahlung radiation
(b) Characteristic radiation
(c) Leakage radiation
(d) None of the above

Ans. (a). Textbook of Radiology for Residents & Technicians, 5th ed., S.K. Bhargava & Sumeet Bhargava, p. 159.

78. With increase in the atomic number of the target material

(a) Efficiency of production of Bremsstrahlung radiation increases
(b) High energy X-ray increases
(c) Both
(d) None

Ans. (c). Textbook of Radiology for Residents & Technicians, 5th ed., S.K. Bhargava & Sumeet Bhargava, p. 159.

79. X-ray generator provides

(a) Electric power to energize X-ray tube
(b) Mechanism to select technique appropriate for a given examination
(c) To protect X-ray tube from possible overload situation
(d) All above

Ans. (d). Textbook of Radiology for Residents & Technicians, 5th ed., S.K. Bhargava & Sumeet Bhargava, p. 127.

80. Step-up transformer supply high voltage to X-ray tube as

(a) Increase the voltage and decrease the current
(b) Decrease the voltage and decrease the current
(c) Increase the voltage and increase the current
(d) Decrease the voltage and increase the current

Ans. (a). Textbook of Radiology for Residents & Technicians, 5th ed., S.K. Bhargava & Sumeet Bhargava, p. 124.

81. Voltage change across the transformer is proportional to turn ratio

(a) Directly proportional
(b) Inversely proportional
(c) No relationship
(d) Both

Ans. (a). Textbook of Radiology for Residents & Technicians, 5th ed., S.K. Bhargava & Sumeet Bhargava, p. 124.

82. Autotransformer provide voltage for

(a) X-ray tube filament circuit
(b) To primary of the high voltage transformer
(c) To subsidiary circuit
(d) All

Ans. (d). Textbook of Radiology for Residents & Technicians, 5th ed., S.K. Bhargava & Sumeet Bhargava, p. 125.

83. High voltage rectifier can be

(a) Solid state type
(b) Vacuum type
(c) Both
(d) None

Ans. (c). Textbook of Radiology for Residents & Technicians, 5th ed., S.K. Bhargava & Sumeet Bhargava, p. 129.

84. Function of the grid to

(a) Absorb scatter radiation
(b) Transmit all primary radiation
(c) Both above
(d) None of the above

Ans. (c). Textbook of Radiology for Residents & Technicians, 5th ed., S.K. Bhargava & Sumeet Bhargava, p. 200.

85. The effective device to reduce the scattered radiation is

(a) Grid
(b) Glass tube
(c) Diaphragm
(d) Cone

Ans. (a). Textbook of Radiology for Residents & Technicians, 5th ed., S.K. Bhargava & Sumeet Bhargava, p. 201.

86. Parallel grid is commonly used with

(a) Mobile units in the wards
(b) Conventional radiography units
(c) Both
(d) None

Ans. (a). Textbook of Radiology for Residents & Technicians, 5th ed., S.K. Bhargava & Sumeet Bhargava, p. 201.

87. Grid lines appear on radiograph with

(a) Stationary grid (b) Moving grid
(c) Both (d) None

Ans. (a). *Textbook of Radiology for Residents & Technicians, 5th ed., S.K. Bhargava & Sumeet Bhargava, p. 201.*

88. Disadvantages of the moving grid are

(a) Synchronism
(b) Vibration to set up in X-ray tube
(c) Requires approximately 15% more radiation to the patient
(d) All above

Ans. (d). *Textbook of Radiology for Residents & Technicians, 5th ed., S.K. Bhargava & Sumeet Bhargava, p. 202.*

89. The disadvantages of the moving grid are

(a) Exposure time is longer
(b) Object film distance is increased
(c) Blurring of the film
(d) All above

Ans. (d). *Textbook of Radiology for Residents & Technicians, 5th ed., S.K. Bhargava & Sumeet Bhargava, p. 202.*

90. With high grid ratio, the exposure dose to the patient is

(a) Increased (b) Decreased
(c) Unaffected (d) None

Ans. (a). *Textbook of Radiology for Residents & Technicians, 5th ed., S.K. Bhargava & Sumeet Bhargava, p. 201.*

91. In biplane cerebral angiography, scattered radiation is reduced by

(a) Closed grid (b) Parallel grid
(c) Focused grid (d) None above

Ans. (a). *Textbook of Radiology for Residents & Technicians, 5th ed., S.K. Bhargava & Sumeet Bhargava, p. 201.*

92. Air gap technique is used to

(a) Reduce scattered radiation (b) Magnification radiography
(c) Image sharpness deteriorates (d) All above

Ans. (d). *Textbook of Radiology for Residents & Technicians, 5th ed., S.K. Bhargava & Sumeet Bhargava, p. 205.*

93. The function of the cone in skull radiography is

(a) To limit the field of the radiation
(b) To reduce the exposure

(c) To increase the life of the X-ray tube
(d) All above

Ans. ***(a).*** *Radiological Science for Technologists by Stewart Carlyce Bushang, 9th Ed., Mosby Elsevier, 2008, p. 188-190.*

94. Density of the processed film is proportional to the radiation exposure

(a) Directly proportional
(b) Inversely proportional
(c) Both above
(d) None above

Ans. (a). *Textbook of Radiology for Residents & Technicians, 5th ed., S.K. Bhargava & Sumeet Bhargava, p. 206.*

95. High speed film require

(a) High exposure
(b) Less exposure
(c) Normal exposure
(d) None above

Ans. (b). *Textbook of Radiology for Residents & Technicians, 5th ed., S.K. Bhargava & Sumeet Bhargava, p. 206.*

96. Choice of the exposure (mAS) is decided by

(a) Speed of the intensifying screen
(b) F.F.D.
(c) Grid factor
(d) All above

Ans. (d). *Textbook of Radiology for Residents & Technicians, 5th ed., S.K. Bhargava & Sumeet Bhargava, p. 207.*

97. The advantages of the high KV radiography are

(a) Reduced mAS
(b) Reduced movement of the blur
(c) Reduced radiation dose
(d) All above

Ans. (d). *Textbook of Radiology for Residents & Technicians, 5th ed., S.K. Bhargava & Sumeet Bhargava, p. 207.*

98. The advantages of high KV radiography are

(a) Frequent use of line focus
(b) Greater exposure latitude
(c) Heating of the X-ray tube reduced
(d) All above

Ans. (d). *Textbook of Radiology for Residents & Technicians, 5th ed., S.K. Bhargava & Sumeet Bhargava, p. 207.*

99. The disadvantages of the high KV radiography are

(a) Loss of the bone detail
(b) Poor contrast
(c) Risk of over penetration
(d) All above

Ans. (d). *Textbook of Radiology for Residents & Technicians, 5th ed., S.K. Bhargava & Sumeet Bhargava, p. 207.*

100. In high KV radiography, to reduce the scattered radiation

(a) High grid ratio is used
(b) Air gap technique
(c) Exposure factors are considerably reduced
(d) All above

Ans. (d). *Textbook of Radiology for Residents & Technicians, 5th ed., S.K. Bhargava & Sumeet Bhargava, p. 207.*

101. During fluoroscopy, the X-ray tube is operated at

(a) Less than 2 mA
(b) Less than 5 mA
(c) More than 5 mA
(d) Between 5–10 mA

Ans. (b). *Textbook of Radiology for Residents & Technicians, 5th ed., S.K. Bhargava & Sumeet Bhargava, p. 284.*

102. The disadvantages of conventional fluoroscopy are

(a) More patient dose
(b) Operator has to have dark adaptation
(c) Difficulty in handling the patient
(d) All above

Ans. (d). *Textbook of Radiology for Residents & Technicians, 5th ed., S.K. Bhargava & Sumeet Bhargava, p. 284.*

103. Conventional fluoroscopy works on the principle of

(a) Fluorescence
(b) Phosphorescence
(c) Both
(d) None

Ans. (a). *Textbook of Radiology for Residents & Technicians, 5th ed., S.K. Bhargava & Sumeet Bhargava, p. 284.*

104. Fluorescent material used in Fluoroscopic screen is made-up of

(a) Zn cd sulphide-copper activated
(b) Calcium tungstate
(c) Cesium iodide
(d) Zn sulphide

Ans. (a). *Textbook of Radiology for Residents & Technicians, 5th ed., S.K. Bhargava & Sumeet Bhargava, p. 283.*

105. In modern image intensifier, the input screen is made-up of

(a) Zn cd sulphide-silver activated
(b) Cesium iodide
(c) Calcium tungstate
(d) Zn sulphide

Ans. (b). *Textbook of Radiology for Residents & Technicians, 5th ed., S.K. Bhargava & Sumeet Bhargava, p. 284.*

106. The component of X-ray image intensifier are

(a) Input phosphor, photo cathode, and accelerating anode
(b) Electrostating focusing lines
(c) Output phosphor
(d) All above

Ans. (d). *Textbook of Radiology for Residents & Technicians, 5th ed., S.K. Bhargava & Sumeet Bhargava, p. 284.*

107. CsI as input phosphor is superior because of

(a) The vertical orientation of the crystals
(b) A greater packing capacity
(c) A more favourable effective atomic number
(d) All above

Ans. (d). *Textbook of Radiology for Residents & Technicians, 5th ed., S.K. Bhargava & Sumeet Bhargava, p. 284.*

108. The image intensifier tube works on the principle of

(a) Thermionic emission
(b) Photoemission
(c) Multiple induction
(d) None of the above

Ans. (b). *Textbook of Radiology for Residents & Technicians, 5th ed., S.K. Bhargava & Sumeet Bhargava, p. 284.*

109. The advantages of the image intensification over conventional fluoroscopy are

(a) More congenial working condition with less patient dose.
(b) Better image detail and brightness
(c) Possibility of attaching three viewing system
(d) All above

Ans. (d). *Textbook of Radiology for Residents & Technicians, 5th ed., S.K. Bhargava & Sumeet Bhargava, p. 284-287.*

110. The brightness gain of image intensifier is due to

(a) Minification gain
(b) Flux gain
(c) Both
(d) None

Ans. (c). *Textbook of Radiology for Residents & Technicians, 5th ed., S.K. Bhargava & Sumeet Bhargava, p. 285.*

111. Flux gain increases the brightness of fluoroscopic image by a factor of

(a) Approx. 10 (b) Approx. 25
(c) Approx. 35 (d) Approx. 50

Ans. (d). *Textbook of Radiology for Residents & Technicians, 5th ed., S.K. Bhargava & Sumeet Bhargava, p. 285.*

112. The signals which convey fluoroscopic image from image intensifier to video camera where it is converted into series of electric impulses are known as

(a) Audio signal (b) Video signal
(c) Gamma camera (d) None of the above

Ans. (b). *Textbook of Radiology for Residents & Technicians, 5th ed., S.K. Bhargava & Sumeet Bhargava, p. 286-287.*

113. Ten day rule is for

(a) Women in the reproductive age
(b) Old women
(c) Young women
(d) Pregnant women

Ans. (a). *Textbook of Radiology for Residents & Technicians, 5th ed., S.K. Bhargava & Sumeet Bhargava, p. 188.*

114. Which of the following is the sensitive material in radiology department?

(a) X-ray cassette (b) Developer
(c) Intensifying screens (d) X-ray films

Ans. (d). *Textbook of Radiology for Residents & Technicians, 5th ed., S.K. Bhargava & Sumeet Bhargava, p. 167.*

115. The amount of energy passing per unit area at a point in a beam of electromagnetic radiation is referred as

(a) Wavelength of beam (b) Intensity of the beam
(c) Quality of the beam (d) Quantity of the beam

Ans. (b). *Textbook of Radiology for Residents & Technicians, 5th ed., S.K. Bhargava & Sumeet Bhargava, p. 113.*

116. The function of the collimator attached to the X-ray tube is

(a) Increase exposure (b) Decrease exposure
(c) Restrict primary beam (d) Decrease processing time

Ans. (c). *Textbook of Radiology for Residents & Technicians, 5th ed., S.K. Bhargava & Sumeet Bhargava, p. 123.*

117. The phosphor used in fluorescent screen is

(a) Calcium tungstate
(b) Barium lead sulphide
(c) Zn sulphide
(d) Zn cd sulphide

Ans. (d). *Textbook of Radiology for Residents & Technicians, 5th ed., S.K. Bhargava & Sumeet Bhargava, p. 178.*

118. Frequency of electric supply refers to

(a) Number of cycles per second
(b) Requirement of the machine
(c) Amount of the current available
(d) Voltage

Ans. (a). *Textbook of Radiology for Residents & Technicians, 5th ed., S.K. Bhargava & Sumeet Bhargava, p. 109.*

119. The electric supply of the static machine is

(a) Single phase
(b) Double phase
(c) Three phase
(d) None of the above

Ans. (c). *Textbook of Radiology for Residents & Technicians, 5th ed., S.K. Bhargava & Sumeet Bhargava, p. 109.*

120. The difference in the densities between adjacent areas of the film is known as

(a) Detail
(b) Distortion
(c) Resolution
(d) Contrast

Ans. (d). *Textbook of Radiology for Residents & Technicians, 5th ed., S.K. Bhargava & Sumeet Bhargava, p. 197.*

121. The emission of the electrons resulting from heating of cathode is called as

(a) Light emission
(b) Photoemission
(c) Evaporation
(d) Thermionic emission

Ans. (d). *Textbook of Radiology for Residents & Technicians, 5th ed., S.K. Bhargava & Sumeet Bhargava, p. 121.*

122. Radioactivity was discovered by

(a) Madam Curie
(b) Sir Wilhelm Conrad Roentgen
(c) Einstein
(d) Hounsfield

Ans. (a). *Textbook of Radiology for Residents & Technicians, 5th ed., S.K. Bhargava & Sumeet Bhargava, p. 114.*

123. X-ray was discovered by

(a) Gustav Buckey

(b) Hounsfield
(c) Madam Curie
(d) Sir Wilhelm Conrad Roentgen

Ans. (d). *Textbook of Radiology for Residents & Technicians, 5th ed., S.K. Bhargava & Sumeet Bhargava, p. 115.*

124. Target in the modern rotating anode tube is made-up of

(a) Rhenium-tungsten (b) Pure tungsten
(c) Tin (d) Copper

Ans. (a). *Textbook of Radiology for Residents & Technicians, 5th ed., S.K. Bhargava & Sumeet Bhargava, p. 122.*

125. The percentage of energy from cathode stream utilized in X-ray formation is

(a) Less than 1% (b) 80–90%
(c) 10–20% (d) 50%

Ans. (a). *Textbook of Radiology for Residents & Technicians, 5th ed., S.K. Bhargava & Sumeet Bhargava, p. 121.*

126. Chest radiography of pregnant women should be avoided during

(a) First trimester (b) Second trimester
(c) Third trimester (d) All of the above

Ans. (a). *Textbook of Radiology for Residents & Technicians, 5th ed., S.K. Bhargava & Sumeet Bhargava, p. 147-157.*

127. Which of the following fluoresce when X-ray fall on it

(a) Silver bromide (b) Lead sulphate
(c) Zn cd sulphide (d) Calcium carbonate

Ans. (c). *Textbook of Radiology for Residents & Technicians, 5th ed., S.K. Bhargava & Sumeet Bhargava, p. 178.*

128. Ultrasound waves are produced by

(a) Fluorescent material (b) Thermo-electrode
(c) Magnetic material (d) Piezoelectric materials

Ans. (d). *Textbook of Radiology for Residents & Technicians, 5th ed., S.K. Bhargava & Sumeet Bhargava, p. 346.*

129. The normal frequency of ultrasound waves used in medical diagnostic units range from

(a) 20,000–50,000 Hz (b) 50,000 – less than 1 MHz
(c) 1 MHz to 20 MHz (d) Above 20 MHz

Ans. (c). *Textbook of Radiology for Residents & Technicians, 5th ed., S.K. Bhargava & Sumeet Bhargava, p. 343.*

130. In X-ray tube, the increase in filament current, the tube current

(a) Increases
(b) Equal
(c) Decreases
(d) None

Ans. (a). *Textbook of Radiology for Residents & Technicians, 5th ed., S.K. Bhargava & Sumeet Bhargava, p. 121.*

131. Compound filter is made-up of

(a) Copper and aluminium
(b) Copper and lead
(c) Lead and aluminium
(d) Aluminium and tin

Ans. (a). *Textbook of Radiology for Residents & Technicians, 5th ed., S.K. Bhargava & Sumeet Bhargava, p. 166.*

132. Anode is blackened in rotating anode tube to

(a) Promote radiation
(b) To absorb excess radiation
(c) Both above
(d) None above

Ans. (a). *Textbook of Radiology for Residents & Technicians, 5th ed., S.K. Bhargava & Sumeet Bhargava, p. 122.*

133. Efficiency of the X-ray production in rotating anode tube is

(a) 1%
(b) 5%
(c) 10%
(d) 20%

Ans. (a). *Textbook of Radiology for Residents & Technicians, 5th ed., S.K. Bhargava & Sumeet Bhargava, p. 122.*

134. Anode in rotating anode X-ray tube is made-up of

(a) Tungsten-nickel alloy
(b) Tungsten-rhenium alloy
(c) Nickel-tin alloy
(d) Tungsten-aluminium alloy

Ans. (b). *Textbook of Radiology for Residents & Technicians, 5th ed., S.K. Bhargava & Sumeet Bhargava, p. 122.*

135. Pin hole diameter of focal spot in X-ray tube is

(a) 0.003 mm
(b) 0.006 mm
(c) 0.009 mm
(d) 0.012 mm

Ans. (a). *Textbook of Radiology for Residents & Technicians, 5th ed., S.K. Bhargava & Sumeet Bhargava, p. 119.*

136. In rotating anode tube, heat produced in target, contribute to incident energy equal to

(a) 70%
(b) 80%
(c) 90%
(d) 99%

Ans. (d). *Textbook of Radiology for Residents & Technicians, 5th ed., S.K. Bhargava & Sumeet Bhargava, p. 122.*

137. Filament in X-ray tube emits electron by process

(a) Space charge effect (b) Thermionic emission
(c) Both above (d) None above

Ans. (b). *Textbook of Radiology for Residents & Technicians, 5th ed., S.K. Bhargava & Sumeet Bhargava, p. 121.*

138. Inherent filtration in X-ray tube is 0.5-1 mm of

(a) Lead equivalent (b) Nickel equivalent
(c) Aluminium equivalent (d) None of the above

Ans. (c). *Textbook of Radiology for Residents & Technicians, 5th ed., S.K. Bhargava & Sumeet Bhargava, p. 123.*

139. Filament current in X-ray tube is about

(a) 5–10 amp (b) 10–15 amp
(c) 0–5 amp (d) 8–12 amp

Ans. (a). *Textbook of Radiology for Residents & Technicians, 5th ed., S.K. Bhargava & Sumeet Bhargava, p. 121.*

140. Tube current in X-ray tube range between

(a) 1–100 mA (b) 1–300 mA
(c) 1–500 mA (d) 1–1000 mA

Ans. (d). *Textbook of Radiology for Residents & Technicians, 5th ed., S.K. Bhargava & Sumeet Bhargava, p. 122.*

141. High frequency generator has ripple factor

(a) 100% (b) 12%
(c) 4% (d) Negligible

Ans. (d). *Textbook of Radiology for Residents & Technicians, 5th ed., S.K. Bhargava & Sumeet Bhargava, p. 134.*

142. Advantage of 3-phase generator over single phase is

(a) Short exposure time and high tube rating
(b) Large exposure time and high tube rating
(c) Large exposure time and low tube rating
(d) Short exposure time and low tube rating

Ans. (a). *Textbook of Radiology for Residents & Technicians, 5th ed., S.K. Bhargava & Sumeet Bhargava, p. 133.*

143. Modern X-Ray tubes used in diagnostic radiology has

(a) Vacuum (b) Helium gas
(c) Carbon dioxide (d) None

Ans. (a). *Textbook of Radiology for Residents & Technicians, 5th ed., S.K. Bhargava & Sumeet Bhargava, p. 120.*

144. In modern X-ray tube, the amount of electrons utilized in producing X-rays are

(a) 99% (b) 50%
(c) 10% (d) 1%

Ans. (d). *Textbook of Radiology for Residents & Technicians, 5th ed., S.K. Bhargava & Sumeet Bhargava, p. 120.*

145. The envelope in modern X-ray vaccumatic tube is made-up of

(a) Borosilicate glass envelope (b) Metal envelope
(c) Lead envelope (d) None

Ans. (a). *Textbook of Radiology for Residents & Technicians, 5th ed., S.K. Bhargava & Sumeet Bhargava, p. 120.*

146. The size of actual focal spot as compare to effective focal spot is

(a) Larger (b) Smaller
(c) Equal (d) None

Ans. (a). *Textbook of Radiology for Residents & Technicians, 5th ed., S.K. Bhargava & Sumeet Bhargava, p. 119.*

147. The requirement of the ideal material for anode is

(a) High atomic number, so high conversion efficiency for electrons into X-rays
(b) High melting point
(c) High specific heat and high thermal conductivity
(d) All of the above

Ans. (d). *Textbook of Radiology for Residents & Technicians, 5th ed., S.K. Bhargava & Sumeet Bhargava, p. 122.*

148. Tungsten is the ideal material for anode because it has

(a) High atomic number (74)
(b) High melting point (3370°C)
(c) High specific heat and high thermal conductivity
(d) All of the above

Ans. (d). *Textbook of Radiology for Residents & Technicians, 5th ed., S.K. Bhargava & Sumeet Bhargava, p. 122.*

149. The "heel effect" is

(a) Higher on cathode side than anode side
(b) Higher on anode side than cathode side
(c) Equal on both on cathode and anode side

Ans. (a). *Textbook of Radiology for Residents & Technicians, 5th ed., S.K. Bhargava & Sumeet Bhargava, p. 137.*

150. "Heel effect" depends on

(a) Anode angle (b) Size of the anode
(c) Shape of the anode (d) None above

Ans. (a). *Textbook of Radiology for Residents & Technicians, 5th ed., S.K. Bhargava & Sumeet Bhargava, p. 137.*

151. Which statement is correct?

(a) Smaller the anode angle, larger the heel effect
(b) Smaller the anode angle, smaller the heel effect
(c) Anode angle has no effect on heel effect
(d) The larger the anode angle, larger the heel effect

Ans. (a). *Textbook of Radiology for Residents & Technicians, 5th ed., S.K. Bhargava & Sumeet Bhargava, p. 122.*

152. The quality of X-rays depends on

(a) Anode angle (b) Atomic number
(c) KVP (d) All above

Ans. (d). *Textbook of Radiology for Residents & Technicians, 5th ed., S.K. Bhargava & Sumeet Bhargava, p. 122.*

153. The quality of X-rays depends upon

(a) Waveform (b) mAs
(c) Exposure time (d) None

Ans. (a). *Textbook of Radiology for Residents & Technicians, 5th ed., S.K. Bhargava & Sumeet Bhargava, p. 122.*

154. The quality of X-rays depends on

(a) Filtration (b) mAs
(c) Exposure time (d) None

Ans. (a). *Textbook of Radiology for Residents & Technicians, 5th ed., S.K. Bhargava & Sumeet Bhargava, p. 118.*

155. Anode heel effect can be used

(a) Thicker parts of the body towards cathode
(b) Thicker parts of the body towards anode
(c) No effect
(d) None of the statement above is true

Ans. (a). *Textbook of Radiology for Residents & Technicians, 5th ed., S.K. Bhargava & Sumeet Bhargava, p. 137.*

156. Rating of the X-ray tube is directly proportional to

(a) kV_p (b) Size of the focus
(c) Rotation of the tube (d) All of the above

Ans. (d). *Textbook of Radiology for Residents & Technicians, 5th ed., S.K. Bhargava & Sumeet Bhargava, p. 139.*

157. Rating of the X-ray tube is highest in

(a) 3-pulse rectification
(b) 6-pulse rectification
(c) 12-pulse rectification
(d) None above

Ans. (c). *Textbook of Radiology for Residents & Technicians, 5th ed., S.K. Bhargava & Sumeet Bhargava, p. 139.*

158. With high KV, patient dose

(a) Increases
(b) Reduced
(c) No effect
(d) None of the above is true

Ans. (b). *Textbook of Radiology for Residents & Technicians, 5th ed., S.K. Bhargava & Sumeet Bhargava, p. 126.*

159. With high KV, contrast of film

(a) Reduced
(b) Increased
(c) No effect
(d) None of the above is true

Ans. (a). *Textbook of Radiology for Residents & Technicians, 5th ed., S.K. Bhargava & Sumeet Bhargava, p. 126.*

160. Size of the focal spot can be measured at

(a) Edge of X-ray beam
(b) Peripheral part of the X-ray beam
(c) Central part of the X-ray beam
(d) In any part of the X-ray beam

Ans. (c). *Textbook of Radiology for Residents & Technicians, 5th ed., S.K. Bhargava & Sumeet Bhargava, p. 119.*

161. Effective focal spot of X-ray tube increases with

(a) High mA
(b) Low kV_p
(c) Increase in anode angle
(d) All above

Ans. (d). *Textbook of Radiology for Residents & Technicians, 5th ed., S.K. Bhargava & Sumeet Bhargava, p. 119.*

162. Modern X-ray tubes has got a dual focus of

(a) 1.2 mm & 2 mm
(b) 0.6 mm & 1.2 mm
(c) 0.3 mm & 2 mm
(d) All above true

Ans. (d). *Textbook of Radiology for Residents & Technicians, 5th ed., S.K. Bhargava & Sumeet Bhargava, p. 121.*

163. Percentage (%) of rhenium mixed in tungsten for anode is

(a) 1–2%
(b) 5–6%
(c) 10–12%
(d) 15–20%

Ans. (b). Textbook of Radiology for Residents & Technicians, 5th ed., S.K. Bhargava & Sumeet Bhargava, p. 122.

164. Rhenium is added in anode tungsten because of
(a) High thermal capacity, thus prevent cracks
(b) High conductivity
(c) High melting point
(d) High atomic number

Ans. (a). Textbook of Radiology for Residents & Technicians, 5th ed., S.K. Bhargava & Sumeet Bhargava, p. 122.

165. Magnification in radiography obtained
(a) Small S.I.R.D. (Source Image Receptor Distance)
(b) Large O.I.D (Object Image Distance)
(c) Small focal spot
(d) All above

Ans. (d). Textbook of Radiology for Residents & Technicians, 5th ed., S.K. Bhargava & Sumeet Bhargava, p. 198.

166. The stem of the rotating anode disc is made-up of molybdenum due to
(a) Good thermal conductivity
(b) Poor thermal conductivity
(c) Good heat storage capacity
(d) No heat storage capacity

Ans. (b). Textbook of Radiology for Residents & Technicians, 5th ed., S.K. Bhargava & Sumeet Bhargava, p. 122.

167. Parallel grid in radiography is frequently used with
(a) Stationary units
(b) Mobile units
(c) Mammography units
(d) Dental units

Ans. (b). Textbook of Radiology for Residents & Technicians, 5th ed., S.K. Bhargava & Sumeet Bhargava, p. 201.

168. Maximum "grid cut-off" is most common in
(a) Parallel grid
(b) Focussed grid
(c) Cross grid
(d) Moving grid

Ans. (a). Textbook of Radiology for Residents & Technicians, 5th ed., S.K. Bhargava & Sumeet Bhargava, p. 201.

169. Which of the statement is not true about grid?
(a) High grid ratio gives high patient dose
(b) High grid ratio gives better grid function
(c) With increase in grid ratio, the contrast improvement factor increases
(d) Primary transmission increase with increasing grid ratio

Ans. (d). Textbook of Radiology for Residents & Technicians, 5th ed., S.K. Bhargava & Sumeet Bhargava, p. 202.

170. Lead strips in grid usually have thickness of

(a) 0.5 mm
(b) 1 mm
(c) 5 mm
(d) 0.05 mm

Ans. (d). Textbook of Radiology for Residents & Technicians, 5th ed., S.K. Bhargava & Sumeet Bhargava, p. 200.

171. Contrast can be improved by

(a) Grid
(b) Air gap technique
(c) kV_p
(d) All

Ans. (d). Textbook of Radiology for Residents & Technicians, 5th ed., S.K. Bhargava & Sumeet Bhargava, p. 202.

172. Which of the following are true for moving grid?

(a) Costly
(b) Gives approx. 15% more radiation to the patient
(c) The distance between patient and film is increased
(d) All above

Ans. (d). Textbook of Radiology for Residents & Technicians, 5th ed., S.K. Bhargava & Sumeet Bhargava, p. 201.

173. Grid ratio is the

(a) Height of lead strip by distance between them
(b) Distance between lead strips by height
(c) Height of the lead strip multiplied by the distance
(d) None of the above

Ans. (a). Textbook of Radiology for Residents & Technicians, 5th ed., S.K. Bhargava & Sumeet Bhargava, p. 201.

174. Interspace material can be made-up of

(a) Aluminium
(b) Card board
(c) Carbon fiber
(d) Any of the above

Ans. (d). Textbook of Radiology for Residents & Technicians, 5th ed., S.K. Bhargava & Sumeet Bhargava, p. 201.

175. Usual contrast improvement factor is

(a) Less than 2
(b) Between 2 and 5
(c) Between 6 and 10
(d) More than 10

Ans. (b). Textbook of Radiology for Residents & Technicians, 5th ed., S.K. Bhargava & Sumeet Bhargava, p. 205.

176. Mostly grids have frequencies in the range of

(a) 1–50 lines per inch
(b) 60–110 lines per inch

(c) 120–160 lines per inch (d) 170–210 lines per inch

Ans. (b). *Textbook of Radiology for Residents & Technicians, 5th ed., S.K. Bhargava & Sumeet Bhargava, p. 202.*

177. Mostly grids have line density of

(a) 1–20 lines per cm (b) 25–45 lines per cm
(c) 50–70 lines per cm (d) 75–90 lines per cm

Ans. (b). *Textbook of Radiology for Residents & Technicians, 5th ed., S.K. Bhargava & Sumeet Bhargava, p. 202.*

178. The main purpose of the interspace material in the grid is to

(a) Absorb scatter radiation (b) Support thin lead strip
(c) Absorb primary radiation (d) None of the above

Ans. (b). *Textbook of Radiology for Residents & Technicians, 5th ed., S.K. Bhargava & Sumeet Bhargava, p. 201.*

179. Patient exposure is higher when material used in grid interspace

(a) Aluminium interspace (b) Carbon fiber
(c) Card board (d) None

Ans. (a). *Textbook of Radiology for Residents & Technicians, 5th ed., S.K. Bhargava & Sumeet Bhargava, p. 202.*

180. "Grid cut-off" can be reduced to

(a) Focussed grid (b) Unfocussed grid
(c) High grid ratio (d) None of the above

Ans. (d). *Textbook of Radiology for Residents & Technicians, 5th ed., S.K. Bhargava & Sumeet Bhargava, p. 202.*

181. By using grids, contrast is

(a) improved (b) decreased
(c) no effect (d) None of the above

Ans. (a). *Textbook of Radiology for Residents & Technicians, 5th ed., S.K. Bhargava & Sumeet Bhargava, p. 201.*

182. Grids are generally used in

(a) Fatty person (b) Thin person
(c) Children (d) Pregnant women

Ans. (a). *Textbook of Radiology for Residents & Technicians, 5th ed., S.K. Bhargava & Sumeet Bhargava, p. 202.*

183. "Grid cut-off" can be reduced

(a) High grid ratio
(b) Longer F.F.D when using unfocussed grids
(c) Shorter F.F.D when using unfocussed grids

(d) None

Ans. (b). *Textbook of Radiology for Residents & Technicians, 5th ed., S.K. Bhargava & Sumeet Bhargava, p. 202.*

184. Which is not true about moving grids

(a) Blur out shadow cast by lead strips
(b) Increase patient dose
(c) Decrease cut-off
(d) More costly than stationary grids

Ans. (c). *Textbook of Radiology for Residents & Technicians, 5th ed., S.K. Bhargava & Sumeet Bhargava, p. 201.*

185. X-ray are identified by

(a) Energy
(b) Wavelength
(c) Frequency
(d) None

Ans. (a). *Radiological Science for Technologists by Stewart Carlyce Bushang, 9th Ed., Mosby Elsevier, 2008, p. 63.*

186. Visible length is identified by

(a) Energy
(b) Wavelength
(c) Frequency
(d) None

Ans. (b). *Radiological Science for Technologists by Stewart Carlyce Bushang, 9th Ed., Mosby Elsevier, 2008, p. 63.*

187. Conductor is a substance in which

(a) Electrons flow easily
(b) Electrons do not allow electrons to flow
(c) Sometimes allow and sometimes does not allow
(d) None

Ans. (a). *Radiological Science for Technologists by Stewart Carlyce Bushang, 9th Ed., Mosby Elsevier, 2008, p. 79.*

188. Insulators are the substance in which

(a) Electrons flow easily
(b) Electrons do not allow electrons to flow
(c) Sometimes allow and sometimes does not allow
(d) None

Ans. (b). *Radiological Science for Technologists by Stewart Carlyce Bushang, 9th Ed., Mosby Elsevier, 2008, p. 79.*

189. The magnitude of the induced current depends on

(a) The strength and velocity of the magnetic field
(b) The angle of the conductor to the magnetic field
(c) The number of the turns in the conductor

(d) All above

Ans. (d). *Radiological Science for Technologists by Stewart Carlyce Bushang, 9th Ed., Mosby Elsevier, 2008, p. 91*

190. The ideal table top required for X-ray table is

(a) Carbon fiber (b) Plastic
(c) Wood (d) None

Ans. (a). *Radiological Science for Technologists by Stewart Carlyce Bushang, 9th Ed., Mosby Elsevier, 2008, p. 101.*

191. The carbon fiber table top is used in X-ray table due to

(a) Strong
(b) Absorb little X-ray radiation
(c) Reduce patient radiation dose
(d) All above

Ans. (d). *Radiological Science for Technologists by Stewart Carlyce Bushang, 9th Ed., Mosby Elsevier, 2008, p. 101.*

192. kV_p determines the

(a) Quality of the X-ray beam (b) Quantity of the X-ray beam
(c) Both (d) None

Ans. (a). *Radiological Science for Technologists by Stewart Carlyce Bushang, 9th Ed., Mosby Elsevier, 2008, p. 106.*

193. Autotransformer operates on the principle of

(a) Induction (b) Conduction
(c) Both (d) None

Ans. (a). *Radiological Science for Technologists by Stewart Carlyce Bushang, 9th Ed., Mosby Elsevier, 2008, p. 105.*

194. The voltage in autotransformer received and then it provides (the secondary voltage) is _______ proportional to the number of turns.

(a) Directly (b) Inversely
(c) Both (d) None

Ans. (a). *Radiological Science for Technologists by Stewart Carlyce Bushang, 9th Ed., Mosby Elsevier, 2008, p. 105.*

195. Artifacts on the radiograph are due to

(a) Exposure (b) Processing
(c) Handling (d) All above

Ans. (d). *Radiological Science for Technologists by Stewart Carlyce Bushang, 9th Ed., Mosby Elsevier, 2008, p. 298.*

196. The effective atomic number of fat is

(a) 6.3
(b) 7.4
(c) 13.8
(d) None

Ans. (a). *Radiological Science for Technologists by Stewart Carlyce Bushang, 9th Ed., Mosby Elsevier, 2008, p. 167.*

197. The effective atomic number of soft tissue/lung is

(a) 6.3
(b) 7.4
(c) 13.8
(d) None

Ans. (b). *Radiological Science for Technologists by Stewart Carlyce Bushang, 9th Ed., Mosby Elsevier, 2008, P. 167.*

198. The effective atomic number of bone is

(a) 6.3
(b) 7.4
(c) 13.8
(d) None

Ans. (c). *Radiological Science for Technologists by Stewart Carlyce Bushang, 9th Ed., Mosby Elsevier, 2008, p. 167.*

199. Xeroradiography has got better detail and contrast because of

(a) High kV_p
(b) High mAs
(c) Edge enhancement
(d) None

Ans. (c). *Radiological Science for Technologists by Stewart Carlyce Bushang, 9th Ed., Mosby Elsevier, 2008, p. 319.*

200. Screening mammography is indicated in

(a) Symptomatic patients
(b) Patients with high or elevated risk factors
(c) Asymptomatic patients
(d) None

Ans. (c). *Radiological Science for Technologists by Stewart Carlyce Bushang, 9th Ed., Mosby Elsevier, 2008, p. 320.*

201. Diagnostic mammography involves

(a) Mediolateral view
(b) Craniocaudal view
(c) Lateral view
(d) All

Ans. (d). *Radiological Science for Technologists by Stewart Carlyce Bushang, 9th Ed., Mosby Elsevier, 2008, p. 320.*

202. Screening mammography involves

(a) Mediolateral view
(b) Craniocaudal view
(c) Lateral view
(d) All

Ans. (a). *Radiological Science for Technologists by Stewart Carlyce Bushang, 9th Ed., Mosby Elsevier, 2008, p. 320.*

203. In breast, most sensitive tissue to cancer by radiation is

(a) Fibrous
(b) Glandular
(c) Adipose (fat)
(d) All tissues

Ans. (b). *Radiological Science for Technologists by Stewart Carlyce Bushang, 9th Ed., Mosby Elsevier, 2008, p. 320.*

204. Dedicated mammography tube should have

(a) High frequency generator with flexibility in patient's positioning and automatic exposure control
(b) Low grid ratio with microfocus X-ray tube
(c) Single emulsion screen film image receptor
(d) All above

Ans. (d). *Radiological Science for Technologists by Stewart Carlyce Bushang, 9th Ed., Mosby Elsevier, 2008, p. 321.*

205. Compression in mammography is important due to

(a) Improved spatial resolution
(b) Improved contrast resolution
(c) Reduced patient dose
(d) All above

Ans. (d). *Radiological Science for Technologists by Stewart Carlyce Bushang, 9th Ed., Mosby Elsevier, 2008, p. 326.*

206. The function of the Automatic Exposure Control (AEC) is to

(a) Measure the X-ray intensity
(b) Improve image quality by improving spatial resolution
(c) Minimize object to image (OID) receptor distance
(d) All above

Ans. (d). *Radiological Science for Technologists by Stewart Carlyce Bushang, 9th Ed., Mosby Elsevier, 2008, p. 327.*

207. The target of mammography tube is made-up of

(a) Tungsten (W)
(b) Molybdenum (Mo)
(c) Rhodium (Rh)
(d) Any of the above

Ans. (d). *Radiological Science for Technologists by Stewart Carlyce Bushang, 9th Ed., Mosby Elsevier, 2008, p. 322.*

208. The characteristic of the small focal spot in mammography to obtain higher spatial resolution is

(a) Effective focal spot sizes (large/small of 0.3/0.1 mm)
(b) Approximate 23^0 angle
(c) 6 degree X-ray tube
(d) All above

Ans. (d). *Radiological Science for Technologists by Stewart Carlyce Bushang, 9th Ed., Mosby Elsevier, 2008, p. 323.*

209. During fluoroscopy

(a) Real time dynamic viewing (b) Spot film taken
(c) Contrast studies (d) All above

Ans. (d). *Radiological Science for Technologists by Stewart Carlyce Bushang, 9th Ed., Mosby Elsevier, 2008, p. 347.*

210. During fluoroscopy, the X-ray tube operates at

(a) Less than 5 mA (b) 10–15 mA
(c) 25–35 mA (d) Above 60 mA

Ans. (a). *Radiological Science for Technologists by Stewart Carlyce Bushang, 9th Ed., Mosby Elsevier, 2008, p. 347.*

211. The patient dose during fluoroscopy as compare to radiography is

(a) Much high (b) Low
(c) Equal (d) None above

Ans. (a). *Radiological Science for Technologists by Stewart Carlyce Bushang, 9th Ed., Mosby Elsevier, 2008, p. 347.*

212. Illumination level during fluoroscopy is measured in

(a) Luminance per square meter or lux
(b) Ampere
(c) Watt
(d) None of the above

Ans. (a). *Radiological Science for Technologists by Stewart Carlyce Bushang, 9th Ed., Mosby Elsevier, 2008, p. 347.*

213. 100–1000 lux is required to visualize the

(a) Radiograph
(b) Image intensified fluoroscopy
(c) Both (a) and (b)
(d) None

Ans. (c). *Radiological Science for Technologists by Stewart Carlyce Bushang, 9th Ed., Mosby Elsevier, 2008, p. 347.*

214. The emission of electron from photocathode to anode is by the process of

(a) Photoemission (b) Thermionic emission
(c) Electroemission (d) None

Ans. (a). *Radiological Science for Technologists by Stewart Carlyce Bushang, 9th Ed., Mosby Elsevier, 2008, p. 350.*

215. Brightness gain in image intensifier is

(a) Minification gain × flux gain

(b) Minification gain ÷ flux gain
(c) Minification gain + flux gain
(d) Minification gain – flux gain

Ans. (a). *Radiological Science for Technologists by Stewart Carlyce Bushang, 9th Ed., Mosby Elsevier, 2008, p. 351.*

216. Minification gain is

(a) Diameter of input phosphor divided by diameter of the output phosphor
(b) Diameter of the input phosphor multiplied by diameter of the output phosphor
(c) Diameter of the input phosphor plus diameter of the output phosphor
(d) Diameter of the input phosphor minus the diameter of the output phosphor

Ans. (a). *Radiological Science for Technologists by Stewart Carlyce Bushang, 9th Ed., Mosby Elsevier, 2008, p. 351.*

217. Flux gain is

(a) Number of output light photon divided by number of input X-ray photons
(b) Number of output light photons multiplied by number of input X-ray photons
(c) Number of output light photons plus number of input X-ray photons
(d) Number of output light photons minus number of input X-ray photons

Ans. (a). *Radiological Science for Technologists by Stewart Carlyce Bushang, 9th Ed., Mosby Elsevier, 2008, p. 351.*

218. Magnification mode results in

(a) Better spatial resolution
(b) Better contrast resolution
(c) Higher patient dose
(d) All above

Ans. (d). *Radiological Science for Technologists by Stewart Carlyce Bushang, 9th Ed., Mosby Elsevier, 2008, p. 352.*

219. The advantage of image intensifier over conventional fluoroscopy are

(a) Increase brightness and contrast
(b) Allows storage of image in its electronic form for later play back and image manipulation
(c) No dark room and adaptation

(d) All above

Ans. (d). Radiological Science for Technologists by Stewart Carlyce Bushang, 9th Ed., Mosby Elsevier, 2008, p. 353.

220. Photospot has the following
(a) Provide adequate image quality over cassette spot
(b) Increase patient dose compare the cassette spot
(c) 105 mm film image is minified as compare to life speed cassette image
(d) All above

Ans. (d). Radiological Science for Technologists by Stewart Carlyce Bushang, 9th Ed., Mosby Elsevier, 2008, p. 358.

221. The cardinal principal of radiation protection are
(a) Keep the time of exposure to radiation as short as possible
(b) Maintain as a large distance as possible between source of radiation and the exposed person
(c) Insert shielding material between the radiation source and the exposed persons
(d) All of the above

Ans. (d). Radiological Science for Technologists by Stewart Carlyce Bushang, 9th Ed., Mosby Elsevier, 2008, p. 572.

222. The leakage radiation at a distance of 1 mm from protective housing must be less than
(a) 100 mR/Hr (b) 200 mR/Hr
(c) 300 mR/Hr (d) 50 mR/Hr

Ans. (a). Radiological Science for Technologists by Stewart Carlyce Bushang, 9th Ed., Mosby Elsevier, 2008, p. 581.

223. The X-ray beam and the light beam must coincide within ______ % of the SID (Surface to Image Receptor Distance).
(a) 2% (b) 5%
(c) 10% (d) 20%

Ans. (a). Radiological Science for Technologists by Stewart Carlyce Bushang, 9th Ed., Mosby Elsevier, 2008, p. 581.

224. The general purpose diagnostic X-ray tubes operated above 70 kV_p must have a total filtration (inherent plus added)
(a) At least 2.5 mm Al (b) At least 1.5 mm Al
(c) At least 0.5 mm Al (d) At least 0.25 mm Al

Ans. (a). Radiological Science for Technologists by Stewart Carlyce Bushang, 9th Ed., Mosby Elsevier, 2008, p. 581.

225. The general purpose diagnostic X-ray tubes operated between 50–70 kV_p must have a total filtration (inherent plus added)

(a) At least 2.5 mm Al (b) At least 1.5 mm Al
(c) At least 0.5 mm Al (d) At least 0.25 mm Al

Ans. (b). *Radiological Science for Technologists by Stewart Carlyce Bushang, 9th Ed., Mosby Elsevier, 2008, p. 581.*

226. The general purpose diagnostic X-ray tubes operated below 50 kV_p must have a total filtration (inherent plus added)

(a) At least 2.5 mm Al (b) At least 1.5 mm Al
(c) At least 0.5 mm Al (d) At least 0.25 mm Al

Ans. (c). *Radiological Science for Technologists by Stewart Carlyce Bushang, 9th Ed., Mosby Elsevier, 2008, p. 581.*

227. During designing of the barriers of an X-ray room, the radiations are to be considered

(a) Leakage radiation (b) Primary radiation
(c) Scattered radiation (d) All above

Ans. (d). *Radiological Science for Technologists by Stewart Carlyce Bushang, 9th Ed., Mosby Elsevier, 2008, p. 581.*

228. In stationary fluoroscopy, the Source to Skin Distance (SSD) must not be less than

(a) 38 cm (b) 25 cm
(c) 15 cm (d) 10 cm

Ans. (a). *Radiological Science for Technologists by Stewart Carlyce Bushang, 9th Ed., Mosby Elsevier, 2008, p. 581.*

229. Change in exposure factors are required for

(a) Fiber glass cast (b) Plaster cast
(c) Both (d) None

Ans. (b). *Textbook of Radiology for Residents & Technicians, 5th ed., S.K. Bhargava & Sumeet Bhargava, p. 194.*

230. To increase the exposure factor for dry cast, mAs should be increased

(a) 2 times (b) 5 times
(c) 7 times (d) No need to increase mAs

Ans. (a). *Textbook of Radiology for Residents & Technicians, 5th ed., S.K. Bhargava & Sumeet Bhargava, p. 194.*

231. Increase in mAs required is greater for

(a) Dry cast (b) Wet cast
(c) Same for both casts (d) No need to increase mAs

Ans. (b). *Textbook of Radiology for Residents & Technicians, 5th ed., S.K. Bhargava & Sumeet Bhargava, p. 194.*

232. Which of the following should be done in case of radiograph of a patient with plaster cast?
(a) Increase in mAs
(b) Increase in kVp
(c) Increase in both mAs and kVp
(d) Decrease in both mAs and kVp

Ans. (a). *Textbook of Radiology for Residents & Technicians, 5th ed., S.K. Bhargava & Sumeet Bhargava, p. 194.*

233. Isotopes have
(a) Same atomic number but different atomic mass
(b) Same atomic number but same atomic mass
(c) Different atomic number but different atomic mass
(d) Different atomic number but same atomic mass

Ans. (a). *Radiological Science for Technologists by Stewart Carlyce Bushang, 9th Ed., Mosby Elsevier, 2008, p. 46.*

234. Isobars have
(a) Same atomic mass but different atomic numbers
(b) Same atomic mass but same atomic number
(c) Different atomic mass but different atomic number
(d) Different atomic mass but same atomic number

Ans. (a). *Radiological Science for Technologists by Stewart Carlyce Bushang, 9th Ed., Mosby Elsevier, 2008, p. 47.*

235. Which of the following are the ionizing radiation
(a) Alpha radiation
(b) Beta radiation
(c) Gamma and X-rays
(d) All of the above

Ans. (d). *Radiological Science for Technologists by Stewart Carlyce Bushang, 9th Ed., Mosby Elsevier, 2008, p. 52.*

236. Alpha particles is a helium that contain
(a) Two protons and two neutrons
(b) Two protons and one neutron
(c) One proton and two neutrons
(d) One proton and one neutron

Ans. (a). *Radiological Science for Technologists by Stewart Carlyce Bushang, 9th Ed., Mosby Elsevier, 2008, p. 53.*

237. Beta particle is
(a) Electron emitted from nucleus of a radioactive atom

(b) Electron emitted from nucleus of an atom
(c) Electron emitted from nucleus of an atom
(d) None above

Ans. (a). *Textbook of Radiology for Residents & Technicians, 5th ed., S.K. Bhargava & Sumeet Bhargava, p. 97-99.*

238. Which of the following is highly ionizing radiation with very short range in matter?

(a) Alpha particle (b) Beta particle
(c) X-rays (d) None

Ans. (a). *Radiological Science for Technologists by Stewart Carlyce Bushang, 9th Ed., Mosby Elsevier, 2008, p. 54.*

239. Which of the following are called photons?

(a) X-rays
(b) Gamma rays
(c) Alpha rays
(d) Both X-rays and gamma rays

Ans. (d). *Radiological Science for Technologists by Stewart Carlyce Bushang, 9th Ed., Mosby Elsevier, 2008, p. 53.*

240. Characteristics of the photons are

(a) No mass
(b) No charge
(c) Travel at speed of light ($C = 3 \times 10^8$ m/s) and loses intensity with distance
(d) All above

Ans. (d). *Radiological Science for Technologists by Stewart Carlyce Bushang, 9th Ed., Mosby Elsevier, 2008, p. 53.*

241. At a given velocity, wavelength and frequency are

(a) Inversely proportional (b) Directly proportional
(c) Equal (d) None

Ans. (a). *Radiological Science for Technologists by Stewart Carlyce Bushang, 9th Ed., Mosby Elsevier, 2008, p. 59.*

242. X-rays are emitted

(a) From electrons cloud of an atom that has stimulated artificially
(b) From inside the electrons of an radioactive atom
(c) Both
(d) None

Ans. (a). *Radiological Science for Technologists by Stewart Carlyce Bushang, 9th Ed., Mosby Elsevier, 2008, p. 63.*

243. Gamma rays are emitted

(a) From electrons cloud of an atom that has stimulated artificially
(b) From inside the electrons of an radioactive atom
(c) Both
(d) None

Ans. (b). *Radiological Science for Technologists by Stewart Carlyce Bushang, 9th Ed., Mosby Elsevier, 2008, p. 63.*

244. An exposure was made using 600 mA and 18 mA . If the mA is changed to 400, which of the following exposure times would most closely approximate the original radiographic density?

(a) 16 ms
(b) 0.16 second
(c) 27 ms
(d) 0.27 second

Ans. (c). *Textbook of Radiology for Residents & Technicians, 5th ed., S.K. Bhargava & Sumeet Bhargava, p. 197.*

245. If the exposure rate to a body standing 3 feet from a radiation source is 12 mR/min., what will be the exposure rate to that body at a distance of 7 feet from the source?

(a) 2.2 mR/min
(b) 5.1 mR/min
(c) 28 mR/min
(d) 36 mR/min

Ans. (a). *Textbook of Radiology for Residents & Technicians, 5th ed., S.K. Bhargava & Sumeet Bhargava, p. 197.*

246. The effective energy of X-ray beam is unrelated by

(a) Filtration
(b) Kilovoltage
(c) Milliampere
(d) All of the above

Ans. (c). *Textbook of Radiology for Residents & Technicians, 5th ed., S.K. Bhargava & Sumeet Bhargava, p. 111.*

247. The effective energy of the X-ray beam is increased by increasing the

(a) Milliampere
(b) Added filtration
(c) Second
(d) None above

Ans. (b). *Textbook of Radiology for Residents & Technicians, 5th ed., S.K. Bhargava & Sumeet Bhargava, p. 111.*

248. The effective energy of the X-ray beam is increased by increasing the

(a) Kilovoltage
(b) Seconds
(c) Milliampere
(d) None of the above

Ans. (a). *Textbook of Radiology for Residents & Technicians, 5th ed., S.K. Bhargava & Sumeet Bhargava, p. 111.*

249. Geometric unsharpness is most likely to be greater

(a) At long side
(b) At the anode end of image
(c) With small focal spot size
(d) At the cathode end of image

Ans. (d). *Textbook of Radiology for Residents & Technicians, 5th ed., S.K. Bhargava & Sumeet Bhargava, p. 196.*

250. Which of the following waveform has the 100% voltage drop between peak voltages?

(a) Single phase
(b) Three phase, 6 pulse
(c) Three phase, 12 pulse
(d) High frequency

Ans. (a). *Textbook of Radiology for Residents & Technicians, 5th ed., S.K. Bhargava & Sumeet Bhargava, p. 130.*

251. Which of the following waveform has about 13% voltage drop between peak voltages?

(a) Single phase
(b) Three phase, 6 pulse
(c) Three phase, 12 pulse
(d) High frequency

Ans. (b). *Textbook of Radiology for Residents & Technicians, 5th ed., S.K. Bhargava & Sumeet Bhargava, p. 130.*

252. Which of the following waveform has about 4% voltage drop between peak voltages?

(a) Single phase
(b) Three phase, 6 pulse
(c) Three phase, 12 pulse
(d) High frequency

Ans. (c). *Textbook of Radiology for Residents & Technicians, 5th ed., S.K. Bhargava & Sumeet Bhargava, p. 130.*

253. Which of the following waveforms have almost negligible (less than 1% voltage ripple)

(a) High frequency
(b) Single phase
(c) Three phase, 6 pulse
(d) Three phase, 12 pulse

Ans. (a). *Textbook of Radiology for Residents & Technicians, 5th ed., S.K. Bhargava & Sumeet Bhargava, p. 130.*

254. All of the following statements regarding three phase current are true except

(a) Three phase current is constant potential direct current
(b) Three phase equipment produce more X-rays per mAs
(c) Three phase produces higher – average energy X-rays than single phase
(d) The three phase wave form has less ripple than single phase

Ans. (a). *Textbook of Radiology for Residents & Technicians, 5th ed., S.K. Bhargava & Sumeet Bhargava, p. 130.*

255. Optical density is measured directly by

(a) Sensitometer
(b) Densitometer
(c) Penetrometer
(d) H & D curve

Ans. (b). *Textbook of Radiology for Residents & Technicians, 5th ed., S.K. Bhargava & Sumeet Bhargava, p. 206.*

256. When X-ray photons interacts with matter and disappear as an photoelectric effect is termed as

(a) Absorption
(b) Scattering
(c) Attenuation
(d) Divergence

Ans. (a). *Textbook of Radiology for Residents & Technicians, 5th ed., S.K. Bhargava & Sumeet Bhargava, p. 159.*

257. Change in direction of X-ray photons occurs when there is partial transfer of energy to matters (as in compton effect)

(a) Absorption
(b) Scattering
(c) Attenuation
(d) Divergence

Ans. (b). *Textbook of Radiology for Residents & Technicians, 5th ed., S.K. Bhargava & Sumeet Bhargava, p. 161.*

258. The reduction in X-ray photon intensity as the photon passes through the material is termed as

(a) Absorption
(b) Scattering
(c) Attenuation
(d) Divergence

Ans. (c). *Textbook of Radiology for Residents & Technicians, 5th ed., S.K. Bhargava & Sumeet Bhargava, p. 158.*

259. Inherent and added filtration in the X-ray tube function to

(a) Reduce patient skin dose
(b) Reduce contrast
(c) Reduce scattered radiation
(d) Soften the X-ray beam

Ans. (a). *Textbook of Radiology for Residents & Technicians, 5th ed., S.K. Bhargava & Sumeet Bhargava, p. 166.*

260. If the entrance of the particular radiograph is 320 mR, the radiation exposure at 1 metre from patient will be approximately

(a) 32 mR
(b) 3.2 mR
(c) 0.32 mR
(d) 0.032 mR

Ans. (c). *Textbook of Radiology for Residents & Technicians, 5th ed., S.K. Bhargava & Sumeet Bhargava, p. 166-168.*

261. The primary function of filtration is to reduce

(a) Patient skin dose
(b) Operator dose
(c) Image noise
(d) Scattered radiation

Ans. (a). *Textbook of Radiology for Residents & Technicians, 5th ed., S.K. Bhargava & Sumeet Bhargava, p. 166-168.*

262. Increase in mA is obtained by
(a) Increase in speed of the anode rotation
(b) Increasing the transformer turn ratio
(c) Using three phase rectification
(d) Increasing the heat of the filament

Ans. (d). *Textbook of Radiology for Residents & Technicians, 5th ed., S.K. Bhargava & Sumeet Bhargava, p. 122.*

263. The image density arising from factors other than the light of the radiation is called
(a) Fog
(b) Log relative exposure
(c) Optical density
(d) Artifacts

Ans. (a). *Textbook of Radiology for Residents & Technicians, 5th ed., S.K. Bhargava & Sumeet Bhargava, p. 206.*

264. The law that governs the force between electric charge is called
(a) Ampere's law
(b) Coulomb's law
(c) Faraday's law
(d) Ohm's law

Ans. (b). *Textbook of Radiology for Residents & Technicians, 5th ed., S.K. Bhargava & Sumeet Bhargava, p. 97-114.*

265. In a charged capacitor, the energy is stored in
(a) the field between the plates
(b) the positive charges
(c) the negative charges
(d) None of the above

Ans. (a). *Textbook of Radiology for Residents & Technicians, 5th ed., S.K. Bhargava & Sumeet Bhargava, p. 97-114.*

266. Which of the following relations is correct?
(a) $v = q/c$
(b) $c = qv$
(c) $v = cq$
(d) $q = v/c$

Ans. (a). *Textbook of Radiology for Residents & Technicians, 5th ed., S.K. Bhargava & Sumeet Bhargava, p. 97-114.*

267. The energy stored in a capacitor of capacity *C* and potential *V* is given by
(a) $CV/2$
(b) $CV^2/2$
(c) $C^2V/2$
(d) $C^2V^2/2$

Ans. (b). *Textbook of Radiology for Residents & Technicians, 5th ed., S.K. Bhargava & Sumeet Bhargava, p. 97-114.*

268. When the temperature of a metallic conductor is increased its resistance

(a) always decreases
(b) always increases
(c) may be increased or decreased
(d) remains the same

Ans. (b). *Textbook of Radiology for Residents & Technicians, 5th ed., S.K. Bhargava & Sumeet Bhargava, p. 97-114.*

269. Heat produced in a conductor is

(a) directly proportional to its resistance
(b) inversely proportional to its resistance
(c) Both (a) and (b)
(d) None of the above

Ans. (a). *Textbook of Radiology for Residents & Technicians, 5th ed., S.K. Bhargava & Sumeet Bhargava, p. 97-114.*

270. The unit of magnetic induction *B* is

(a) weber
(b) weber/metre^2
(c) newton/(amp × metre)
(d) newton/metre

Ans. (b). *Textbook of Radiology for Residents & Technicians, 5th ed., S.K. Bhargava & Sumeet Bhargava, p. 97-114.*

271. Lenz's law is a statement of

(a) law of conservation of energy
(b) law of conservation of charge
(c) law of conservation of mass
(d) law of conservation of linear momentum

Ans. (a). *Textbook of Radiology for Residents & Technicians, 5th ed., S.K. Bhargava & Sumeet Bhargava, p. 97-114.*

272. A moving conductor coil produces an induced emf, this is in accordance with

(a) Lenz's law
(b) Faraday's law
(c) Coulomb's law
(d) Ampere's law

Ans. (b). *Textbook of Radiology for Residents & Technicians, 5th ed., S.K. Bhargava & Sumeet Bhargava, p. 97-114.*

273. Whenever current is changed in a coil, there is produced an induced emf in the same coil. This property of the coil is due to

(a) mutual induction
(b) self-induction
(c) eddy current
(d) hysteresis

Ans. (b). *Textbook of Radiology for Residents & Technicians, 5th ed., S.K. Bhargava & Sumeet Bhargava, p. 97-114.*

274. If the number of turns per unit length of a coil of a solenoid is doubled, the self-inductance of the solenoid will

(a) remain unchanged (b) be halved
(c) be doubled (d) become four times

Ans. (d). *Textbook of Radiology for Residents & Technicians, 5th ed., S.K. Bhargava & Sumeet Bhargava, p. 115-146.*

275. Which of the following are not EMW?

(a) Cosmic rays (b) Gamma rays
(c) Beta rays (d) X-rays

Ans. (c). *Textbook of Radiology for Residents & Technicians, 5th ed., S.K. Bhargava & Sumeet Bhargava, p. 97-114.*

276. Diode valves can be used as

(a) demodulator (b) amplifier
(c) an oscillator (d) a rectifier

Ans. (d). *Textbook of Radiology for Residents & Technicians, 5th ed., S.K. Bhargava & Sumeet Bhargava, p. 97-114.*

277. In which of the following the width of the forbidden band is small?

(a) Good conductors (b) Semiconductors
(c) Insulators (d) None of the above

Ans. (b). *Textbook of Radiology for Residents & Technicians, 5th ed., S.K. Bhargava & Sumeet Bhargava, p. 97-114.*

278. In insulators

(a) the valence band is partially filled with electrons.
(b) the conduction band is partially filled with electrons.
(c) the conduction band is filled with electrons and valence band is empty.
(d) the conduction band is empty and valence band is filled with electrons.

Ans. (d). *Textbook of Radiology for Residents & Technicians, 5th ed., S.K. Bhargava & Sumeet Bhargava, p. 97-114.*

279. X-ray were discovered by

(a) Madam Curie (b) W.C. Roentgen
(c) Van Laue (d) Rutherford

Ans. (b). *Textbook of Radiology for Residents & Technicians, 5th ed., S.K. Bhargava & Sumeet Bhargava, p. 97-114.*

280. X-rays are produced

(a) during electric discharge at low pressure.
(b) during nuclear explosions.

(c) when cathode rays are reflected from the target.
(d) when electron from higher energy state comes back to lower energy state.

Ans. (d). *Textbook of Radiology for Residents & Technicians, 5th ed., S.K. Bhargava & Sumeet Bhargava, p. 97-114.*

281. X-rays are produced due to
(a) break-up of molecules.
(b) changes in atomic energy level.
(c) changes in nuclear energy level.
(d) radioactive disintegration.

Ans. (b). *Textbook of Radiology for Residents & Technicians, 5th ed., S.K. Bhargava & Sumeet Bhargava, p. 97-114.*

282. The maximum frequency of X-ray is determined by
(a) current in filament.
(b) potential difference across filament.
(c) potential difference across cathode and anticathode.
(d) current from high tension.

Ans. (c). *Textbook of Radiology for Residents & Technicians, 5th ed., S.K. Bhargava & Sumeet Bhargava, p. 115-146.*

283. X-rays
(a) are deflected in magnetic field.
(b) are deflected in electric field.
(c) remain undeflected by both a and b.
(d) are deflected in both the fields.

Ans. (c). *Textbook of Radiology for Residents & Technicians, 5th ed., S.K. Bhargava & Sumeet Bhargava, p. 97-114.*

284. In radiotherapy, X-rays are used to
(a) detect bone fracture
(b) treat cancer
(c) detect full in radio receiver
(d) detect heart diseases

Ans. (b). *Textbook of Radiology for Residents & Technicians, 5th ed., S.K. Bhargava & Sumeet Bhargava, p. 537-577.*

285. The shortest wavelength of X-rays emitted from X-ray tube depends on
(a) the current in the tube.
(b) voltage applied to the tube.
(c) the nature of the glass in tube.
(d) the atomic number of the target material.

Ans. (b). *Textbook of Radiology for Residents & Technicians, 5th ed., S.K. Bhargava & Sumeet Bhargava, p. 115-146.*

286. In an X-ray tube, the intensity of the emitted X-ray beam is increased by

(a) increase in filament current (b) decrease in filament current
(c) increase in target potential (d) decrease in target potential

Ans. (a). *Textbook of Radiology for Residents & Technicians, 5th ed., S.K. Bhargava & Sumeet Bhargava, p. 115-146.*

287. Moseley's law relates

(a) wavelength and angle of scattering.
(b) wavelength and intensity of X-ray.
(c) frequency and atomic number.
(d) frequency and applied voltage.

Ans. (c). *Textbook of Radiology for Residents & Technicians, 5th ed., S.K. Bhargava & Sumeet Bhargava, p. 97-114.*

288. When high speed electrons hit target of high atomic number

(a) only heat is produced.
(b) only continuous X-rays are produced.
(c) only continuous and characteristic X-rays are produced.
(d) heat is produced and simultaneously continuous and characteristic X-rays are produced.

Ans. (d). *Textbook of Radiology for Residents & Technicians, 5th ed., S.K. Bhargava & Sumeet Bhargava, p. 115-146.*

289. On increasing number of electrons striking the anode of an X-ray tube, which one of the following parameters of resulting X-ray would increase

(a) penetration power (b) frequency
(c) wavelength (d) intensity

Ans. (d). *Textbook of Radiology for Residents & Technicians, 5th ed., S.K. Bhargava & Sumeet Bhargava, p. 115-146.*

290. The difference between soft and hard X-rays is of

(a) velocity (b) intensity
(c) frequency (d) polarization

Ans. (c). *Textbook of Radiology for Residents & Technicians, 5th ed., S.K. Bhargava & Sumeet Bhargava, p. 97-114.*

291. When two coils are placed very close, the magnetic flux change in one coil induces an emf in the other coil, this phenomenon is known as

(a) mutual induction (b) self-induction
(c) Eddy current (d) AC generator

Ans. ***(a).*** *Textbook of Radiology for Residents & Technicians, 5th ed., S.K. Bhargava & Sumeet Bhargava, p. 97-114.*

292. Faraday's law state that

(a) magnitude of the induced emf is inversely proportional to the rate of change of magnetic flux.
(b) direction of induced emf is always opposite to the change of magnetic flux.
(c) magnetic flux of the induced emf is proportional to the rate of change of magnetic flux.
(d) magnetic flux of the induced emf is proportional to the rate of change of electric flux.

Ans. ***(c).*** *Textbook of Radiology for Residents & Technicians, 5th ed., S.K. Bhargava & Sumeet Bhargava, p. 97-114.*

293. The direction of current produced can be found by using

(a) Lenz's law (b) Faraday's law
(c) Fleming right hand rule (d) None of the above

Ans. ***(c).*** *Textbook of Radiology for Residents & Technicians, 5th ed., S.K. Bhargava & Sumeet Bhargava, p. 97-114.*

294. Who was W.C. Roentgen?

(a) Canadian technologist (b) Australian radiologist
(c) German physicist (d) Farmer

Ans. ***(c).*** *Textbook of Radiology for Residents & Technicians, 5th ed., S.K. Bhargava & Sumeet Bhargava, p. 97-114.*

295. Roentgen received the first Noble Prize in Physics in

(a) 1896 (b) 1901
(c) 1905 (d) 1921

Ans. ***(b).*** *Textbook of Radiology for Residents & Technicians, 5th ed., S.K. Bhargava & Sumeet Bhargava, p. 97-114.*

296. X-ray photons, which are produced by an X-ray tube, are

(a) homogeneous in energy (d) heterogeneous
(c) Both (a) and (b) (d) None of the above

Ans. ***(b).*** *Textbook of Radiology for Residents & Technicians, 5th ed., S.K. Bhargava & Sumeet Bhargava, p. 115-146.*

297. Melting point of tungsten target is

(a) 1480° C (b) 2800° C
(c) 2000° C (d) 3370° C

Ans. ***(d).*** *Textbook of Radiology for Residents & Technicians, 5th ed., S.K. Bhargava & Sumeet Bhargava, p. 115-146.*

298. Diagnostic X-ray tubes have an anode angle between

(a) 20° to 25° angles (b) 3° to 9° angles
(c) 12° to 15° angles (d) 15° to 25° angles

Ans. (c). *Textbook of Radiology for Residents & Technicians, 5th ed., S.K. Bhargava & Sumeet Bhargava, p. 115-146.*

299. A small anode angle (6°) is used for special technique such as

(a) CECT (b) angiography
(c) dacryocystography (d) hepatic biliary system

Ans. (b). *Textbook of Radiology for Residents & Technicians, 5th ed., S.K. Bhargava & Sumeet Bhargava, p. 115-146.*

300. The cloud of electron is known as

(a) heel effect (b) line focus principle
(c) space charge (d) effective focal spot

Ans. (c). *Textbook of Radiology for Residents & Technicians, 5th ed., S.K. Bhargava & Sumeet Bhargava, p. 115-146.*

301. In the X-ray tube, how much percentage of the electrical power supplied is converted to X-rays?

(a) 15% (b) Less than 1%
(c) More than 1% (d) 99.9%

Ans. (b). *Textbook of Radiology for Residents & Technicians, 5th ed., S.K. Bhargava & Sumeet Bhargava, p. 115-146.*

302. In which year the rotating anode X-ray tube was invented?

(a) 1898 (b) 1905
(c) 1920 (d) 1933

Ans. (d). *Textbook of Radiology for Residents & Technicians, 5th ed., S.K. Bhargava & Sumeet Bhargava, p. 115-146.*

303. Anode rotates at a speed of about

(a) 100 revolution per minute (rpm)
(b) 10,000–20,000 revolution per minute (rpm)
(c) 3,000–9000 revolution per minute (rpm)
(d) 18,000–25,000 revolution per minute (rpm)

Ans. (c). *Textbook of Radiology for Residents & Technicians, 5th ed., S.K. Bhargava & Sumeet Bhargava, p. 115-146.*

304. Dental X-ray units system use

(a) rotating anode tube (b) stationary anode tube
(c) gas tube (d) Both (a) and (b)

Ans. (b). *Textbook of Radiology for Residents & Technicians, 5th ed., S.K. Bhargava & Sumeet Bhargava, p. 115-146.*

305. The reduced intensity of the X-ray beam towards the anode side this phenomenon is known as

(a) line focus principle (b) heel effect
(c) off-focus radiation (d) space charge effect

Ans. (b). Textbook of Radiology for Residents & Technicians, 5th ed., S.K. Bhargava & Sumeet Bhargava, p. 115-146.

306. The tube housing is internally shielded with

(a) aluminium (b) lead
(c) nickel (d) molybdenum

Ans. (b). Textbook of Radiology for Residents & Technicians, 5th ed., S.K. Bhargava & Sumeet Bhargava, p. 115-146.

307. The major advantage of 3-phase generator over single-phase generator is

(a) X-ray energy is lower
(b) produces a pulsating potential
(c) produces a nearly constant potential
(d) lower tube rating

Ans. (c). Textbook of Radiology for Residents & Technicians, 5th ed., S.K. Bhargava & Sumeet Bhargava, p. 158-165.

308. Now-a-days 3-phase generators are available to withstand a tube current of

(a) 500 ma (b) 800 ma
(c) 1000 ma (d) 2000 ma

Ans. (d). Textbook of Radiology for Residents & Technicians, 5th ed., S.K. Bhargava & Sumeet Bhargava, p. 158-165.

309. If a circuit produces 12 pulses per cycle, it is known as

(a) 3-pulse generator (b) 6-pulse generator
(c) 9-pulse generator (d) 12-pulse generator

Ans. (d). Textbook of Radiology for Residents & Technicians, 5th ed., S.K. Bhargava & Sumeet Bhargava, p. 158-165.

310. Coherent scattering contributes _______ in diagnostic radiology.

(a) less than 5% (b) less than 90%
(c) more than 33% (d) more than 90%

Ans. (a). Textbook of Radiology for Residents & Technicians, 5th ed., S.K. Bhargava & Sumeet Bhargava, p. 158-165.

311. The maximum photon energy in a X-ray beam is determined by

(a) atomic number of the target.
(b) atomic number of the X-ray beam filter.

(c) voltage across the X-ray tube.
(d) total exposure time.

Ans. (c). *Textbook of Radiology for Residents & Technicians, 5th ed., S.K. Bhargava & Sumeet Bhargava, p. 115-146.*

312. X-ray tube output is increased most strongly by increasing the

(a) voltage across the tube (kV_p) (b) anode diameter
(c) atomic number of the target (d) filtration

Ans. (a). *Textbook of Radiology for Residents & Technicians, 5th ed., S.K. Bhargava & Sumeet Bhargava, p. 115-146.*

313. The number of electrons accelerated across an X-ray tube is determined by

(a) anode speed (b) focal spot size
(c) filament current (d) X-ray tube filtration

Ans. (c). *Textbook of Radiology for Residents & Technicians, 5th ed., S.K. Bhargava & Sumeet Bhargava, p. 115-146.*

314. The line focus principle may be explained as

(a) apparent focus is smaller than exposed target region.
(b) another name for the heel effect.
(c) image magnification.
(d) reduction in intensity at anode edge.

Ans. (a). *Textbook of Radiology for Residents & Technicians, 5th ed., S.K. Bhargava & Sumeet Bhargava, p. 115-146.*

315. Beam hardening is affected primarily by

(a) filament current (b) tube current
(c) exposure time (d) filtration

Ans. (d). *Textbook of Radiology for Residents & Technicians, 5th ed., S.K. Bhargava & Sumeet Bhargava, p. 115-146.*

316. Stray radiation is the sum of

(a) primary and transmitted (b) primary and scatter
(c) scatter and leakage (d) primary and leakage

Ans. (c). *Textbook of Radiology for Residents & Technicians, 5th ed., S.K. Bhargava & Sumeet Bhargava, p. 166-168.*

317. Step-up transformers

(a) increase current (b) decrease voltage
(c) increase voltage (d) Both (b) and (c)

Ans. (c). *Textbook of Radiology for Residents & Technicians, 5th ed., S.K. Bhargava & Sumeet Bhargava, p. 115-146.*

318. The focal spot size enlarges as milliamperes increase owing to the repulsion of adjacent electrons. This effect is called

(a) heel effect (b) blooming effect
(c) line focus effect (d) space charge

Ans. (b). *Textbook of Radiology for Residents & Technicians, 5th ed., S.K. Bhargava & Sumeet Bhargava, p. 115-146.*

319. A small focal spot is preferred when _______ is a priority.

(a) spatial resolution (b) short exposure time
(c) larger heat loading (d) All of the above

Ans. (a). *Textbook of Radiology for Residents & Technicians, 5th ed., S.K. Bhargava & Sumeet Bhargava, p. 115-146.*

320. The intensity of scattered radiation is typically

(a) 90% of the intensity incident on a patient.
(b) 45% of the intensity incident on a patient.
(c) 99.9% of the intensity incident on a patient.
(d) 0.1% of the intensity incident on a patient.

Ans. (d). *Textbook of Radiology for Residents & Technicians, 5th ed., S.K. Bhargava & Sumeet Bhargava, p. 158-165.*

321. X-ray tubes are surrounded by _______ to absorb unwanted radiation.

(a) lead (b) glass
(c) aluminium (d) oil

Ans. (a). *Textbook of Radiology for Residents & Technicians, 5th ed., S.K. Bhargava & Sumeet Bhargava, p. 115-146.*

322. Cooling of the anode and housing is described by

(a) angiographic rating chart (b) thermal characteristic chart
(c) anode heating chart (d) radiographic rating chart

Ans. (b). *Textbook of Radiology for Residents & Technicians, 5th ed., S.K. Bhargava & Sumeet Bhargava, p. 158-165.*

323. The threshold energy for pair production is

(a) 3.45 MeV (b) 5.11 MeV
(c) 6.88 MeV (d) 1.022 MeV

Ans. (d). *Textbook of Radiology for Residents & Technicians, 5th ed., S.K. Bhargava & Sumeet Bhargava, p. 158-165.*

324. The attenuation coefficient for diagnostic X-ray photons in soft tissue

(a) decreases continuously with increasing energy.
(b) decreases to about 25 keV, then rises again.

(c) increases continuously with energy.
(d) depends on the molecular structure.

Ans. (a). *Textbook of Radiology for Residents & Technicians, 5th ed., S.K. Bhargava & Sumeet Bhargava, p. 158-165.*

325. Quenching gases are used in

(a) ionization chambers
(b) pocket chambers
(c) TLDs
(d) Geiger Muller counter

Ans. (d). *Textbook of Radiology for Residents & Technicians, 5th ed., S.K. Bhargava & Sumeet Bhargava, p. 599-602.*

326. Film badges

(a) cannot distinguish between low and high energy X-rays.
(b) can measure doses of 0.01 mGy.
(c) are insensitive to heat.
(d) estimate the dose from the film optical density.

Ans. (d). *Textbook of Radiology for Residents & Technicians, 5th ed., S.K. Bhargava & Sumeet Bhargava, p. 145-146.*

327. When heated, TLDs emit

(a) X-rays
(b) characteristic X-rays
(c) photoelectron
(d) light

Ans. (d). *Textbook of Radiology for Residents & Technicians, 5th ed., S.K. Bhargava & Sumeet Bhargava, p. 145-146.*

328. What describes the electron cloud created by heating the filament?

(a) Thermionic emission
(b) Subatomic emission
(c) Hysteresis
(d) Saturation current

Ans. (a). *Textbook of Radiology for Residents & Technicians, 5th ed., S.K. Bhargava & Sumeet Bhargava, p. 115-146.*

329. At what temperature does an X-ray tube filament exhibit significant thermionic emission?

(a) 500° C
(b) 1000° C
(c) 2500° C
(d) 10000° C

Ans. (c). *Textbook of Radiology for Residents & Technicians, 5th ed., S.K. Bhargava & Sumeet Bhargava, p. 115-146.*

330. Which of the following generators produces the smallest ripple in exposure output from a diagnostic X-ray tube?

(a) Single-phase, 2-pulse
(b) Three-phase, 6-pulse
(c) Three-phase, 12-pulse
(d) High frequency at 12 kHz

Ans. (d). *Textbook of Radiology for Residents & Technicians, 5th ed., S.K. Bhargava & Sumeet Bhargava, p. 115-146.*

331. In 1913 _______ invented a new type of X-ray tube.

(a) W.D. Coolidge (b) Sir W.C. Roentgen
(c) Madam Curie (d) Madam Bartha

Ans. (b). *Textbook of Radiology for Residents & Technicians, 5th ed., S.K. Bhargava & Sumeet Bhargava, p. 115-146.*

332. The distance between the filament and target is _______ to _______ cm.

(a) 3, 5 (b) 1, 3
(c) 3, 4 (d) 4, 5

Ans. (b). *Textbook of Radiology for Residents & Technicians, 5th ed., S.K. Bhargava & Sumeet Bhargava, p. 122.*

333. The binding energy of an electron in the K-shell of the tungsten is about _______.

(a) 80 keV (b) 60 keV
(c) 90 keV (d) 70 keV

Ans. (d). *Textbook of Radiology for Residents & Technicians, 5th ed., S.K. Bhargava & Sumeet Bhargava, p. 158-165.*

334. Anode angle vary from _______ degree.

(a) 6–20 degree (b) 20–30 degree
(c) 30–40 degree (d) 40–50 degree

Ans. (a). *Textbook of Radiology for Residents & Technicians, 5th ed., S.K. Bhargava & Sumeet Bhargava, p. 122.*

335. The anode and the cathode are enclosed in a _______.

(a) Borosilicate glass (b) Plastic
(c) Steel (d) Iron

Ans. (a). *Textbook of Radiology for Residents & Technicians, 5th ed., S.K. Bhargava & Sumeet Bhargava, p. 120.*

336. The leakage radiation measured at a distance of _______ meter from the source shall not exceed _______ mR in _______ hour when the tube is operated at its maximum current for the maximum rated tube potential.

(a) 3, 1000, 1 (b) 1, 100, 1
(c) 2, 10, 1 (d) 5, 1, 1

Ans. (b). *Textbook of Radiology for Residents & Technicians, 5th ed., S.K. Bhargava & Sumeet Bhargava, p. 147-157.*

337. Special _______ shaped filters are used in CT imaging systems to compensate for the shape of head or body.

(a) Wedge
(b) Bilateral wedge
(c) Trough
(d) Bow tie

Ans. (d). *Radiological Science for Technologists by Stewart Carlyce Bushang, 9th Ed., Mosby Elsevier, 2008, p. 158.*

338. An _______ particle is a helium nucleus that contains two protons and two neutrons.

(a) Alpha
(b) Beta
(c) Gamma
(d) Neutron

Ans. (a). *Radiological Science for Technologists by Stewart Carlyce Bushang, 9th Ed., Mosby Elsevier, 2008, p. 53.*

339. _______ allows electrons to the flow in the only one direction.

(a) Resistor
(b) Diode
(c) Ammeter
(d) Voltmeter

Ans. (b). *Radiological Science for Technologists by Stewart Carlyce Bushang, 9th Ed., Mosby Elsevier, 2008, p. 80.*

340. The degree to which a material can be the magnetized is its _______.

(a) Magnetic susceptibility
(b) Magnetic dipole moment
(c) Magnetic induction
(d) Magnetic field

Ans. (a). *Radiological Science for Technologists by Stewart Carlyce Bushang, 9th Ed., Mosby Elsevier, 2008, p. 86.*

341. A transformer with a turns ratio greater than 1 is a _______.

(a) Step-down transformer
(b) Isolation transformer
(c) Step-up transformer
(d) Autotransformer

Ans. (c). *Radiological Science for Technologists by Stewart Carlyce Bushang, 9th Ed., Mosby Elsevier, 2008, p. 94.*

342. The _______ measures the voltage provided to the X-ray imaging system and adjusts that voltage to precisely 220 V.

(a) Line compensator
(b) Voltmeter
(c) Rheostat
(d) Resistor

Ans. (a). *Radiological Science for Technologists by Stewart Carlyce Bushang, 9th Ed., Mosby Elsevier, 2008, p. 104.*

343. Three-phase, 12-pulse power results in only _______ ripple.

(a) 14%
(b) 4%
(c) 20%
(d) 30%

Ans. (b). *Radiological Science for Technologists by Stewart Carlyce Bushang, 9th Ed., Mosby Elsevier, 2008, p. 115.*

344. Filament of X-ray tube is usually made up of _______.

(a) Molybdenum (b) Carbon
(c) Nickel (d) Thoriated tungsten

Ans. (d). *Radiological Science for Technologists by Stewart Carlyce Bushang, 9th Ed., Mosby Elsevier, 2008, p. 122.*

345. When a smaller image receptor is used the anode angle can be _______.

(a) Perpendicular to the target (b) Steeper
(c) Slopy (d) 120 degree to the target

Ans. (b). *Radiological Science for Technologists by Stewart Carlyce Bushang, 9th Ed., Mosby Elsevier, 2008, p. 129.*

346. Only the _______ characteristics X-rays of tungsten are useful for imaging.

(a) K (b) L
(c) M (d) N

Ans. (a). *Radiological Science for Technologists by Stewart Carlyce Bushang, 9th Ed., Mosby Elsevier, 2008, p. 141.*

347. _______ X-rays have precisely fixed (discrete) energies and form a discrete emission spectrum.

(a) Bremsstrahlung (b) Characteristic
(c) Both (d) None

Ans. (b). *Radiological Science for Technologists by Stewart Carlyce Bushang, 9th Ed., Mosby Elsevier, 2008, p. 144.*

348. In the diagnostic range a 15% increase in kV_p is equivalent to _______ the mAs.

(a) Quarter (b) Doubling
(c) Half (d) 60 degree

Ans. (b). *Radiological Science for Technologists by Stewart Carlyce Bushang, 9th Ed., Mosby Elsevier, 2008, p. 147.*

349. An increase in voltage ripple, a _______ in quantity and quality.

(a) Increase (b) Decrease
(c) No effect (d) None of these

Ans. (b). *Radiological Science for Technologists by Stewart Carlyce Bushang, 9th Ed., Mosby Elsevier, 2008, p. 149.*

350. The HVL of an X-ray beam is the thickness of absorbing material necessary to reduce the X-ray intensity to _______ of its original value.

(a) Half (b) Double

(c) 1/4 (d) 1/16

Ans. (a). Radiological Science for Technologists by Stewart Carlyce Bushang, 9th Ed., Mosby Elsevier, 2008, p. 155.

351. K-shell binding energies for tungsten is _______ keV.

(a) 1.56 (b) 6.04
(c) 37.4 (d) 69.5

Ans. (d). Principles of Radiographic Imaging, 5th ed., Richard R. Carlton, p. 194.

352. K-shell binding energies for molybdenum is _______ keV.

(a) 20.0 (b) 33.2
(c) 37.4 (d) 69.5

Ans. (a). Principles of Radiographic Imaging, 5th ed., Richard R. Carlton, p. 194.

353. Coherent scattering occurs in a very _______ X-ray energy range.

(a) High (b) Medium
(c) Low (d) All of the above

Ans. (c). Principles of Radiographic Imaging, 5th ed., Richard R. Carlton, p. 196.

354. Thomson scattering involves a _______ electron in the interaction.

(a) Double (b) Single
(c) Inner shell (d) All of the above

Ans. (b). Principles of Radiographic Imaging, 5th ed., Richard R. Carlton, p. 197.

355. _______ occurs when an incident X-ray photon interacts with a loosely bound outer shell electron, removes the electron from its shell in a different direction as a scattered photon.

(a) Coherent scattering (b) Compton scattering
(c) Photoelectric absorption (d) Pair production

Ans. (b). Principles of Radiographic Imaging, 5th ed., Richard R. Carlton, p. 197.

356. As density of absorbed increases _______.

(a) Less photoelectric effect (b) More photoelectric effect
(c) No effect (d) All of the above

Ans. (b). Textbook of Radiology for Residents & Technicians, 5th ed., S.K. Bhargava & Sumeet Bhargava, p. 158-166.

357. Compton scattering does not depend upon the _______.

(a) Density

(b) X-ray energy
(c) Atomic number of absorbing material
(d) None of the above

Ans. ***(c).*** *Textbook of Radiology for Residents & Technicians, 5th ed., S.K. Bhargava & Sumeet Bhargava, p. 158-166.*

358. Linear attenuation coefficient of coherent scattering is directly proportional to

(a) Square of energy
(b) Square of atomic number
(c) Half of atomic energy
(d) Energy

Ans. ***(b).*** *Textbook of Radiology for Residents & Technicians, 5th ed., S.K. Bhargava & Sumeet Bhargava, p. 589-590.*

359. _______ does not occur during X-ray imaging.

(a) Coherent scattering
(b) Compton scattering
(c) Photoelectric absorption
(d) Pair production

Ans. ***(d).*** *Radiological Science for Technologists by Stewart Carlyce Bushang, 9th Ed., Mosby Elsevier, 2008, p. 168.*

360. The incident photon must have atleast _______ of energy in pair production interaction.

(a) 0.51 MeV
(b) 10 keV
(c) 1.02 MeV
(d) 2.04 MeV

Ans. ***(c).*** *Radiological Science for Technologists by Stewart Carlyce Bushang, 9th Ed., Mosby Elsevier, 2008, p. 169.*

361. The positron unites with a free electron and the mass of both particles is converted to energy in a process called _______.

(a) Annihilation radiation
(b) Photoelectric absorption
(c) Coherent scattering
(d) Rayleigh scattering

Ans. ***(a).*** *Radiological Science for Technologists by Stewart Carlyce Bushang, 9th Ed., Mosby Elsevier, 2008, p. 169.*

362. Pair-production is important in _______ modality.

(a) CT
(b) MRI
(c) PET
(d) Ultrasound

Ans. ***(c).*** *Radiological Science for Technologists by Stewart Carlyce Bushang, 9th Ed., Mosby Elsevier, 2008, p. 169.*

363. _______ interaction occurs in X-rays with energy above approximately 10 MeV.

(a) Pair-production
(b) Photoelectric absorption
(c) Photo disintegration
(d) None of the above

Ans. (c). Radiological Science for Technologists by Stewart Carlyce Bushang, 9th Ed., Mosby Elsevier, 2008, p. 169.

364. Differential absorption controls the _______ of an X-ray image.

(a) Sharpness
(b) Resolution
(c) Noise
(d) Contrast

Ans. (d). Radiological Science for Technologists by Stewart Carlyce Bushang, 9th Ed., Mosby Elsevier, 2008, p. 176.

365. The _______ is the fraction of X-ray removed from a beam per unit thickness of attenuating medium.

(a) Linear attenuation coefficient
(b) Infrared radiation
(c) Transmitted radiation
(d) Incident radiation

Ans. (a). Textbook of Radiology for Residents & Technicians, 5th ed., S.K. Bhargava & Sumeet Bhargava, p. 589-590.

366. _______ interaction enhances the natural tissue contrast.

(a) Coherent scattering
(b) Photoelectric absorption
(c) Compton scattering
(d) Pair-production

Ans. (b). Textbook of Radiology for Residents & Technicians, 5th ed., S.K. Bhargava & Sumeet Bhargava, p. 158-165.

367. Collimation reduces _______ and improves _______.

(a) Contrast resolution, Patient dose
(b) Patient dose, Contrast resolution
(c) Resolution, contrast
(d) SID, Scattered radiation

Ans. (b). Radiological Science for Technologists by Stewart Carlyce Bushang, 9th Ed., Mosby Elsevier, 2008, p. 232.

368. The use of high-frequency grids results in _______ patient radiation dose.

(a) Higher
(b) Lower
(c) Half
(d) No effect

Ans. (a). Radiological Science for Technologists by Stewart Carlyce Bushang, 9th Ed., Mosby Elsevier, 2008, p. 233.

369. The higher the grid ratio, the _______ is the bucky factor.

(a) Higher
(b) Lower
(c) Half
(d) No effect

Ans. (b). Radiological Science for Technologists by Stewart Carlyce Bushang, 9th Ed., Mosby Elsevier, 2008, p. 235.

370. The bucky factor _______ with increasing kV_p.

(a) Increases (b) Decreases
(c) Halves (d) Quarter

Ans. (a). *Radiological Science for Technologists by Stewart Carlyce Bushang, 9th Ed., Mosby Elsevier, 2008, p. 235.*

371. As the bucky factor increases, patient dose _______ proportionately.

(a) Decreases (b) Increases
(c) Halves (d) No effect

Ans. (b). *Radiological Science for Technologists by Stewart Carlyce Bushang, 9th Ed., Mosby Elsevier, 2008, p. 235.*

372. High-ratio grids are used for _______ examinations.

(a) Low kV_p (b) High kV_p
(c) Both (d) None of the above

Ans. (b). *Radiological Science for Technologists by Stewart Carlyce Bushang, 9th Ed., Mosby Elsevier, 2008, p. 241.*

CHAPTER

3

Processing Room

1. The usual thickness of the radiographic film is about

(a) 0.05 mm (b) 0.25 mm
(c) 0.75 mm (d) 1.00 mm

Ans. (b). *Textbook of Radiology for Residents & Technicians, 5th ed., S.K. Bhargava & Sumeet Bhargava, p. 171.*

2. Which is not the material used in base of X-ray film?

(a) Cellulose triacetate (b) Polyester
(c) Card board (d) None of the above

Ans. (c). *Textbook of Radiology for Residents & Technicians, 5th ed., S.K. Bhargava & Sumeet Bhargava, p. 171.*

3. The silver halide crystal used in emulsion of X-ray film is

(a) Silver bromide (b) Silver nitrate
(c) Silver iodide (d) Silver chloride

Ans. (a) & (d). *Textbook of Radiology for Residents & Technicians, 5th ed., S.K. Bhargava & Sumeet Bhargava, p. 171.*

4. Which of the following is not the advantage of double coated-ray film?

(a) With less exposure, better contrast
(b) Stability of film
(c) Prevent curling of film
(d) None of the above

Ans. (d). *Textbook of Radiology for Residents & Technicians, 5th ed., S.K. Bhargava & Sumeet Bhargava, p. 171.*

5. Which of the following is not true for double-coated film

(a) Crystal is 1 micrometer in size
(b) Each crystal can have 10 to the power 6 silver atoms
(c) Effected by mechanical pressure
(d) Emulsion is not sensitive to visible light

Ans. (d). *Textbook of Radiology for Residents & Technicians, 5th ed., S.K. Bhargava & Sumeet Bhargava, p. 171.*

6. Which is true for ideal processing (dark room)

(a) 100 sq. feet floor and 11 feet ceiling height
(b) 150 sq. feet floor and 15 feet ceiling height
(c) 50 sq. feet floor and 20 feet ceiling height
(d) 125 sq. feet floor and 15 feet ceiling height

Ans. (a). *Textbook of Radiology for Residents & Technicians, 5th ed., S.K. Bhargava & Sumeet Bhargava, p. 170.*

7. Wall of the dark room should be lined with lead sheet or some substance equivalent to

(a) 1.5 mm thickness of lead or lead equivalent
(b) 2.5 mm thickness of lead or lead equivalent
(c) 0.5 mm thickness of lead or lead equivalent
(d) 4.0 mm thickness of lead or lead equivalent

Ans. (a). *Textbook of Radiology for Residents & Technicians, 5th ed., S.K. Bhargava & Sumeet Bhargava, p. 169.*

8. Safe light distance from the processing tank should not be less than

(a) 1.2 metres (b) 0.5 metre
(c) 0.8 metre (d) 1.0 metre

Ans. (a). *Textbook of Radiology for Residents & Technicians, 5th ed., S.K. Bhargava & Sumeet Bhargava, p. 169.*

9. Which is not true for green sensitive films?

(a) Less stable sensitometric response
(b) Improve image quality and sharpness
(c) Low replacement rates needed
(d) Better resistance to scratches

Ans. (a). *Textbook of Radiology for Residents & Technicians, 5th ed., S.K. Bhargava & Sumeet Bhargava, p. 173.*

10. Which is not true for green sensitive films?

(a) Uses T-grain silver halide
(b) Antistatic layer present
(c) With less exposure, more sharp image

(d) Does not require green light emitting screens

Ans. (d). *Textbook of Radiology for Residents & Technicians, 5th ed., S.K. Bhargava & Sumeet Bhargava, p. 173.*

11. K-edge of 70 keV is characteristic of

(a) Tungsten (b) Barium
(c) Molybdenum (d) Lanthanum

Ans. (a). *Textbook of Radiology for Residents & Technicians, 5th ed., S.K. Bhargava & Sumeet Bhargava, p. 167.*

12. K-edge of 40 keV is characteristic of

(a) Tungsten (b) Gadolinium
(c) Molybdenum (d) Barium

Ans. (b). *Textbook of Radiology for Residents & Technicians, 5th ed., S.K. Bhargava & Sumeet Bhargava, p. 167.*

13. Molybdenum has a K-edge of

(a) 17.5 keV (b) 19.6 keV
(c) 70 keV (d) 40 keV

Ans. (a) & (b). *Textbook of Radiology for Residents & Technicians, 5th ed., S.K. Bhargava & Sumeet Bhargava, p. 167.*

14. Which is not true for the latent image of X-ray film to form?

(a) Sensitivity specks
(b) Silver ion is reduced to silver atoms
(c) Latent image forms after exposure of film
(d) Latent image forms after development of film

Ans. (d). *Textbook of Radiology for Residents & Technicians, 5th ed., S.K. Bhargava & Sumeet Bhargava, p. 171.*

15. Which is not true when using intensifying screens

(a) Improve film gamma
(b) Improves quantum mottle
(c) Resolution is less
(d) Base is made-up of card board

Ans. (d). *Textbook of Radiology for Residents & Technicians, 5th ed., S.K. Bhargava & Sumeet Bhargava, p. 177.*

16. X-ray radiation contribute to form latent image is

(a) 1% (b) 2%
(c) 3.6% (d) 30%

Ans. (c). *Textbook of Radiology for Residents & Technicians, 5th ed., S.K. Bhargava & Sumeet Bhargava, p. 172.*

17. Which of the following phosphor not used in intensifying screen

(a) Calcium tungstate (b) Zinc cadmium sulfide
(c) Terbium (d) Thulium blue

Ans. (b). *Textbook of Radiology for Residents & Technicians, 5th ed., S.K. Bhargava & Sumeet Bhargava, p. 176.*

18. Which is not true about X-ray cassettes?

(a) Keep film screen in close
(b) Front side of the cassette is made-up of aluminium
(c) Is a light tight box
(d) Back side of the cassette is made-up of carbon fiber

Ans. (d). *Textbook of Radiology for Residents & Technicians, 5th ed., S.K. Bhargava,. p. 175.*

19. Which is not true for developer?

(a) Mettol and hydroquinone acts as an reducing agent
(b) Potassium bromide acts as an antifogging agent
(c) Sodium sulphite acts as preservative
(d) Developer solution is acidic

Ans. (d). *Textbook of Radiology for Residents & Technicians, 5th ed., S.K. Bhargava & Sumeet Bhargava, p. 178.*

20. Which is not true in the statement that replenisher differ from developer because of

(a) No bromide
(b) Higher concentration of hydroquinone
(c) Replenisher has lower pH
(d) It does not act to supplement the quantity of developing solution

Ans. (d). *Textbook of Radiology for Residents & Technicians, 5th ed., S.K. Bhargava & Sumeet Bhargava, p. 179.*

21. Which is not true for fixer?

(a) Sodium/Ammonium thiosulphate act as fixing agent
(b) Sodium sulphite act as preservative
(c) Chrome alum/potassium alum acts as hardener
(d) Fixer solution is alkaline

Ans. (d). *Textbook of Radiology for Residents & Technicians, 5th ed., S.K. Bhargava & Sumeet Bhargava, p. 179.*

22. Which is not true about processing?

(a) Turn out of the X-ray films is less in automatic than conventional
(b) Improper washing after fixation would lead to brownish discoloration due to retained hypo
(c) Film should be washed after developer and fixer

(d) Process of fixing a developed film, dissolves out the silver ions from the film leaving behind metallic silver atoms

Ans. (a). *Textbook of Radiology for Residents & Technicians, 5th ed., S.K. Bhargava & Sumeet Bhargava, p. 179.*

23. Which is not true about rare earth screens?
(a) Faster than tungsten screen
(b) Less exposure than tungsten screen to achieve same density film
(c) Conversion efficiency is better than tungsten
(d) It is cheaper than tungsten screen

Ans. (d). *Textbook of Radiology for Residents & Technicians, 5th ed., S.K. Bhargava & Sumeet Bhargava, p. 184.*

24. Which is not true about safe light?
(a) Distance between safe light and processing tank should not be less than 1.2 meters
(b) Amber safe light filter is used with calcium tungsten screens
(c) Should be sufficient not to fog the unexposed films
(d) Bulb used in safe light is more than 15 watts

Ans. (d). *Textbook of Radiology for Residents & Technicians, 5th ed., S.K. Bhargava & Sumeet Bhargava, p. 170.*

25. Which is not true about the optical density of the film?
(a) Density of the film is the sum of the densities on each side
(b) Inversely proportional to the number of the atoms in that area
(c) Directly proportional to the weight of the silver ions in that area
(d) Equal to the log 10 transmitted light – incident light

Ans. (d). *Textbook of Radiology for Residents & Technicians, 5th ed., S.K. Bhargava & Sumeet Bhargava, p. 197.*

26. Which is not correct for characteristic curve of the film?
(a) Graph density against logarithm of the X-ray exposure
(b) Exposure on Y-axis and density on X-axis
(c) A & B of the curve represent normal density without exposure of the base density
(d) None of the above

Ans. (d). *Textbook of Radiology for Residents & Technicians, 5th ed., S.K. Bhargava & Sumeet Bhargava, p. 206.*

27. Amber safe light is compatible with films having
(a) Blue sensitive film
(b) Green sensitive film
(c) Yellow sensitive film
(d) None of the above

Ans. (a). *Textbook of Radiology for Residents & Technicians, 5th ed., S.K. Bhargava & Sumeet Bhargava, p. 170.*

28. Red safe light is compatible with films having

(a) Green sensitive films (b) Blue sensitive films
(c) Yellow sensitive films (d) None of the above

Ans. (a). *Textbook of Radiology for Residents & Technicians, 5th ed., S.K. Bhargava & Sumeet Bhargava, p. 170.*

29. Which is not true about intensifying screens?

(a) Does not convert the energy of X-ray film to visible light
(b) Terbium acts as activator
(c) Addition of certain dyes extends sensitivity of the film
(d) Decrease the resolution of the image

Ans. (a). *Textbook of Radiology for Residents & Technicians, 5th ed., S.K. Bhargava & Sumeet Bhargava, p. 176.*

30. Fluorescence signifies

(a) Light emitted by screen within 10^{-8} sec
(b) Light emitted by screen after 10^{-8} sec
(c) Light emitted by screen at 10^{-8} sec
(d) None

Ans. (a). *Textbook of Radiology for Residents & Technicians, 5th ed., S.K. Bhargava & Sumeet Bhargava, p. 178.*

31. Phosphorescence signifies

(a) Light emitted by screen within 10^{-8} sec
(b) Light emitted by screen after 10^{-8} sec
(c) Light emitted by screen at 10^{-8} sec
(d) None

Ans. (b). *Textbook of Radiology for Residents & Technicians, 5th ed., S.K. Bhargava & Sumeet Bhargava, p. 178.*

32. Silver halide in emulsion of X-ray films are

(a) 90% silver iodide and 10% silver bromide
(b) 90% silver bromide and 10% silver iodide
(c) 90% silver bromide and 10% silver chloride
(d) None of the above

Ans. (b). *Textbook of Radiology for Residents & Technicians, 5th ed., S.K. Bhargava & Sumeet Bhargava, p. 171.*

33. Inherent film fog is

(a) D = 0.2 (b) D = 0.12
(c) D = 0.4 (d) D = 0.5

Ans. (b). *Textbook of Radiology for Residents & Technicians, 5th ed., S.K. Bhargava & Sumeet Bhargava, p. 208.*

34. With accidental exposure to X-rays film fog

(a) Increases (b) Decreases
(c) No effect

Ans. (a). *Textbook of Radiology for Residents & Technicians, 5th ed., S.K. Bhargava & Sumeet Bhargava, p. 206.*

35. Characteristic curve signifies about

(a) Film gamma (b) Density of the film
(c) Intensification factor (d) All above

Ans. (d). *Textbook of Radiology for Residents & Technicians, 5th ed., S.K. Bhargava & Sumeet Bhargava, p. 206.*

36. Which is not true about film contrast?

(a) Inversely proportional to object film distance
(b) Inversely proportional to filtration
(c) Inversely proportional to film size
(d) Inversely proportional to focal spot size

Ans. (d). *Textbook of Radiology for Residents & Technicians, 5th ed., S.K. Bhargava & Sumeet Bhargava, p. 198.*

37. Which is not true about intensifying screens?

(a) Reduce patient dose
(b) Decrease spatial resolution
(c) Reduce blurring
(d) Increase loading of X-ray tube

Ans. (d). *Textbook of Radiology for Residents & Technicians, 5th ed., S.K. Bhargava & Sumeet Bhargava, p. 200.*

38. Which is not true about intensifying screen?

(a) Increase patient dose
(b) Speed is inversely proportional to exposure
(c) Intensification factor is the ratio of the exposure required to produce the same film density without screen/with screen
(d) Improve film gamma thus contrast and sharpness

Ans. (d). *Textbook of Radiology for Residents & Technicians, 5th ed., S.K. Bhargava & Sumeet Bhargava, p. 200.*

39. Which is not true about film latitude?

(a) Is range of exposures to produce useful range of densities
(b) Normal latitude of film-screen is 40:1
(c) Film latitude and gamma are directly related
(d) High film latitude requires for chest X-rays

Ans. (c). *Textbook of Radiology for Residents & Technicians, 5th ed., S.K. Bhargava & Sumeet Bhargava, p. 201.*

40. Which is not true about Intensification Factor (IF)

(a) IF increased by increasing thickness and size of the phosphor
(b) IF increased by increasing kV
(c) Increase in IF increases the patient dose
(d) IF gives idea of the speed of the screen

Ans. (c). *Textbook of Radiology for Residents & Technicians, 5th ed., S.K. Bhargava & Sumeet Bhargava, p. 177.*

41. Which is not true about film?

(a) Parallax effect does not occur with double-coated film
(b) Base is blue tinted
(c) Each grain is about 1 micron in size
(d) Crossed over in double coated film increases unsharpness

Ans. (a). *Textbook of Radiology for Residents & Technicians, 5th ed., S.K. Bhargava & Sumeet Bhargava, p. 177.*

42. The phosphor used in manufacturing the X-ray films are

(a) Silver nitrate (b) Silver bromide
(c) Calcium tungstate (d) Sodium sulphite

Ans. (b). *Textbook of Radiology for Residents & Technicians, 5th ed., S.K. Bhargava & Sumeet Bhargava, p. 177.*

43. The cellulose acetate based films are _______ films.

(a) Inflammable (b) Not flammable
(c) Safer (d) Breakable

Ans. (a). *Textbook of Radiology for Residents & Technicians, 5th ed., S.K. Bhargava & Sumeet Bhargava, p. 177.*

44. The substratum layer or binding layer is made-up

(a) Silver bromide crystals
(b) Gelatin plus acetone and water
(c) Gelatin
(d) None of the above

Ans. (b). *Textbook of Radiology for Residents & Technicians, 5th ed., S.K. Bhargava & Sumeet Bhargava, p. 177.*

45. The super coating is made-up of

(a) Cellulose chloride
(b) Varnish
(c) Gelatin
(d) Silver iodide

Ans. (a). *Textbook of Radiology for Residents & Technicians, 5th ed., S.K. Bhargava & Sumeet Bhargava, p. 177.*

46. Monochromatic films are sensitive to colors of the spectrum

(a) One color (b) Two color
(c) Three color (d) All colors

Ans. (a). Textbook of Radiology for Residents & Technicians, 5th ed., S.K. Bhargava & Sumeet Bhargava, p. 176.

47. Green yellow spectrum is sensitive to

(a) Monochromatic film (b) Orthochromatic film
(c) Panchromatic film (d) None of the above

Ans. (a). Textbook of Radiology for Residents & Technicians, 5th ed., S.K. Bhargava & Sumeet Bhargava, p. 176.

48. Blackness of the exposed film after processing is called as

(a) Resolution (b) Sharpness
(c) Density (d) Contrast

Ans. (c). Textbook of Radiology for Residents & Technicians, 5th ed., S.K. Bhargava & Sumeet Bhargava, p. 197.

49. Single coated films are used for

(a) Mammography (b) Ultrasound
(c) CT (d) All above

Ans. (d). Textbook of Radiology for Residents & Technicians, 5th ed., S.K. Bhargava & Sumeet Bhargava, p. 177.

50. The device to keep the X-ray film for exposure

(a) X-ray cassette (b) X-ray magazine
(c) X-ray box (d) X-ray container

Ans. (a). Textbook of Radiology for Residents & Technicians, 5th ed., S.K. Bhargava & Sumeet Bhargava, p. 177.

51. The graph showing relationship between density and log of exposure is known as

(a) H & D curve (b) Density and exposure curve
(c) Characteristic curve (d) All above

Ans. (d). Textbook of Radiology for Residents & Technicians, 5th ed., S.K. Bhargava & Sumeet Bhargava, p. 206.

52. Density is proportional to

(a) Increase in exposure
(b) Increase in amount of silver present
(c) Increase in developing time
(d) All of the above

Ans. (d). Textbook of Radiology for Residents & Technicians, 5th ed., S.K. Bhargava & Sumeet Bhargava, p. 206.

53. Non-screen films are used for

(a) Thin part of the body (b) Thick part of the body
(c) Less exposure technique (d) None

Ans. (a). *Textbook of Radiology for Residents & Technicians, 5th ed., S.K. Bhargava & Sumeet Bhargava, p. 201.*

54. The film boxes are arranged vertically upon the shelf in store room

(a) To avoid pressure on the film (b) To avoid light leaking
(c) To minimize the space (d) For convenience

Ans. (a). *Textbook of Radiology for Residents & Technicians, 5th ed., S.K. Bhargava & Sumeet Bhargava, p. 201.*

55. Fluorescent material used in intensifying screen is

(a) Silver bromide (b) Calcium tungstate
(c) Calcium carbonate (d) Potassium bromide

Ans. (b). *Textbook of Radiology for Residents & Technicians, 5th ed., S.K. Bhargava & Sumeet Bhargava, p. 176.*

56. The characteristic of the phosphor used in the intensifying screen should be

(a) High atomic number (absorbing more radiation)
(b) High X-ray conversion efficiency (produce more light)
(c) Minimum after glow
(d) None of the above

Ans. (d). *Textbook of Radiology for Residents & Technicians, 5th ed., S.K. Bhargava & Sumeet Bhargava, p. 178.*

57. The speed of the intensifying screen primarily depends upon

(a) Type of the film
(b) Size of the focal spot
(c) Size of the phosphor crystals
(d) Material used for the cassette

Ans. (c). *Textbook of Radiology for Residents & Technicians, 5th ed., S.K. Bhargava & Sumeet Bhargava, p. 176.*

58. Poor screen film contact results in

(a) Increase object–film distance
(b) Magnification of the image
(c) Blurring of the image
(d) Black streaks on the edges

Ans. (c). *Textbook of Radiology for Residents & Technicians, 5th ed., S.K. Bhargava & Sumeet Bhargava, p. 176.*

59. Curved cassettes are used in

(a) OPG (Orthopentogram)
(b) Knee joint (arthritis, severe fibrosis)
(c) Axial view of the shoulder
(d) All above

Ans. (d). *Textbook of Radiology for Residents & Technicians, 5th ed., S.K. Bhargava & Sumeet Bhargava, p. 176.*

60. Dark Room should be located

(a) Near the radiographic room
(b) Away from the radiographic room
(c) In the center of the radiographic room
(d) None of the above

Ans. (c). *Textbook of Radiology for Residents & Technicians, 5th ed., S.K. Bhargava & Sumeet Bhargava, p. 169.*

61. The ideal temperature of the dark room (processing room) should be

(a) 70° to 80° F (b) 23° to 27° C
(c) 16° to 22° C (d) None of the above

Ans. (c). *Textbook of Radiology for Residents & Technicians, 5th ed., S.K. Bhargava & Sumeet Bhargava, p. 169.*

62. The material used to make the floor of the dark room should be

(a) Resistance to chemicals and staining
(b) Non-porous
(c) Non-slippery
(d) All of the above

Ans. (d). *Textbook of Radiology for Residents & Technicians, 5th ed., S.K. Bhargava & Sumeet Bhargava, p. 169.*

63. The visible image is formed on the exposed film

(a) By donation of the electron from developer
(b) By liberation of the electron from the film
(c) By donation of the electron from fixer
(d) None of the above

Ans. (a). *Textbook of Radiology for Residents & Technicians, 5th ed., S.K. Bhargava & Sumeet Bhargava, p. 178.*

64. Which of the following is the accelerator in the developer?

(a) Sodium carbonate and sodium hydroxide
(b) Potassium carbonate
(c) Ammonium bromide
(d) None of the above

Ans. (a). *Textbook of Radiology for Residents & Technicians, 5th ed., S.K. Bhargava & Sumeet Bhargava, p. 179.*

65. The function of the accelerators in the developer is

(a) To stop the development
(b) To decrease the rate of the development
(c) To increase the rate of the development
(d) None of the above

Ans. (c). *Textbook of Radiology for Residents & Technicians, 5th ed., S.K. Bhargava & Sumeet Bhargava, p. 179.*

66. The fastest reducing agent responsible to produce low contrast film is

(a) Phenidione (b) Hydroquinone
(c) Sodium sulphate (d) Potassium bromide

Ans. (a). *Textbook of Radiology for Residents & Technicians, 5th ed., S.K. Bhargava & Sumeet Bhargava, p. 179.*

67. The preservative in the developing solution is for

(a) To stop the development
(b) To decrease the rate of the development
(c) To prolong the effective life span of the developer
(d) None of the above

Ans. (c). *Textbook of Radiology for Residents & Technicians, 5th ed., S.K. Bhargava & Sumeet Bhargava, p. 179.*

68. Film is agitated during development

(a) To increase the development
(b) To maintain uniform development of film
(c) To maintain the uniform temperature of solution
(d) All above

Ans. (d). *Textbook of Radiology for Residents & Technicians, 5th ed., S.K. Bhargava & Sumeet Bhargava, p. 179.*

69. The replenisher solution does not contain

(a) Metal (b) Hydroquinone
(c) Phenidione (d) Potassium bromide

Ans. (d). *Textbook of Radiology for Residents & Technicians, 5th ed., S.K. Bhargava & Sumeet Bhargava, p. 179.*

70. The range of concentration of pH in the developing chemicals are

(a) 10.0 to 11.5 (b) 7.0 to 10.0
(c) 5.0 to 7.0 (d) 12.0 to 15.0

Ans. ***(a).*** *Textbook of Radiology for Residents & Technicians, 5th ed., S.K. Bhargava & Sumeet Bhargava, p. 179.*

71. The reduction in the level of developing chemicals in tanks depends upon

(a) Number of the films developed
(b) The method of the development
(c) Size and type of the film used
(d) All above

Ans. ***(d).*** *Textbook of Radiology for Residents & Technicians, 5th ed., S.K. Bhargava & Sumeet Bhargava, p. 179.*

72. The first automatic film processor was developed in England without drying section by

(a) Kodak
(b) Siemens
(c) GE
(d) Potter

Ans. ***(a).*** *Textbook of Radiology for Residents & Technicians, 5th ed., S.K. Bhargava & Sumeet Bhargava, p. 180.*

73. The radiation dose of the patient can be reduced by

(a) Radiography without screen
(b) Standard film and screen
(c) Low speed screen and films
(d) High speed screen and films

Ans. ***(d).*** *Textbook of Radiology for Residents & Technicians, 5th ed., S.K. Bhargava & Sumeet Bhargava, p. 176.*

74. The kilovoltage determines the film

(a) Density
(b) Contrast
(c) Detail
(d) Distortion

Ans. ***(b).*** *Textbook of Radiology for Residents & Technicians, 5th ed., S.K. Bhargava & Sumeet Bhargava, p. 200.*

75. The action of the developer on unexposed silver bromide crystals of emulsion as

(a) Dissolved
(b) Oxidized
(c) Washed away
(d) Unaffected

Ans. ***(d).*** *Textbook of Radiology for Residents & Technicians, 5th ed., S.K. Bhargava & Sumeet Bhargava, p. 178.*

76. The concentration, temperature of solution along with agitation of film determines the

(a) Rate of development of the film
(b) Technique of the development of the film
(c) Rate of the fixing of the film
(d) None of the above

Ans. ***(a).*** *Textbook of Radiology for Residents & Technicians, 5th ed., S.K. Bhargava & Sumeet Bhargava, p. 178.*

77. Cassette front should have an aluminium equivalent of

(a) 1.4 mm (b) 1.6 mm
(c) 1.4 cm (d) 1.6 cm

Ans. ***(b).*** *Textbook of Radiology for Residents & Technicians, 5th ed., S.K. Bhargava & Sumeet Bhargava, p. 175.*

78. Lead equivalent of the cassette back is

(a) 0.18 mm (b) 0.18 cm
(c) 0.12 mm (d) 0.12 cm

Ans. ***(c).*** *Textbook of Radiology for Residents & Technicians, 5th ed., S.K. Bhargava & Sumeet Bhargava, p. 175.*

79. Single screen cassettes are used in

(a) Mammography (b) Angiography
(c) Orthodontic radiography (d) Ultrasound

Ans. ***(a).*** *Textbook of Radiology for Residents & Technicians, 5th ed., S.K. Bhargava & Sumeet Bhargava, p. 175.*

80. In obtaining the intercondylar view of knee the cassette used is

(a) Gridded (b) Curved
(c) Formatter (d) Multisection

Ans. ***(b).*** *Textbook of Radiology for Residents & Technicians, 5th ed., S.K. Bhargava & Sumeet Bhargava, p. 175.*

81. Cassette used for imaging from a cathode ray tube or TV monitors

(a) Formatter (b) Multisection
(c) Angiography (d) Photofluorography

Ans. ***(a).*** *Textbook of Radiology for Residents & Technicians, 5th ed., S.K. Bhargava & Sumeet Bhargava, p. 175.*

82. Examples of the formatter cassette includes all, except

(a) Ultrasound
(b) Digital subtraction angiography
(c) Computed tomography
(d) Mammography

Ans. ***(d).*** *Textbook of Radiology for Residents & Technicians, 5th ed., S.K. Bhargava & Sumeet Bhargava, p. 297.*

83. In CR cassette the photostimulable phosphor used is

(a) Europium activated barium fluorohalide
(b) Yttrium activated barium fluorohalide

(c) Both
(d) None

Ans. (a). Textbook of Radiology for Residents & Technicians, 5th ed., S.K. Bhargava & Sumeet Bhargava, p. 579.

84. Intensifying screens are not used in

(a) Mammography
(b) Ultrasound
(c) Both
(d) None

Ans. (b). Textbook of Radiology for Residents & Technicians, 5th ed., S.K. Bhargava & Sumeet Bhargava, p. 175.

85. Locking methods in cassettes

(a) Spring clips
(b) Sliding-lock bars
(c) None
(d) Both

Ans. (d). Textbook of Radiology for Residents & Technicians, 5th ed., S.K. Bhargava & Sumeet Bhargava, p. 175.

86. True about formatter cassettes

(a) Single emulsion film used
(b) No intensifying screens needed
(c) Both
(d) None

Ans. (c). Textbook of Radiology for Residents & Technicians, 5th ed., S.K. Bhargava & Sumeet Bhargava, p. 297.

87. True about care of the cassettes

(a) Should be kept horizontal one above the other
(b) To avoid contacts with the fluids
(c) None of the above
(d) Both

Ans. (b). Textbook of Radiology for Residents & Technicians, 5th ed., S.K. Bhargava & Sumeet Bhargava, p. 175.

88. Clips are present on

(a) Front of the cassette
(b) Back of the cassette
(c) On the sides
(d) Any of the above

Ans. (b). Textbook of Radiology for Residents & Technicians, 5th ed., S.K. Bhargava & Sumeet Bhargava, p. 175.

89. The purpose of the lead lining at the back of the cassettes is to

(a) Prevent back scatter of radiation
(b) To decrease the radiation dose of the patient
(c) None
(d) Both

Ans. (a). *Textbook of Radiology for Residents & Technicians, 5th ed., S.K. Bhargava & Sumeet Bhargava, p. 175.*

90. Features of the ideal cassette includes all, except

(a) Light weight
(b) Easy to close and open
(c) Regular thickness
(d) Maximum beam attenuation

Ans. (d). *Textbook of Radiology for Residents & Technicians, 5th ed., S.K. Bhargava & Sumeet Bhargava, p. 175.*

91. Function of the cassettes

(a) To hold intensifying screens and protect them from damage
(b) To exclude all lights from entering the cassette and fogging the film
(c) To maintain a close and uniform contact between film and screen
(d) All of the above

Ans. (d). *Textbook of Radiology for Residents & Technicians, 5th ed., S.K. Bhargava & Sumeet Bhargava, p. 175.*

92. Angiography cassettes are

(a) EOT system
(b) PUCK system
(c) Both
(d) None

Ans. (c). *Textbook of Radiology for Residents & Technicians, 5th ed., S.K. Bhargava & Sumeet Bhargava, p. 481.*

93. Loading and unloading of the cassettes

(a) Should take place under safe light conditions
(b) Should be done gently
(c) Unexposed film is lightly lowered into the cassette well
(d) All of the above

Ans. (d). *Textbook of Radiology for Residents & Technicians, 5th ed., S.K. Bhargava & Sumeet Bhargava, p. 175.*

94. Filmless cassettes are used in

(a) Computed tomography
(b) Computed radiography
(c) Mammography
(d) Angiography

Ans. (b). *Textbook of Radiology for Residents & Technicians, 5th ed., S.K. Bhargava & Sumeet Bhargava, p. 578.*

95. Conventional film screen systems have

(a) Front intensifying screen
(b) Back intensifying screen
(c) None
(d) Both

Ans. (d). *Textbook of Radiology for Residents & Technicians, 5th ed., S.K. Bhargava & Sumeet Bhargava, p. 176.*

96. True about the ideal cassette

(a) Front to be of uniform thickness and density and have no irregularities
(b) Back of the cassette lined with lead
(c) None
(d) Both

Ans. (d). *Textbook of Radiology for Residents & Technicians, 5th ed., S.K. Bhargava & Sumeet Bhargava, p. 175.*

97. The front surface of the cassette should be made-up of

(a) Plastic (b) Copper
(c) Lead (d) Iron

Ans. (a). *Textbook of Radiology for Residents & Technicians, 5th ed., S.K. Bhargava & Sumeet Bhargava, p. 175.*

98. The back cover of the cassette is made-up of

(a) Carbon (b) Plastic
(c) Lead (d) Iron

Ans. (c). *Textbook of Radiology for Residents & Technicians, 5th ed., S.K. Bhargava & Sumeet Bhargava, p. 175.*

99. The X-rays after transmission through the film screen combination undergo following interaction in the back cover of the cassette

(a) Compton (b) Photoelectric
(c) Elastic scatter (d) Pair production

Ans. (b). *Textbook of Radiology for Residents & Technicians, 5th ed., S.K. Bhargava & Sumeet Bhargava, p. 159.*

100. The tint of the film is of the _______ color.

(a) Red (b) Green
(c) Blue (d) Yellow

Ans. (c). *Textbook of Radiology for Residents & Technicians, 5th ed., S.K. Bhargava & Sumeet Bhargava, p. 172.*

101. The film fog is

(a) 0.30–0.40 (b) 0.40–0.50
(c) 0.12–0.20 (d) 0.50–0.60

Ans. (c). *Textbook of Radiology for Residents & Technicians, 5th ed., S.K. Bhargava & Sumeet Bhargava, p. 186.*

102. Characteristic curve gives information regarding all except

(a) Quantum mottle

(b) Intensification factor
(c) Film gamma
(d) Spatial resolution

Ans. (a). *Textbook of Radiology for Residents & Technicians, 5th ed., S.K. Bhargava & Sumeet Bhargava, p. 206.*

103. Which of the following is not the type of film

(a) Metal film
(b) Mammography film
(c) Duplicating film
(d) Dental film

Ans. (a). *Textbook of Radiology for Residents & Technicians, 5th ed., S.K. Bhargava & Sumeet Bhargava, p. 172.*

104. The emulsion of the film consists of the mixture of

(a) Gelatin
(b) Silver halide crystal
(c) Both
(d) None

Ans. (c). *Textbook of Radiology for Residents & Technicians, 5th ed., S.K. Bhargava & Sumeet Bhargava, p. 173.*

105. Polyester is superior to cellulose triacetate for the manufacture of the film base because

(a) Dimensional stability is superior
(b) It is stronger
(c) More resistant
(d) All of the above

Ans. (a). *Textbook of Radiology for Residents & Technicians, 5th ed., S.K. Bhargava & Sumeet Bhargava, p. 173.*

106. The filter in the dark room used for the blue sensitive film is

(a) Amber
(b) Red
(c) Green
(d) White

Ans. (a). *Textbook of Radiology for Residents & Technicians, 5th ed., S.K. Bhargava & Sumeet Bhargava, p. 170.*

107. Very low humidity in the dark room can lead to

(a) Crinkle marks
(b) Static electric discharges
(c) Excessive emulsion swellings
(d) Chemical fog

Ans. (b). *Textbook of Radiology for Residents & Technicians, 5th ed., S.K. Bhargava & Sumeet Bhargava, p. 172.*

108. Uniform density of the radiograph is obtained by

(a) Grid
(b) Penetrometer
(c) Intensifying screens
(d) Compensating filters

Ans. (d). *Textbook of Radiology for Residents & Technicians, 5th ed., S.K. Bhargava & Sumeet Bhargava, p. 166.*

109. In the dark room, there is

(a) Complete darkness
(b) Safe light
(c) Bright light
(d) Sun light

Ans. (b). *Textbook of Radiology for Residents & Technicians, 5th ed., S.K. Bhargava & Sumeet Bhargava, p. 170.*

110. The floor space in dark room should be

(a) 100 square feet
(b) 200 square feet
(c) 300 square feet
(d) 400 square feet

Ans. (a). *Textbook of Radiology for Residents & Technicians, 5th ed., S.K. Bhargava & Sumeet Bhargava, p. 170.*

111. Ceiling height in the dark room should be

(a) 41 feet
(b) 31 feet
(c) 21 feet
(d) 11 feet

Ans. (d). *Textbook of Radiology for Residents & Technicians, 5th ed., S.K. Bhargava & Sumeet Bhargava, p. 170.*

112. The dry side in the dark room has

(a) Loading bench
(b) Processing tank
(c) Replenishing solution
(d) Running water

Ans. (a). *Textbook of Radiology for Residents & Technicians, 5th ed., S.K. Bhargava & Sumeet Bhargava, p. 170.*

113. The wet side of the dark room has

(a) Loading bench
(b) Processing tank
(c) Replenishing solution
(d) Unused films

Ans. (b). *Textbook of Radiology for Residents & Technicians, 5th ed., S.K. Bhargava & Sumeet Bhargava, p. 170.*

114. The wall of the dark room be lined with lead equivalent thickness

(a) 2.5 mm
(b) 1.5 mm
(c) 3.5 mm
(d) 4.5 mm

Ans. (b). *Textbook of Radiology for Residents & Technicians, 5th ed., S.K. Bhargava & Sumeet Bhargava, p. 169.*

115. Most suitable location of pass box is near

(a) Gate
(b) Processing solution
(c) Loading bench
(d) Window

Ans. (c). *Textbook of Radiology for Residents & Technicians, 5th ed., S.K. Bhargava & Sumeet Bhargava, p. 170.*

116. Types of the entrances of the dark room are

(a) Electrically interlocked doors
(b) Maze
(c) Revolving door
(d) All of the above

Ans. (d). *Textbook of Radiology for Residents & Technicians, 5th ed., S.K. Bhargava & Sumeet Bhargava, p. 170.*

117. The working distance from the safe light to the film should not be less than

(a) 0.10 metre
(b) 1.2 metres
(c) 5 metres
(d) 15 metres

Ans. (b). *Textbook of Radiology for Residents & Technicians, 5th ed., S.K. Bhargava & Sumeet Bhargava, p. 170.*

118. Safe light should preferably be less than

(a) 100 watts
(b) 200 watts
(c) 45 watts
(d) 15 watts

Ans. (d). *Textbook of Radiology for Residents & Technicians, 5th ed., S.K. Bhargava & Sumeet Bhargava, p. 170.*

119. A screen converts

(a) Energy of the light to X-ray beam
(b) Energy of the X-ray beam to light
(c) Energy of the light to UV rays
(d) Energy of the UV to light rays

Ans. (b). *Textbook of Radiology for Residents & Technicians, 5th ed., S.K. Bhargava & Sumeet Bhargava, p. 170.*

120. A phosphor should have

(a) Low atomic number
(b) Low atomic mass
(c) High atomic mass
(d) High atomic number

Ans. (d). *Textbook of Radiology for Residents & Technicians, 5th ed., S.K. Bhargava & Sumeet Bhargava, p. 176.*

121. All of the following are phosphor material except

(a) Rare earth materials used for making screens
(b) Calcium tungstate
(c) Silver bromide
(d) Caesium iodide

Ans. (c). *Textbook of Radiology for Residents & Technicians, 5th ed., S.K. Bhargava & Sumeet Bhargava, p. 176.*

122. Large crystal size of phosphor in screen causes the following change in speed

(a) Increases
(b) Decreases
(c) No change
(d) Initially decreases than increases

Ans. (a). *Textbook of Radiology for Residents & Technicians, 5th ed., S.K. Bhargava & Sumeet Bhargava, p. 176.*

123. Intensifying screens are made-up of

(a) Iron (b) Carbon
(c) Polyester (d) Aluminium

Ans. (c). *Textbook of Radiology for Residents & Technicians, 5th ed., S.K. Bhargava & Sumeet Bhargava, p. 170.*

124. Calcium tungstate emits

(a) Blue light (b) Green light
(c) Yellow light (d) Red light

Ans. (a). *Textbook of Radiology for Residents & Technicians, 5th ed., S.K. Bhargava & Sumeet Bhargava, p. 170.*

125. Characteristic curve can be derived by the instrument

(a) Dosimeter (b) Potentiometer
(c) Electrometer (d) Sensitometer

Ans. (d). *Textbook of Radiology for Residents & Technicians, 5th ed., S.K. Bhargava & Sumeet Bhargava, p. 206.*

126. Rare earth screen are all except of the following

(a) Lanthanum oxybromide (b) Lanthanum oxysulphide
(c) Calcium tungstate (d) Gadolinium oxysulphide

Ans. (c). *Textbook of Radiology for Residents & Technicians, 5th ed., S.K. Bhargava & Sumeet Bhargava, p. 189.*

127. When a relatively small X-ray exposure produces a given output of light and causes certain darkening of the film, the screen is said to be

(a) Slow (b) Fast
(c) Both (d) None

Ans. (b). *Textbook of Radiology for Residents & Technicians, 5th ed., S.K. Bhargava & Sumeet Bhargava, p. 170.*

128. An increase in KV causes the screen speed to

(a) Increase (b) Decrease
(c) Both (d) None

Ans. ***(d).*** *Textbook of Radiology for Residents & Technicians, 5th ed., S.K. Bhargava & Sumeet Bhargava, p. 170.*

129. The main function of the developer is

(a) To reduce calcium tungstate to calcium
(b) To oxidize iodine
(c) To reduce exposed silver halide to metallic silver
(d) To reduce calcium to calcium tungstate

Ans. ***(c).*** *Textbook of Radiology for Residents & Technicians, 5th ed., S.K. Bhargava & Sumeet Bhargava, p. 178.*

130. Reducing agents used in developing solutions is

(a) Sodium carbonate
(b) Sodium chloride
(c) Sodium sulphite
(d) Hydroquinone

Ans. ***(d).*** *Textbook of Radiology for Residents & Technicians, 5th ed., S.K. Bhargava & Sumeet Bhargava, p. 178.*

131. Optimum temperature for film development is

(a) 30–40 degree C
(b) 20–24 degree C
(c) 40–50 degree C
(d) 10–20 degree C

Ans. ***(b).*** *Textbook of Radiology for Residents & Technicians, 5th ed., S.K. Bhargava & Sumeet Bhargava, p. 178.*

132. Purpose of the fixing is

(a) To remove unexposed silver halides
(b) To remove silver ions
(c) To make the film soft
(d) To make the film more thick

Ans. ***(a).*** *Textbook of Radiology for Residents & Technicians, 5th ed., S.K. Bhargava & Sumeet Bhargava, p. 179.*

133. Fixing agents used is

(a) Sulphuric acid
(b) Sodium sulphite
(c) Sodium thiosulphite
(d) Sodium chloride

Ans. ***(c).*** *Textbook of Radiology for Residents & Technicians, 5th ed., S.K. Bhargava & Sumeet Bhargava, p. 178.*

134. The solution used for fixation is

(a) Acidic
(b) Alkaline
(c) Neutral
(d) Highly alkaline

Ans. ***(a).*** *Textbook of Radiology for Residents & Technicians, 5th ed., S.K. Bhargava & Sumeet Bhargava, p. 178.*

135. Washing during processing of the film should be done under

(a) Stagnant water
(b) Using detergents

(c) Using running water (d) Using petrol

Ans. (c). Textbook of Radiology for Residents & Technicians, 5th ed., S.K. Bhargava & Sumeet Bhargava, p. 179.

136. The concentration of hydroquinone in replenisher solution is

(a) Lower (b) Higher
(c) Same (d) None

Ans. (b). Textbook of Radiology for Residents & Technicians, 5th ed., S.K. Bhargava & Sumeet Bhargava, p. 179.

137. Film should be kept in a place which is

(a) Hot
(b) Cool
(c) Wet
(d) Exposed to various chemicals

Ans. (b). Textbook of Radiology for Residents & Technicians, 5th ed., S.K. Bhargava & Sumeet Bhargava, p. 169.

138. Unexposed silver halide has an electrostatic charge

(a) Positive (b) Neutral
(c) Negative (d) None

Ans. (c). Textbook of Radiology for Residents & Technicians, 5th ed., S.K. Bhargava & Sumeet Bhargava, p. 170.

139. Most commonly used photosensitive agents is

(a) silver chloride (b) silver bromide
(c) silver iodide (d) None of the above

Ans. (b). Textbook of Radiology for Residents & Technicians, 5th ed., S.K. Bhargava & Sumeet Bhargava, p. 169-187.

140. Which of these provide formation of latent image?

(a) Gurney Mott theory (b) Reciprocate law
(c) Both of (a) and (b) (d) None of the above

Ans. (a). Textbook of Radiology for Residents & Technicians, 5th ed., S.K. Bhargava & Sumeet Bhargava, p. 169-187.

141. Silver halide is a product of chemical reaction between

(a) silver nitrate and alkali halide
(b) silver bromide and potassium nitrate
(c) Either of the above
(d) None of the above

Ans. (a). Textbook of Radiology for Residents & Technicians, 5th ed., S.K. Bhargava & Sumeet Bhargava, p. 169-187.

142. Which helps to bind emulsion to the base?

(a) Subbing layer (b) Supercoat
(c) Both of the above (d) None of the above

Ans. (a). Textbook of Radiology for Residents & Technicians, 5th ed., S.K. Bhargava & Sumeet Bhargava, p. 169-187.

143. In duplitized film

(a) single intensifying screen is used
(b) double intensifying screen is used
(c) Both of the above
(d) None of the above

Ans. (b). Textbook of Radiology for Residents & Technicians, 5th ed., S.K. Bhargava & Sumeet Bhargava, p. 169-187.

144. Optical density in most transparent part is

(a) 0.2 (b) 1.0
(c) 0.8 (d) 5.0

Ans. (a). Textbook of Radiology for Residents & Technicians, 5th ed., S.K. Bhargava & Sumeet Bhargava, p. 169-187.

145. Fog due to unavoidable exposure of the film to natural background radiation is

(a) age veil (b) storage fog
(c) chemical fog (d) safelight fog

Ans. (b). Textbook of Radiology for Residents & Technicians, 5th ed., S.K. Bhargava & Sumeet Bhargava, p. 169-187.

146. Optical density can be measured by

(a) densitometer (b) sensitometer
(c) survey meter (d) gyrometer

Ans. (a). Textbook of Radiology for Residents & Technicians, 5th ed., S.K. Bhargava & Sumeet Bhargava, p. 169-187.

147. Those films which are sensitive to green light are

(a) monochromatic (b) orthochromatic
(c) panchromatic (d) None of the above

Ans. (a). Textbook of Radiology for Residents & Technicians, 5th ed., S.K. Bhargava & Sumeet Bhargava, p. 169-187.

148. Medical X-ray sheet film has base thickness of

(a) 0.18 mm (b) 0.03 mm
(c) 1.5 mm (d) 0.0001 mm

Ans. (a). Textbook of Radiology for Residents & Technicians, 5th ed., S.K. Bhargava & Sumeet Bhargava, p. 169-187.

149. Cross-over effect occurs with

(a) intensifying screen
(b) without intensifying screen
(c) Either of the above
(d) None of the above

Ans. (a). *Textbook of Radiology for Residents & Technicians, 5th ed., S.K. Bhargava & Sumeet Bhargava, p. 169-187.*

150. Polyurethane is contained in which of the following layers?

(a) Supercoat
(b) Phosphor layer
(c) Base
(d) None of the above

Ans. (b). *Textbook of Radiology for Residents & Technicians, 5th ed., S.K. Bhargava & Sumeet Bhargava, p. 169-187.*

151. Why we need intensifying screen?

(a) To use lower exposure
(b) It permits short exposure time
(c) Give high contrast image
(d) All of the above

Ans. (d). *Textbook of Radiology for Residents & Technicians, 5th ed., S.K. Bhargava & Sumeet Bhargava, p. 169-187.*

152. Lead equivalent of cassette back is

(a) 1.6 mm
(b) 0.12 mm
(c) 2.0 mm
(d) 2.3 mm

Ans. (b). *Textbook of Radiology for Residents & Technicians, 5th ed., S.K. Bhargava & Sumeet Bhargava, p. 169-187.*

153. The pH of fixing agent is

(a) 9.5–10.7
(b) 3.3–5.5
(c) 4.0–5.0
(d) 1.0–2.3

Ans. (c). *Textbook of Radiology for Residents & Technicians, 5th ed., S.K. Bhargava & Sumeet Bhargava, p. 169-187.*

154. The pH of developing agent is

(a) 9.5–10.7
(b) 1.7–3.3
(c) 4.0–5.0
(d) 7.4–8.3

Ans. (a). *Textbook of Radiology for Residents & Technicians, 5th ed., S.K. Bhargava & Sumeet Bhargava, p. 169-187.*

155. Which of the following is solvent in processing cycle?

(a) Potassium carbonate
(b) Phenidone
(c) Water
(d) None of the above

Ans. (c). *Textbook of Radiology for Residents & Technicians, 5th ed., S.K. Bhargava & Sumeet Bhargava, p. 169-187.*

156. Why preservative is used in developer?

(a) To reduce oxidation of developing agents
(b) To prevent excessive swallowing
(c) Both (a) and (b)
(d) None of the above

Ans. (a). *Textbook of Radiology for Residents & Technicians, 5th ed., S.K. Bhargava & Sumeet Bhargava, p. 169-187.*

157. EDTA

(a) Ethylene Dimethyl Tetramine Acetic acid
(b) Ethylene Diamine Tetra Acetic acid
(c) Ethane Dimethyl Tetramine Acetic acid
(d) None of the above

Ans. (b). *Textbook of Radiology for Residents & Technicians, 5th ed., S.K. Bhargava & Sumeet Bhargava, p. 169-187.*

158. Rollers of automatic processor are made-up of

(a) rubber
(b) metal
(c) paper
(d) cloth

Ans. (a). *Textbook of Radiology for Residents & Technicians; 5th ed., S.K. Bhargava & Sumeet Bhargava, p. 169-187.*

159. Typical temperature of developer in automatic processor is

(a) 20°C
(b) 50°C
(c) 90°C
(d) 35°C

Ans. (d). *Textbook of Radiology for Residents & Technicians, 5th ed., S.K. Bhargava & Sumeet Bhargava, p. 169-187.*

160. Silver recovery is done from

(a) developer
(b) rinser
(c) fixer
(d) washing

Ans. (c). *Textbook of Radiology for Residents & Technicians, 5th ed., S.K. Bhargava & Sumeet Bhargava, p. 169-187.*

161. Tree static, crown static, crow's feet are the type of artifact due to

(a) finge marks
(b) static marks
(c) chemical staining
(d) radiographic artifacts

Ans. (b). *Textbook of Radiology for Residents & Technicians, 5th ed., S.K. Bhargava & Sumeet Bhargava, p. 169-187.*

162. What intercepts light and redirects it to film?

(a) Phosphor layer
(b) Base layer

(c) Protective layer
(d) Reflexive layer

Ans. (d). *Textbook of Radiology for Residents & Technicians, 5th ed., S.K. Bhargava & Sumeet Bhargava, p. 169-187.*

163. What do you do to clean intensifying screen?

(a) You do not do anything
(b) Use soft lint-free cloth
(c) Windex and paper towel
(d) Sterilize and wash it

Ans. (b). *Textbook of Radiology for Residents & Technicians, 5th ed., S.K. Bhargava & Sumeet Bhargava, p. 169-187.*

164. To reduce artifact, cleaning must be done

(a) once annually
(b) once in a month
(c) twice in a week
(d) once in a day

Ans. (b). *Textbook of Radiology for Residents & Technicians, 5th ed., S.K. Bhargava & Sumeet Bhargava, p. 169-187.*

165. Rigid holder that contains the intensifying screen and film

(a) beam restrictor
(b) radiographic cassette
(c) compressive cassette
(d) folder

Ans. (b). *Textbook of Radiology for Residents & Technicians, 5th ed., S.K. Bhargava & Sumeet Bhargava, p. 169-187.*

166. Restricts the useful X-ray beam to the part of the body being imaged, thereby reducing the level of scatter radiation and unnecessary exposure

(a) collimator
(b) filter
(c) emulsion
(d) base

Ans. (a). *Textbook of Radiology for Residents & Technicians, 5th ed., S.K. Bhargava & Sumeet Bhargava, p. 169-187.*

167. Absorb low energy X-ray before reaching the patient

(a) collimator
(b) filter
(c) emulsion
(d) base

Ans. (b). *Textbook of Radiology for Residents & Technicians, 5th ed., S.K. Bhargava & Sumeet Bhargava, p. 169-187.*

168. Safe film handling time in darkroom is

(a) 20–40 sec
(b) 60–80 sec
(c) 100–120 sec
(d) 3 min

Ans. (a). *Textbook of Radiology for Residents & Technicians, 5th ed., S.K. Bhargava & Sumeet Bhargava, p. 169-187.*

169. If you get a chemical in your eyes, what should you do?

(a) Wash your eyes immediately under running water
(b) Rub the chemical out of your eyes
(c) Blot your eyes with a tissue
(d) None of the above

Ans. (a). *Textbook of Radiology for Residents & Technicians, 5th ed., S.K. Bhargava & Sumeet Bhargava, p. 169-187.*

170. To absorb backscatter, the back of most cassettes is lined with

(a) lead (b) felt
(c) intensifying screen (d) X-ray film

Ans. (a). *Textbook of Radiology for Residents & Technicians, 5th ed., S.K. Bhargava & Sumeet Bhargava, p. 169-187.*

171. The main advantage of today's rare earth-coated intensifying screen is

(a) its emmision of light is the blue region of UV spectrum
(b) its ability to convert a latent image into visible image
(c) they are easy and inexpensive to separate from earth
(d) they have a higher X-ray to light conversion efficiency

Ans. (d). *Textbook of Radiology for Residents & Technicians, 5th ed., S.K. Bhargava & Sumeet Bhargava, p. 169-187.*

172. Which of the following are appropriate storage conditions for radiographic film?

(a) 10° to 15°C, 40% to 60% humidity
(b) 1° to 15°C, 40% to 80% humidity
(c) 10° to 20°C, 40% to 0% humidity
(d) None of the above

Ans. (a). *Textbook of Radiology for Residents & Technicians, 5th ed., S.K. Bhargava & Sumeet Bhargava, p. 169-187.*

173. The walls of darkroom should be white or cream-coloured because

(a) it is easier to keep those colours clean
(b) these colours help to detect light leaks
(c) more reflection of safelight is produced, producing a more visible working environment
(d) None of the above

Ans. (c). *Textbook of Radiology for Residents & Technicians, 5th ed., S.K. Bhargava & Sumeet Bhargava, p. 169-187.*

174. Which of the following film are more sensitive?

(a) Exposed film (b) Unexposed film

(c) Developed film (d) Both (a) and (b)

Ans. (a). *Textbook of Radiology for Residents & Technicians, 5th ed., S.K. Bhargava & Sumeet Bhargava, p. 169-187.*

175. What is rinser?

(a) Remaining chemicals are washed from the film.
(b) Remove excess developer from the emulsion, stop the development process.
(c) Convert invisible image into visible image.
(d) None of the above

Ans. (b). *Textbook of Radiology for Residents & Technicians, 5th ed., S.K. Bhargava & Sumeet Bhargava, p. 169-187.*

176. The conversion of X-radiation into visible light occur via

(a) double emulsion film (b) processor
(c) intensifying screen (d) cassette

Ans. (c). *Textbook of Radiology for Residents & Technicians, 5th ed., S.K. Bhargava & Sumeet Bhargava, p. 169-187.*

177. Which of the following is completely dry, non-chemical process?

(a) Xeroradiography (b) Conventional radiography
(c) Mammography (d) All of the above

Ans. (a). *Textbook of Radiology for Residents & Technicians, 5th ed., S.K. Bhargava & Sumeet Bhargava, p. 169-187.*

178. Which of the following is also known as edge gradient?

(a) Geometric unsharpness (b) Movement unsharpness
(c) Absorption unsharpness (d) Screen unsharpness

Ans. (a). *Textbook of Radiology for Residents & Technicians, 5th ed., S.K. Bhargava & Sumeet Bhargava, p. 169-187.*

179. What is the difference between photographic density of exposed and unexposed adjacent parts of the image?

(a) Resolution (b) Contrast
(c) Unsharpness (d) Fog

Ans. (b). *Textbook of Radiology for Residents & Technicians, 5th ed., S.K. Bhargava & Sumeet Bhargava, p. 169-187.*

180. How to reduce geometrical unsharpness?

(a) Put object as close as possible (b) Use long FFD
(c) Use small focal spot (d) All of the above

Ans. (d). *Textbook of Radiology for Residents & Technicians, 5th ed., S.K. Bhargava & Sumeet Bhargava, p. 169-187.*

181. Modern X-ray developers use a combination of two developing agents, which are

(a) phenidone and hydroquinone
(b) phenidone and ammonium sulphate
(c) ammonium sulphate and sodium thiosulphate
(d) hydroquinone and boric acid

Ans. (a). *Textbook of Radiology for Residents & Technicians, 5th ed., S.K. Bhargava & Sumeet Bhargava, p. 169-187.*

182. Cross-over effect occurs in

(a) single emulsion film
(b) double emulsion film
(c) Both (a) and (b)
(d) None of the above

Ans. (b). *Textbook of Radiology for Residents & Technicians, 5th ed., S.K. Bhargava & Sumeet Bhargava, p. 169-187.*

183. Film blackening depends on

(a) mAS
(b) kV_p
(c) FFD
(d) SID

Ans. (a). *Textbook of Radiology for Residents & Technicians, 5th ed., S.K. Bhargava & Sumeet Bhargava, p. 169-187.*

184. Intensification factor (IF) =

(a) IF = Exposure without screen × Exposure with screen
(b) IF = Exposure without screen × Exposure with screen / 1000
(c) IF = Exposure without screen / Exposure with screen
(d) None of the above

Ans. (c). *Textbook of Radiology for Residents & Technicians, 5th ed., S.K. Bhargava & Sumeet Bhargava, p. 169-187.*

185. The darkroom should be lined with

(a) lead
(b) aluminium
(c) molybdenum
(d) steel

Ans. (a). *Textbook of Radiology for Residents & Technicians, 5th ed., S.K. Bhargava & Sumeet Bhargava, p. 169-187.*

186. The lead equivalent for darkroom wall thickness is

(a) 1.5 mm
(b) 2.5 mm
(c) 0.5 mm
(d) None of the above

Ans. (a). *Textbook of Radiology for Residents & Technicians, 5th ed., S.K. Bhargava & Sumeet Bhargava, p. 169-187.*

187. Which film uses T-grain technology?

(a) Green sensitive
(b) Blue sensitive
(c) Red sensitive
(d) None of the above

Ans. (a). *Textbook of Radiology for Residents & Technicians, 5th ed., S.K. Bhargava & Sumeet Bhargava, p. 169-187.*

188. Advantage of T-grain technology over conventional halide grains is

(a) improved image quality
(b) compatibility with processing cycle
(c) Both (a) and (b)
(d) None of the above

Ans. (c). *Textbook of Radiology for Residents & Technicians, 5th ed., S.K. Bhargava & Sumeet Bhargava, p. 169-187.*

189. Rare earth has conversion efficiency of

(a) 40–50% (b) 5–10%
(c) 20–25% (d) 80–90%

Ans. (c). *Textbook of Radiology for Residents & Technicians, 5th ed., S.K. Bhargava & Sumeet Bhargava, p. 169-187.*

190. Light emitted after 10^{-8} sec is called

(a) fluorescence (b) phosphorescence
(c) scintillation (d) All of the above

Ans. (b). *Textbook of Radiology for Residents & Technicians, 5th ed., S.K. Bhargava & Sumeet Bhargava, p. 169-187.*

191. Which is more sensitive to aerial oxidation?

(a) Hydroquinone (b) Phenidone
(c) Both (a) and (b) (d) None of the above

Ans. (a). *Textbook of Radiology for Residents & Technicians, 5th ed., S.K. Bhargava & Sumeet Bhargava, p. 169-187.*

192. Oxidized developer attains which colour?

(a) Brownish (b) Greenish
(c) Bluish (d) Either of them

Ans. (a). *Textbook of Radiology for Residents & Technicians, 5th ed., S.K. Bhargava & Sumeet Bhargava, p. 169-187.*

193. Which is processor artifact?

(a) Water spots (b) Shoe mark
(c) Roller mark (d) All of the above

Ans. (d). *Textbook of Radiology for Residents & Technicians, 5th ed., S.K. Bhargava & Sumeet Bhargava, p. 169-187.*

194. Rare earth screen is made-up of elements which have atomic numbers

(a) 57–71 (b) 12–20
(c) 52 –60 (d) None of the above

Ans. (a). *Textbook of Radiology for Residents & Technicians, 5th ed., S.K. Bhargava & Sumeet Bhargava, p. 169-187.*

195. In rare earth screen, thallium produces which colour?

(a) Green (b) Blue
(c) Red (d) All of the above

Ans. (b). *Textbook of Radiology for Residents & Technicians, 5th ed., S.K. Bhargava & Sumeet Bhargava, p. 169-187.*

196. Why foreign particle should be removed from screen?

(a) It will produce area of under-exposure.
(b) It will eliminate light spot on screen.
(c) Both (a) and (b)
(d) None of the above

Ans. (c). *Textbook of Radiology for Residents & Technicians, 5th ed., S.K. Bhargava & Sumeet Bhargava, p. 169-187.*

197. Carbon fibre cassettes are used to _______.

(a) Reduce patient dose
(b) Increase patient dose
(c) Use high kV_p
(d) None of the above

Ans. (a). *Textbook of Radiology for Residents & Technicians, 5th ed., S.K. Bhargava & Sumeet Bhargava, p. 169-187.*

198. Vacuum cassettes are made from _______.

(a) Flexible vinyl material (b) 0.5 mm Al equivalent
(c) Carbon fibre (d) Cassette tunnel

Ans. (a). *Textbook of Radiology for Residents & Technicians, 5th ed., S.K. Bhargava & Sumeet Bhargava, p. 169-187.*

199. In _______ cassette, no intensifying screen is used.

(a) Mammography (b) Vacuum
(c) Formatter (d) Multisection

Ans. (c). *Textbook of Radiology for Residents & Technicians, 5th ed., S.K. Bhargava & Sumeet Bhargava, p. 169-187.*

200. Developers used in radiography are _______.

(a) Alkaline (b) Acidic
(c) Neutral (d) None of the above

Ans. (a). *Textbook of Radiology for Residents & Technicians, 5th ed., S.K. Bhargava & Sumeet Bhargava, p. 169-187.*

201. Fixing solutions are used in radiography are _______.

(a) Alkaline (b) Acidic

(c) Neutral (d) None of the above

Ans. (b). *Textbook of Radiology for Residents & Technicians, 5th ed., S.K. Bhargava & Sumeet Bhargava, p. 169-187.*

202. _______ stage converts the invisible image into visible image in automatic processing.

(a) Development (b) Fixing

(c) Washing (d) Drying

Ans. (a). *Textbook of Radiology for Residents & Technicians, 5th ed., S.K. Bhargava & Sumeet Bhargava, p. 169-187.*

203. _______ begins to accumulate in the developer causing its pH to fall.

(a) Hydroquinone (b) Metol

(c) Hydrobromic acid (d) Sodium carbonate

Ans. (c). *Textbook of Radiology for Residents & Technicians, 5th ed., S.K. Bhargava & Sumeet Bhargava, p. 169-187.*

204. If the developer temperature is too warm, then it produces _______.

(a) Developmental fog (b) Safelight fog

(c) Chemical fog (d) Oxidation fog

Ans. (c). *Textbook of Radiology for Residents & Technicians, 5th ed., S.K. Bhargava & Sumeet Bhargava, p. 169-187.*

205. _______ is the activator which is used in manual processing to swell the emulsion layer.

(a) Potassium bromide

(b) Potassium iodide

(c) Sodium sulfite

(d) Sodium carbonate

Ans. (d). *Textbook of Radiology for Residents & Technicians, 5th ed., S.K. Bhargava & Sumeet Bhargava, p. 169-187.*

206. _______ is the antifogging agent which is used in manual processing.

(a) Sodium carbonate

(b) Sodium hydroxide

(c) Potassium bromide and potassium iodide

(d) Hydroquinone and metol

Ans. (c). *Textbook of Radiology for Residents & Technicians, 5th ed., S.K. Bhargava & Sumeet Bhargava, p. 169-187.*

207. _______ protects the reducing agents from oxidation by the air in manual processing

(a) Sodium sulfite (b) Sodium carbonate
(c) Sodium hydroxide (d) Hydroquinone

Ans. (a). *Textbook of Radiology for Residents & Technicians, 5th ed., S.K. Bhargava & Sumeet Bhargava, p. 169-187.*

208. Contamination by the developer would quickly deprive the fixer of its effectiveness and give rise to _______ fog.

(a) Developmental (b) Chemical
(c) Colour (d) Safelight fog

Ans. (c). *Textbook of Radiology for Residents & Technicians, 5th ed., S.K. Bhargava & Sumeet Bhargava, p. 169-187.*

209. _______ protects the fixing agent from decomposition.

(a) Sodium sulfite (b) Sodium thiosulphate
(c) Sodium carbonate (d) Sodium hydroxide

Ans. (a). *Textbook of Radiology for Residents & Technicians, 5th ed., S.K. Bhargava & Sumeet Bhargava, p. 169-187.*

210. _______ hardens the gelatin in the emulsion, thereby protecting it against scratches in manual processing.

(a) Chrome alum or potassium alum
(b) Hypo sodium thiosulphate
(c) Benzotriazole
(d) Sodium carbonate

Ans. (a). *Textbook of Radiology for Residents & Technicians, 5th ed., S.K. Bhargava & Sumeet Bhargava, p. 169-187.*

211. Anti-halation layer is mainly present in _______.

(a) Duplitized film
(b) Intraoral dental film
(c) Kidney surgery film
(d) Single-sided emulsion film

Ans. (d). *Textbook of Radiology for Residents & Technicians, 5th ed., S.K. Bhargava & Sumeet Bhargava, p. 169-187.*

212. Some Kodak X-ray films have a _______ dye added to the surface of the emulsion crystals during manufacture to remove crossover effect.

(a) Red (b) Green
(c) Magenta (d) White

Ans. (c). *Textbook of Radiology for Residents & Technicians, 5th ed., S.K. Bhargava & Sumeet Bhargava, p. 169-187.*

213. Crossover effect is a source of _______.

(a) Sharpness
(b) Unsharpness
(c) Improved contrast
(d) Improved resolution

Ans. (b). *Textbook of Radiology for Residents & Technicians, 5th ed., S.K. Bhargava & Sumeet Bhargava, p. 169-187.*

214. Cine films are _______.

(a) Single emulsion films
(b) Duplitized emulsion films
(c) Envelope wrapped films
(d) Polaroid films

Ans. (a). *Textbook of Radiology for Residents & Technicians, 5th ed., S.K. Bhargava & Sumeet Bhargava, p. 169-187.*

215. Non-screen films are used because of their superior _______ compared to a screen film system.

(a) Resolution
(b) Contrast
(c) Sharpness
(d) Noise

Ans. (a). *Textbook of Radiology for Residents & Technicians, 5th ed., S.K. Bhargava & Sumeet Bhargava, p. 169-187.*

216. Radiation dose is lower when we use _______ film.

(a) Non-screen type
(b) Screen-type
(c) Envelope wrapped
(d) Direct exposure

Ans. (b). *Textbook of Radiology for Residents & Technicians, 5th ed., S.K. Bhargava & Sumeet Bhargava, p. 169-187.*

217. Size of occlusal film used in dental radiography is _______.

(a) 31×41 mm
(b) 57×76 mm
(c) 94×106 mm
(d) 78×94 mm

Ans. (b). *Textbook of Radiology for Residents & Technicians, 5th ed., S.K. Bhargava & Sumeet Bhargava, p. 169-187.*

218. _______ foil insert in the intra-oral dental film which acts as an attenuator of back-scattered radiation.

(a) Aluminium
(b) Copper
(c) Lead
(d) Zinc

Ans. (c). *Textbook of Radiology for Residents & Technicians, 5th ed., S.K. Bhargava & Sumeet Bhargava, p. 169-187.*

219. Green sensitive films are also known as _______.

(a) Monochromatic
(b) Orthochromatic
(c) Panchromatic
(d) None of the above

Ans. (b). *Textbook of Radiology for Residents & Technicians, 5th ed., S.K. Bhargava & Sumeet Bhargava, p. 169-187.*

220. Screen type films having their average gradient is > _____.

(a) 1 (b) 2
(c) 3 (d) 4

Ans. (a). *Textbook of Radiology for Residents & Technicians, 5th ed., S.K. Bhargava & Sumeet Bhargava, p. 169-187.*

221. Stand X-ray film boxes _______ upon the shelves.

(a) Horizontally (b) At an acute angle
(c) Vertically (d) At an 90 degree angle.

Ans. (c). *Textbook of Radiology for Residents & Technicians, 5th ed., S.K. Bhargava & Sumeet Bhargava, p. 169-187.*

222. The recommended relative humidity for a film store room is _______.

(a) 40% (b) 50%
(c) 60% (d) 70%

Ans. (b). *Textbook of Radiology for Residents & Technicians, 5th ed., S.K. Bhargava & Sumeet Bhargava, p. 169-187.*

223. If X-ray films to be stored for more than 3 months, then background radiation should not exceed _______.

(a) 1.29 nC/kg/h (b) 3.30 nC/kg/h
(c) 4.10 nC/kg/h (d) 5.40 nC/kg/h

Ans. (a). *Textbook of Radiology for Residents & Technicians, 5th ed., S.K. Bhargava & Sumeet Bhargava, p. 169-187.*

224. A reflective later in intensifying screen, _______ the speed.

(a) Increases (b) Decreases
(c) No effect on (d) None of the above

Ans. (a). *Textbook of Radiology for Residents & Technicians, 5th ed., S.K. Bhargava & Sumeet Bhargava, p. 169-187.*

225. In a high resolution screen _______ is added to reduce lateral resolution.

(a) Carbon granules (b) Lead granules
(c) Phosphor granules (d) Iron granules

Ans. (a). *Textbook of Radiology for Residents & Technicians, 5th ed., S.K. Bhargava & Sumeet Bhargava, p. 169-187.*

226. Active layer in the intensifying screen is _______.

(a) Base (b) Subbing layer
(c) Phosphor layer (d) Emulsion layer

Ans. (c). *Textbook of Radiology for Residents & Technicians, 5th ed., S.K. Bhargava & Sumeet Bhargava, p. 169-187.*

227. Fluorescent crystals are suspended in a transparent binder such as _______.

(a) Gelatin (b) Polyurethane
(c) Carbon gel (d) Coloured pigment

Ans. (b). *Textbook of Radiology for Residents & Technicians, 5th ed., S.K. Bhargava & Sumeet Bhargava, p. 169-187.*

228. The use of carbon granules thus _______ photographic unsharpness but _______ the speed of the screen.

(a) Minimizes, reduces
(b) Increases, decreases
(c) Decreases, increases
(d) Increases, increases

Ans. (a). *Textbook of Radiology for Residents & Technicians, 5th ed., S.K. Bhargava & Sumeet Bhargava, p. 169-187.*

229. The greater the number of grains in intensifying screen, the _______ the coating weight.

(a) Lesser (b) Greater
(c) Same (d) None of the above

Ans. (b). *Textbook of Radiology for Residents & Technicians, 5th ed., S.K. Bhargava & Sumeet Bhargava, p. 169-187.*

230. Materials which convert invisible radiation into luminous radiation are known as _______.

(a) Carbon granules (b) Polyurethane
(c) Phosphors (d) Acetate

Ans. (c). *Textbook of Radiology for Residents & Technicians, 5th ed., S.K. Bhargava & Sumeet Bhargava, p. 169-187.*

231. Full form of QDE is _______.

(a) Quantum Detection Efficiency
(b) Quantum Detection Effectiveness
(c) Quantum Detailed Efficiency
(d) Quantum Differentiated Effectiveness

Ans. (a). *Textbook of Radiology for Residents & Technicians, 5th ed., S.K. Bhargava & Sumeet Bhargava, p. 169-187.*

232. Gadolinium oxysulphide activated with terbium emits _______ light.

(a) Blue (b) Green
(c) White (d) Orange

Ans. (b). *Textbook of Radiology for Residents & Technicians, 5th ed., S.K. Bhargava & Sumeet Bhargava, p. 169-187.*

233. Yttrium tantalate activated with niobium emits _______ light.

(a) Blue (b) Green
(c) White (d) Violet

Ans. (a). Textbook of Radiology for Residents & Technicians, 5th ed., S.K. Bhargava & Sumeet Bhargava, p. 169-187.

234. If larger phosphor crystal size is used in an intensifying screen then the speed will get _______.

(a) Increased (b) No effect
(c) Decreased (d) None of the above

Ans. (a). Textbook of Radiology for Residents & Technicians, 5th ed., S.K. Bhargava & Sumeet Bhargava, p. 169-187.

235. Accelerators used in automatic process is _______.

(a) Potassium carbonate (b) Sodium carbonate
(c) Sodium hydroxide (d) Sodium sulfite

Ans. (a). Textbook of Radiology for Residents & Technicians, 5th ed., S.K. Bhargava & Sumeet Bhargava, p. 169-187.

236. _______ maintain the pH of the developing solutions in automatic processor.

(a) Accelerators (b) Buffers
(c) Restrainers (d) Sequestering agents

Ans. (b). Textbook of Radiology for Residents & Technicians, 5th ed., S.K. Bhargava & Sumeet Bhargava, p. 169-187.

237. Antifogging agent used in automatic processor is _______.

(a) Carbonates (b) Hydrobromic acid
(c) Benzotriazole (d) Glutaraldehyde

Ans. (c). Textbook of Radiology for Residents & Technicians, 5th ed., S.K. Bhargava & Sumeet Bhargava, p. 169-187.

238. _______ is a commonly used developer preservative in automatic processor.

(a) Potassium sulfite (b) Sodium carbonate
(c) Sodium hydroxide (d) Potassium carbonate

Ans. (a). Textbook of Radiology for Residents & Technicians, 5th ed., S.K. Bhargava & Sumeet Bhargava, p. 169-187.

239. _______ prevents the precipitation of insoluble mineral salts, which tends to occur in hard water.

(a) Glutaraldehyde
(b) EDTA (Ethylene Diamine Tetra Acetic Acid)

(c) Hydroquinone
(d) Phenidone

Ans. (b). *Textbook of Radiology for Residents & Technicians, 5th ed., S.K. Bhargava & Sumeet Bhargava, p. 169-187.*

240. In automatic processor, the developer temperature is _______.

(a) 38–42°C (b) 50–55°C
(c) 18–20°C (d) 25–30°C

Ans. (a). *Textbook of Radiology for Residents & Technicians, 5th ed., S.K. Bhargava & Sumeet Bhargava, p. 169-187.*

241. _______ and _______ are commonly used hardening agents in fixing solutions of automatic processor.

(a) Hydroquinone, Metol
(b) Acetic acid, Sulphuric acid
(c) Aluminium chloride, Aluminium sulphate
(d) Sodium acetate, Boric acid

Ans. (c). *Textbook of Radiology for Residents & Technicians, 5th ed., S.K. Bhargava & Sumeet Bhargava, p. 169-187.*

CHAPTER

4

Imaging Equipments

MRI

Fill in the Blanks

1. To see the adrenal mass, we scan _______ area. (kidney)
2. For MRI purpose we are only concerned with the _______ atom. (hydrogen)
3. The magnet in an MRI system is rated using a unit of measure known as _______. (tesla)
4. The most important component in MRI is _______. (magnet)
5. More the magnetic strength, _______ will be precession frequency. (higher)
6. Whenever there is electric current, there is _______. (magnetic field)
7. Less energy is required to align _______ to external magnetic field. (parallel)
8. Speed at which protons precess is measured as _______. (precession frequency).
9. Larmor equation is given as _______. (w0 = y B0)
10. Spin density images are also known as _______. (proton density)
11. Magnetization of patient is in direction along the external magnetic field is known as _______. (longitudinal magnetization)
12. To get the image we need to send _______ in MRI. (radio-frequency pulse)
13. Energy exchange is possible when protons and radiofrequency pulse have the _______. (same frequency)
14. RF pulse causes longitudinal magnetization to _______ (decrease) and establishes new _______ magnetization. (transversal)

15. Protons at different point precess with _______ frequency due to different field strength. (different)
16. With the help of frequency, signal is assigned to different and certain location. This gives us _______. (spatial information)
17. Relaxation is a _______ process. (continuous)
18. Protons release the excess energy to surroundings. These surrounding area is called _______. (lattice)
19. Longitudinal relaxation is also known as _______. (spin lattice relaxation)
20. Time taken by longitudinal magnetization to recover is called _______ denoted as _______. (longitudinal relaxation time, T_1)
21. The graph between transverse magnetization v/s time is known as _______. (T_2 curve)
22. T_1 is normally _______ than T_2. (longer)
23. T_2 = Time when transversal magnetization decrease to _______ of original value. (37%)
24. Pathological/diseased tissue which has high water content than surrounding normal tissue has _______ relaxation time. (longer)
25. The transversal component of the net magnetization can induce a _______ signal. (T_2)
26. Measuring the relaxation time _______ give tissue characteristics. (does not)
27. Fat has a _______ T_2 than water. (shorter)
28. An RF pulse which tilts the magnetization of 90 degree is called _______. (90° pulse)
29. The net magnetic field is a sum vector with direction _______ longitudinal and transversal field. (midway between).
30. TR is _______ when protons have fully recovered from the effects of first pulse. (long)
31. Longitudinal and transversal relaxation are _______ processes. (independent)
32. If we send in 2nd pulse after shorter TR, the difference in longitudinal magnetization is rather large, so there will be _______ contrast. (better tissue)
33. The loss of phase coherence results in decreasing _______ magnetization. (transversal)
34. T_2 effects are important with _______ sequences. (fast imaging)
35. Time between 90° pulse and spin echo is called _______. (time of echo)
36. The shorter the TE, _______ the signal that we get from a tissue. (stronger)

37. If we use long TE, resulting image should be heavily _______ weighted. (T_2)
38. _______ is the name of contrast media used in MRI. (Gadolinium)
39. Relaxation constants T_1 and T_2 are known as _______ parameters. (tissue)
40. Short TR will gives a _______ weighted image. (T_1)
41. If fluid e.g. CSF or urine is white, image is _______ weighted. (T_2)
42. We experience cross talk when _______ is very small. (slice distance)
43. Smaller the FOV, _______ will be the image resolution. (higher)
44. Permitted no. of slices is higher in _______ weighted image. (T_2)
45. In case of rectangular FOV, SNR _______. (reduces)
46. SAR values are _______ for T_2 than T_1 weighted sequences. (less)
47. When the object to be acquired is larger than the FOV, the signal from stimulated tissue outside FOV produces _______ effect in the image. (wrap around)
48. Echo time which are too long will result in _______ CNR. (decreased)
49. _______ the slice, more intense the signal and so higher the SNR. (Thicker)
50. To get strong T_2 weighted image and good SNR, flip angle need to be _______. (reduced)
51. T_1 and T_2 constants are _______ in infant brain than those of adults. (higher)
52. HASTE is used for sequential acquisition of high resolution _______ weighted image. (T_2)
53. We can achieve flow suppression by means of _______ slab. (presaturation)
54. For breast MRI, patient is positioned _______. (prone)
55. Visualization of pathological lesions is more reliable in _______ weighted image. (T_2)
56. If the slice distances are too small, the signals of adjacent slices affect one another, even if slice distance is 0%. This phenomenon is called _______. (cross talk)

MCQs

1. _______ energy is required by protons to align anti-parallel to external magnetic field.

(a) More (b) Less
(c) Zero (d) None of the above

Ans. (a). *Textbook of Radiology for Residents & Technicians, 5th ed., S.K. Bhargava & Sumeet Bhargava, p. 409.*

2. **For MRI, we need magnetization which is _______ to external magnetic field.**
   (a) Longitudinal to internal magnetic field
   (b) Transversal to internal magnetic field
   (c) Longitudinal to external magnetic field
   (d) Transversal to external magnetic field

   Ans. (d). *Textbook of Radiology for Residents & Technicians, 5th ed., S.K. Bhargava & Sumeet Bhargava, p. 410.*

3. **RF pulse causes longitudinal magnetization to _______ and establishes a new transversal magnetization.**
   (a) Increase (b) Decrease
   (c) Remain unchanged (d) Become zero

   Ans. (b). *Textbook of Radiology for Residents & Technicians, 5th ed., S.K. Bhargava & Sumeet Bhargava, p. 411.*

4. **In absolute terms, in biological tissue T_1 is about.**
   (a) 300–2000 msec (b) 30–2000 msec
   (c) 30–150 msec (d) 150–300 msec

   Ans. (a). *Textbook of Radiology for Residents & Technicians, 5th ed., S.K. Bhargava & Sumeet Bhargava, p. 412.*

5. **In absolute terms, biological tissue T_2 is about.**
   (a) 300–2000 msec (b) 30–2000 msec
   (c) 30–150 msec (d) 150–300 msec

   Ans. (c). *Textbook of Radiology for Residents & Technicians, 5th ed., S.K. Bhargava & Sumeet Bhargava, p. 416.*

6. **T_1 = Time when appox _______ of original longitudinal magnetization is reached.**
   (a) 37% (b) 50%
   (c) 63% (d) 100%

   Ans. (c). *Textbook of Radiology for Residents & Technicians, 5th ed., S.K. Bhargava & Sumeet Bhargava, p. 410.*

7. **T_2 = Time when transversal magnetization decrease to _______ of original value.**
   (a) 37% (b) 50%
   (c) 63% (d) 100%

   Ans. (a). *Textbook of Radiology for Residents & Technicians, 5th ed., S.K. Bhargava & Sumeet Bhargava, p. 416.*

8. **1/ T_1 is also called _______.**
   (a) Longitudinal relaxation rate (b) Longitudinal frequency

(c) Transverse relaxation rate (d) Transverse frequency

Ans. ***(a).*** *Textbook of Radiology for Residents & Technicians, 5th ed., S.K. Bhargava & Sumeet Bhargava, p. 412.*

9. 1/ T_2 is also called _______.

(a) Longitudinal relaxation rate (b) Longitudinal frequency
(c) Transverse relaxation rate (d) Transverse frequency

Ans. ***(c).*** *Textbook of Radiology for Residents & Technicians, 5th ed., S.K. Bhargava & Sumeet Bhargava, p. 416.*

10. Pathological/diseased tissue which has high water content than surrounding normal tissue has _______.

(a) Shorter relaxation time (b) Longer relaxation time
(c) Zero relaxation time (d) None of these

Ans. ***(b).*** *Textbook of Radiology for Residents & Technicians, 5th ed., S.K. Bhargava & Sumeet Bhargava, p. 416.*

11. T_2 of fat is _______ that of water.

(a) Longer than (b) Shorter than
(c) Equal to (d) Inversely proportional to

Ans. ***(b).*** *Textbook of Radiology for Residents & Technicians, 5th ed., S.K. Bhargava & Sumeet Bhargava, p. 416.*

12. We get T_1 weighted image, when TR is _______.

(a) Short (b) Long
(c) Too long to be measured (d) None of these

Ans. ***(a).*** *Textbook of Radiology for Residents & Technicians, 5th ed., S.K. Bhargava & Sumeet Bhargava, p. 412.*

13. TR less than _______ is short.

(a) 100 msec (b) 300 msec
(c) 500 msec (d) 700 msec

Ans. ***(c).*** *Textbook of Radiology for Residents & Technicians, 5th ed., S.K. Bhargava & Sumeet Bhargava, p. 418.*

14. TR more than _______ is long.

(a) 500 msec (b) 700 msec
(c) 1000 msec (d) 1500 msec

Ans. ***(d).*** *Textbook of Radiology for Residents & Technicians, 5th ed., S.K. Bhargava & Sumeet Bhargava, p. 418.*

15. _______ effects are important with fast imaging sequences.

(a) T_1 (b) T_1 & T_2
(c) T_2 (d) All of the above

Ans. (c). *Textbook of Radiology for Residents & Technicians, 5th ed., S.K. Bhargava & Sumeet Bhargava, p. 418.*

16. If we use long TE, resulting image should be heavily _______.
(a) T_1 weighted
(b) T_2 weighted
(c) TR weighted
(d) None of these

Ans. (b). *Textbook of Radiology for Residents & Technicians, 5th ed., S.K. Bhargava & Sumeet Bhargava, p. 419.*

17. If TE is long _______.
(a) Total signal intensity becomes smaller & smaller
(b) Noise is more
(c) Image quality reduces, becomes grainy
(d) All of the above

Ans. (d). *Textbook of Radiology for Residents & Technicians, 5th ed., S.K. Bhargava & Sumeet Bhargava, p. 419.*

18. Long TR is about _______ times as long as short TR.
(a) Two
(b) Three
(c) Five
(d) Ten

Ans. (b). *Textbook of Radiology for Residents & Technicians, 5th ed., S.K. Bhargava & Sumeet Bhargava, p. 419.*

19. TE less than _______ is considered short.
(a) 10 msec
(b) 30 msec
(c) 50 msec
(d) 80 msec

Ans. (b). *Textbook of Radiology for Residents & Technicians, 5th ed., S.K. Bhargava & Sumeet Bhargava, p. 419.*

20. TE greater than _______ is considered to be long.
(a) 30 msec
(b) 50 msec
(c) 80 msec
(d) 100 msec

Ans. (c). *Textbook of Radiology for Residents & Technicians, 5th ed., S.K. Bhargava & Sumeet Bhargava, p. 419.*

21. Image by long TR and short TE is _______.
(a) PD weighted images
(b) T_1 weighted image
(c) T_2 weighted image
(d) No image can be produced

Ans. (a). *Textbook of Radiology for Residents & Technicians, 5th ed., S.K. Bhargava & Sumeet Bhargava, p. 419.*

22. Image by short TR and short TE is _______.
(a) PD weighted images
(b) T_1 weighted image
(c) T_2 weighted image
(d) No image can be produced

Ans. ***(b).*** *Textbook of Radiology for Residents & Technicians, 5th ed., S.K. Bhargava & Sumeet Bhargava, p. 419.*

23. Image by very short TR and very long TE
(a) PD weighted images
(b) T_1 weighted image
(c) T_2 weighted image
(d) No image can be produced

Ans. ***(d).*** *Textbook of Radiology for Residents & Technicians, 5th ed., S.K. Bhargava & Sumeet Bhargava, p. 419.*

24. Strong TR will give a _______.
(a) PD weighted images
(b) T_1 weighted image
(c) T_2 weighted image
(d) No image can be produced

Ans. ***(b).*** *Textbook of Radiology for Residents & Technicians, 5th ed., S.K. Bhargava & Sumeet Bhargava, p. 419.*

25. Long TE gives _______.
(a) PD weighted images
(b) T_1 weighted image
(c) T_2 weighted image
(d) No image can be produced

Ans. ***(c).*** *Textbook of Radiology for Residents & Technicians, 5th ed., S.K. Bhargava & Sumeet Bhargava, p. 419.*

26. If fluid e.g. CSF or urine is white, image _______.
(a) PD weighted images
(b) T_1 weighted image
(c) T_2 weighted image
(d) None of these

Ans. ***(c).*** *Textbook of Radiology for Residents & Technicians, 5th ed., S.K. Bhargava & Sumeet Bhargava, p. 419.*

27. If fluid is darker than solids, we have _______.
(a) PD weighted images
(b) T_1 weighted image
(c) T_2 weighted image
(d) None of these

Ans. ***(a).*** *Textbook of Radiology for Residents & Technicians, 5th ed., S.K. Bhargava & Sumeet Bhargava, p. 419.*

28. If CSF is dark, grey substance is darker (more grey) than white substance, it is a typical _______.
(a) PD weighted images
(b) T_1 weighted image
(c) T_2 weighted image
(d) None of these

Ans. ***(b).*** *Textbook of Radiology for Residents & Technicians, 5th ed., S.K. Bhargava & Sumeet Bhargava, p. 419.*

29. If CSF is dark, grey substance is less grey than white matter in image, the image is _______.
(a) Proton density weighted
(b) T_1 weighted image
(c) T_2 weighted image
(d) None of these

Ans. (a). *Textbook of Radiology for Residents & Technicians, 5th ed., S.K. Bhargava & Sumeet Bhargava, p. 421.*

30. If CSF has higher signal intensity than grey and white substance, picture is _______.

(a) PD weighted images (b) T_1 weighted image
(c) T_2 weighted image (d) None of these

Ans. (c). *Textbook of Radiology for Residents & Technicians, 5th ed., S.K. Bhargava & Sumeet Bhargava, p. 421.*

31. In case of T_1 weighted images, dark color represents _______.

(a) Water (b) Edema
(c) Calcium (d) All of the above

Ans. (d). *Textbook of Radiology for Residents & Technicians, 5th ed., S.K. Bhargava & Sumeet Bhargava, p. 420.*

32. In case of T_1 weighted images, bright represents

(a) Lipid (b) Gadolinium
(c) Both (a) and (b) (d) None

Ans. (c). *Textbook of Radiology for Residents & Technicians, 5th ed., S.K. Bhargava & Sumeet Bhargava, p. 421.*

33. In case of T_2 weighted image, dark color represents

(a) Bone (b) Lipid
(c) Gadolinium (d) None of these

Ans. (a). *Textbook of Radiology for Residents & Technicians, 5th ed., S.K. Bhargava & Sumeet Bhargava, p. 421.*

34. In case of T_2 weighted image, bright color represents

(a) Water (b) Edema
(c) CSF (d) All of the above

Ans. (d). *Textbook of Radiology for Residents & Technicians, 5th ed., S.K. Bhargava & Sumeet Bhargava, p. 415.*

35. In a normal case, air is seen as dark in

(a) T_1 weighted MR image (b) T_2 weighted MR image
(c) CT image (d) All of the above

Ans. (d). *Textbook of Radiology for Residents & Technicians, 5th ed., S.K. Bhargava & Sumeet Bhargava, p. 415.*

36. In a normal case, dense bone is seen dark in

(a) MR image (b) CT image
(c) In both MR & CT image (d) In none of CT or MR image

Ans. (a). *Textbook of Radiology for Residents & Technicians, 5th ed., S.K. Bhargava & Sumeet Bhargava, p. 415.*

37. In a normal case, water is seen bright in

(a) T_1 weighted MR image (b) T_2 weighted MR image
(c) CT image (d) In none of CT or MR image

Ans. (b). *Textbook of Radiology for Residents & Technicians, 5th ed., S.K. Bhargava & Sumeet Bhargava, p. 415.*

38. In a normal case, fat is seen as dark in

(a) MR image (b) CT image
(c) In both (a) and (b) (d) None of these

Ans. (b). *Textbook of Radiology for Residents & Technicians, 5th ed., S.K. Bhargava & Sumeet Bhargava, p. 415.*

39. In case of abnormal tissue, blood is seen as bright in

(a) T_1 weighted image (b) T_2 weighted image
(c) None of these (d) Both (a) and (b)

Ans. (d). *Textbook of Radiology for Residents & Technicians, 5th ed., S.K. Bhargava & Sumeet Bhargava, p. 415.*

40. Infarct is seen dark in

(a) T_1 weighted MR image & T_2 weighted MR image
(b) T_2 weighted MR image & CT image
(c) T_1 weighted MR image & CT image
(d) In all three above

Ans. (c). *Textbook of Radiology for Residents & Technicians, 5th ed., S.K. Bhargava & Sumeet Bhargava, p. 440.*

41. Which one of following is not a pulse parameter?

(a) T_1 (b) T_2
(c) Flip angle (d) TR

Ans. (b). *Textbook of Radiology for Residents & Technicians, 5th ed., S.K. Bhargava & Sumeet Bhargava, p. 418.*

42. If we increase the slice thickness, SNR will

(a) Higher (b) Lower
(c) No change (d) Cannot be determined

Ans. (a). *Textbook of Radiology for Residents & Technicians, 5th ed., S.K. Bhargava & Sumeet Bhargava, p. 411.*

43. Longer TE yields

(a) Decreased SNR
(b) Increased SNR
(c) Decreased T_2 weighting
(d) Increased contrast to noise ratio

Ans. (a). *Textbook of Radiology for Residents & Technicians, 5th ed., S.K. Bhargava & Sumeet Bhargava, p. 419.*

44. Reduced TR yields

(a) Decreased scan time
(b) Reduced SNR
(c) Reduced slice coverage
(d) All of the above

Ans. (d). *Textbook of Radiology for Residents & Technicians, 5th ed., S.K. Bhargava & Sumeet Bhargava, p. 419.*

45. If we reduce FOV, image resolution will _______ and voxel size will reduce.

(a) Increase
(b) Decrease
(c) Will not vary
(d) Become unpredictable

Ans. (a). *Textbook of Radiology for Residents & Technicians, 5th ed., S.K. Bhargava & Sumeet Bhargava, p. 420.*

46. SNR is proportional to

(a) Slice thickness
(b) FOV
(c) Matrix size
(d) All of these

Ans. (d). *Textbook of Radiology for Residents & Technicians, 5th ed., S.K. Bhargava & Sumeet Bhargava, p. 411.*

47. Selected matrix size effect

(a) Measurement time
(b) SNR
(c) Resolution
(d) All of these

Ans. (d). *Textbook of Radiology for Residents & Technicians, 5th ed., S.K. Bhargava & Sumeet Bhargava, p. 422.*

48. If matrix size is reduced to 128 × 128 from 256 × 256, measurement time will

(a) Become half
(b) Become double
(c) Become 1/4th
(d) Remain unchanged

Ans. (a). *Textbook of Radiology for Residents & Technicians, 5th ed., S.K. Bhargava & Sumeet Bhargava, p. 422.*

49. SNR is proportional to

(a) Square root of no. of scans
(b) Voxel volume
(c) Pixel size when slice thickness is constant
(d) All of these

Ans. (d). *Textbook of Radiology for Residents & Technicians, 5th ed., S.K. Bhargava & Sumeet Bhargava, p. 411.*

50. Multiple acquisition improve SNR but measurement time becomes

(a) Shorter (b) Longer
(c) Unchanged (d) Unknown

Ans. (b). *Textbook of Radiology for Residents & Technicians, 5th ed., S.K. Bhargava & Sumeet Bhargava, p. 411.*

51. 3-D spin echo sequences usually have

(a) Very short measurement time
(b) Very long measurement time
(c) Very good resolution
(d) None of these

Ans. (b). *Textbook of Radiology for Residents & Technicians, 5th ed., S.K. Bhargava & Sumeet Bhargava, p. 421.*

52. Faster gradient-echo sequences with breath-hold should be used for MR imaging of

(a) Brain (b) Spine
(c) Abdomen (d) All of these

Ans. (c). *Textbook of Radiology for Residents & Technicians, 5th ed., S.K. Bhargava & Sumeet Bhargava, p. 421.*

53. If we reduce the measurement time

(a) SNR improves
(b) Motion artifacts reduce
(c) Both (a) and (b)
(d) None of these

Ans. (c). *Textbook of Radiology for Residents & Technicians, 5th ed., S.K. Bhargava & Sumeet Bhargava, p. 416.*

54. Specific Absorption Rate (SAR)

(a) Define radiation levels that can be safely absorbed by the body
(b) Measure the thermal effects of radiation for a brief amount of time
(c) Represents the RF absorption rate in body tissues
(d) All of these

Ans. (d). *Textbook of Radiology for Residents & Technicians, 5th ed., S.K. Bhargava & Sumeet Bhargava, p. 416.*

55. Spin Echo Pulse Sequence is not useful for _______ MR imaging.

(a) Brain, orbital cavity, auditory nerves
(b) Orthopedic range
(c) Spinal column
(d) Abdominal, breath hold

Ans. (d). *Textbook of Radiology for Residents & Technicians, 5th ed., S.K. Bhargava & Sumeet Bhargava, p. 421.*

56. Inversion Recovery Sequence has major clinical relevance for

(a) Fat suppression (b) Abdominal, breath hold
(c) Enhancing CSF (d) All of these

Ans. (a). *Textbook of Radiology for Residents & Technicians, 5th ed., S.K. Bhargava & Sumeet Bhargava, p. 421.*

57. In sagittal plane of thoracic spine, a pre-saturation slab is positioned above the heart, perpendicular to image plane so that

(a) Measurement time reduces
(b) Artifacts caused by cardiac motion and blood flow are eliminated.
(c) No. of slices can be reduced
(d) Increase signal contribution from blood flow.

Ans. (b). *Textbook of Radiology for Residents & Technicians, 5th ed., S.K. Bhargava & Sumeet Bhargava, p. 421.*

58. Putting a pre-saturation slab does not give signal from blood

(a) Entering from that direction.
(b) Entering from opposite direction
(c) Entering from any direction

Ans. (a). *Textbook of Radiology for Residents & Technicians, 5th ed., S.K. Bhargava & Sumeet Bhargava, p. 421.*

59. MRIs are made with

(a) Ultrasonic pulse
(b) Radiofrequency pulse
(c) High-energy X-rays
(d) Gamma pulse

Ans. (b). *Textbook of Radiology for Residents & Technicians, 5th ed., S.K. Bhargava & Sumeet Bhargava, p. 408-473.*

60. Who described NMR?

(a) W.C. Roentgen and Felix Bloch
(b) Felix Bloch and Edward Purcell
(c) Edward Purcell and Cormack
(d) Cormark and Hounsfield

Ans. (b). *Textbook of Radiology for Residents & Technicians, 5th ed., S.K. Bhargava & Sumeet Bhargava, p. 408-473.*

61. Who proposed that nucleus behave like a small magnet?

(a) Faraday (b) Bloch
(c) Newton (d) Brewester

Ans. (b). *Textbook of Radiology for Residents & Technicians, 5th ed., S.K. Bhargava & Sumeet Bhargava, p. 408-473.*

62. Who first showed that malignant tissue has a different NMR spectrum than that of normal tissue?

(a) Felix Bloch (b) Purcell
(c) Paul Lauterberg (d) Dramadian

Ans. (d). *Textbook of Radiology for Residents & Technicians, 5th ed., S.K. Bhargava & Sumeet Bhargava, p. 408-473.*

63. Why do magnetic resonance imaging?

(a) To demonstrate dense bone details
(b) Because of higher spatial resolution
(c) There is no chance of claustrophobia
(d) Because it provides excellent soft tissue contrast resolution

Ans. (d). *Textbook of Radiology for Residents & Technicians, 5th ed., S.K. Bhargava & Sumeet Bhargava, p. 408-473.*

64. The drawback of MRI

(a) Inability to demonstrate dense bone details
(b) Takes longer imaging time
(c) Limited spatial resolution
(d) All of the above

Ans. (d). *Textbook of Radiology for Residents & Technicians, 5th ed., S.K. Bhargava & Sumeet Bhargava, p. 408-473.*

65. MRIs are made with RF pulse in the range from

(a) 1–80 MHz (b) 80–100 kHz
(c) 10,000–10^6 MHz (d) 1–20 MHz

Ans. (a). *Textbook of Radiology for Residents & Technicians, 5th ed., S.K. Bhargava & Sumeet Bhargava, p. 408-473.*

66. Atomic nuclei are made-up of

(a) Proton (b) Neutron
(c) Electron (d) Both (a) and (b)

Ans. (d). *Textbook of Radiology for Residents & Technicians, 5th ed., S.K. Bhargava & Sumeet Bhargava, p. 408-473.*

67. Protons have a

(a) Zero charge (b) Positive charge
(c) Negative charge (d) Neutral charge

Ans. (b). *Textbook of Radiology for Residents & Technicians, 5th ed., S.K. Bhargava & Sumeet Bhargava, p. 408-473.*

68. If nuclei are aligned with the external field, they are in

(a) Normal energy state (b) Lower energy state

(c) Higher energy state
(d) Both (b) and (c)

Ans. (b). *Textbook of Radiology for Residents & Technicians, 5th ed., S.K. Bhargava & Sumeet Bhargava, p. 408-473.*

69. The sum of individual magnetic movements aligned parallel to external field is known as

(a) Longitudinal magnetization
(b) Transverse magnetization
(c) Net magnetization
(d) Both (a) and (b)

Ans. (c). *Textbook of Radiology for Residents & Technicians, 5th ed., S.K. Bhargava & Sumeet Bhargava, p. 408-473.*

70. The spinning protons do not align themselves exactly with the main magnetic field but align at an angle of approximately

(a) 45°
(b) 37°
(c) 18°
(d) 59°

Ans. (b). *Textbook of Radiology for Residents & Technicians, 5th ed., S.K. Bhargava & Sumeet Bhargava, p. 408-473.*

71. The rate of precession of protons in magnetic field is characteristic for that element and also depends on the strength of main magnetic field. This is known as

(a) Oscillation frequency
(b) Gyrometric ratio
(c) Larmor frequency
(d) Net magnetization

Ans. (c). *Textbook of Radiology for Residents & Technicians, 5th ed., S.K. Bhargava & Sumeet Bhargava, p. 408-473.*

72. Relaxation is the process that occurs after terminating the

(a) RF pulse
(b) Switch
(c) Pulse sequence
(d) Grid

Ans. (a). *Textbook of Radiology for Residents & Technicians, 5th ed., S.K. Bhargava & Sumeet Bhargava, p. 408-473.*

73. The primary MR signal is called

(a) Transverse magnetization
(b) Longitudinal magnetization
(c) Spin density
(d) Free inductance decay

Ans. (d). *Textbook of Radiology for Residents & Technicians, 5th ed., S.K. Bhargava & Sumeet Bhargava, p. 408-473.*

74. Which flip angle is commonly used in MR imaging?

(a) 30°
(b) 45°
(c) 60°
(d) 90°

Ans. (d). *Textbook of Radiology for Residents & Technicians, 5th ed., S.K. Bhargava & Sumeet Bhargava, p. 408-473.*

75. Higher the concentration of mobile hydrogen nuclei

(a) Stronger the MR signal (b) Higher the resolution
(c) Higher the contrast (d) Reduced scan time

Ans. (a). *Textbook of Radiology for Residents & Technicians, 5th ed., S.K. Bhargava & Sumeet Bhargava, p. 408-473.*

76. The delay time between 180° and 90° RF pulse is

(a) Inversion delay time (b) Time of echo
(c) Time of repetition (d) Time of relaxation

Ans. (a). *Textbook of Radiology for Residents & Technicians, 5th ed., S.K. Bhargava & Sumeet Bhargava, p. 408-473.*

77. Permanent magnets are manufactured from

(a) Paramagnetic materials (b) Ferromagnetic materials
(c) Piezoelectric materials (d) Diamagnet

Ans. (b). *Textbook of Radiology for Residents & Technicians, 5th ed., S.K. Bhargava & Sumeet Bhargava, p. 408-473.*

78. Contraindication for use of NMR technique is

(a) Psychotic patient
(b) Patient on lithium
(c) Intracranial metallic aneurysm clips
(d) Patient receiving radiotherapy

Ans. (c). *Textbook of Radiology for Residents & Technicians, 5th ed., S.K. Bhargava & Sumeet Bhargava, p. 408-473.*

79. Which of the following sequences shows the best anatomical details on MRI?

(a) Inversion recovery (b) Spin echo
(c) Saturation recovery (d) All of the above

Ans. (a). *Textbook of Radiology for Residents & Technicians, 5th ed., S.K. Bhargava & Sumeet Bhargava, p. 408-473.*

80. Which of the following substances is diamagnetic?

(a) Iron (b) Wood
(c) Nickel (d) None of the above

Ans. (d). *Textbook of Radiology for Residents & Technicians, 5th ed., S.K. Bhargava & Sumeet Bhargava, p. 408-473.*

81. When a paramagnetic substance is placed in a magnetic field, the magnetic induction inside the substances

(a) Remains constant (b) Decreases
(c) Increases (d) Reduces to zero

Ans. (c). Textbook of Radiology for Residents & Technicians, 5th ed., S.K. Bhargava & Sumeet Bhargava, p. 408-473.

82. The material used for permanent magnet should have

(a) High retentivity, high coercivity
(b) Low retentivity, low coercivity
(c) Low retentivity, high coercivity
(d) High retentivity, low coercivity

Ans. (a). Textbook of Radiology for Residents & Technicians, 5th ed., S.K. Bhargava & Sumeet Bhargava, p. 408-473.

83. Time interval between initial 180° RF pulse and the 90° RF pulse is known as

(a) Relaxation time
(b) Echo time
(c) Inversion time
(d) Time of repetition

Ans. (c). Textbook of Radiology for Residents & Technicians, 5th ed., S.K. Bhargava & Sumeet Bhargava, p. 408-473.

84. Why the use of a flip angle of less than 90° in gradient echo pulse sequence?

(a) To maintain longitudinal megnetization.
(b) To maintain transverse megnetization.
(c) To maintain both longitudinal and transverse megnetization.
(d) None of the above

Ans. (c). Textbook of Radiology for Residents & Technicians, 5th ed., S.K. Bhargava & Sumeet Bhargava, p. 408-473.

85. The critical temperature required to produce zero resistance for the alloy is

(a) –290°C
(b) –269°C
(c) –273°C
(d) –300°C

Ans. (b). Textbook of Radiology for Residents & Technicians, 5th ed., S.K. Bhargava & Sumeet Bhargava, p. 408-473.

86. Critical temperature is achieved by immersing the coils in

(a) Nitrogen
(b) Oxygen
(c) Liquid helium
(d) Liquid sulphur

Ans. (c). Textbook of Radiology for Residents & Technicians, 5th ed., S.K. Bhargava & Sumeet Bhargava, p. 408-473.

87. ______ magnets require the use of cryogens.

(a) Bar
(b) Resistive
(c) Superconducting
(d) Permanent

Ans. (c). Textbook of Radiology for Residents & Technicians, 5th ed., S.K. Bhargava & Sumeet Bhargava, p. 408-473.

88. The ___ encodes frequencies and phases into the MR echoes.

(a) Gradient coils (b) Host computer
(c) RF coils (d) ADC

***Ans. (a).** Textbook of Radiology for Residents & Technicians, 5th ed., S.K. Bhargava & Sumeet Bhargava, p. 408-473.*

89. A _____ coil is preferable when a very uniform signal intensity level must be achieved throughout a cross-section of anatomy.

(a) volumetric (b) linear
(c) flat array (d) surface

***Ans. (a).** Textbook of Radiology for Residents & Technicians, 5th ed., S.K. Bhargava & Sumeet Bhargava, p. 408-473.*

90. Gadolinium is an example of a

(a) Diamagnetic (b) Paramagnetic
(c) Super-paramagnetic (d) Ferromagnetic

***Ans. (b).** Textbook of Radiology for Residents & Technicians, 5th ed., S.K. Bhargava & Sumeet Bhargava, p. 408-473.*

91. 1 gauss = ___ tesla.

(a) 5×10^2 T (b) 10^{-4} T
(c) 1000 T (d) None of the above

***Ans. (b).** Textbook of Radiology for Residents & Technicians, 5th ed., S.K. Bhargava & Sumeet Bhargava, p. 408-473.*

92. The DB is defined as the _____ of two intensifiers.

(a) Sum (b) Difference
(c) Product (d) Ratio

***Ans. (d).** Textbook of Radiology for Residents & Technicians, 5th ed., S.K. Bhargava & Sumeet Bhargava, p. 342-358.*

93. The receiver band width represents the range of frequencies sampled during the

(a) Phase gradient (b) Slice selection gradient
(c) Frequency encoding gradient (d) Gradient coils

***Ans. (d).** Textbook of Radiology for Residents & Technicians, 5th ed., S.K. Bhargava & Sumeet Bhargava, p. 408-473.*

94. At a field strength of 1.0 tesla, the approximate t_2 relaxation time for spleen tissue is

(a) 60 ms (b) 80 ms
(c) 90 ms (d) 1000 ms

***Ans. (b).** Textbook of Radiology for Residents & Technicians, 5th ed., S.K. Bhargava & Sumeet Bhargava, p. 408-473.*

95. During the acquisition of axial images of the body with the frequency direction L/R, phase encoding is performed by which physical gradient?

(a) X (b) Y
(c) Z (d) X and Y

Ans. (c). *Textbook of Radiology for Residents & Technicians, 5th ed., S.K. Bhargava & Sumeet Bhargava, p. 408-473.*

96. MR resolution is approximately

(a) 1 LP/mm (b) 0.1 LP/mm
(c) 0.3 LP/mm (d) 0.9 LP/mm

Ans. (c). *Textbook of Radiology for Residents & Technicians, 5th ed., S.K. Bhargava & Sumeet Bhargava, p. 408-473.*

CT SCAN

97. Computed tomography invented by

(a) Godfrey Hounsfield
(b) Alan Cormack
(c) Sir Wilhelm Conrad Roentgen
(d) None of the above

Ans. (a). *Radiological Science for Technologists by Stewart Carlyce Bushang, 9th Ed., Mosby Elsevier, 2008, p. 368.*

98. Mathematics used to reconstruct the images was evaluated by

(a) Godfrey Hounsfield
(b) Alan Cormack
(c) Sir Wilhelm Conrad Roentgen
(a) None of the above

Ans. (b). *Radiological Science for Technologists by Stewart Carlyce Bushang, 9th Ed., Mosby Elsevier, 2008, p. 368.*

99. Spatial resolution in CT is

(a) 1 lp mm^{-1} (b) 2 lp mm^{-1}
(c) 4 lp mm^{-1} (d) 10 lp mm^{-1}

Ans. (a). *Radiological Science for Technologists by Stewart Carlyce Bushang, 9th Ed., Mosby Elsevier, 2008, p. 380.*

100. Contrast resolution in CT is

(a) Better than conventional films
(b) Less than conventional films
(c) Same as conventional films
(d) None of the above

Ans. (a). Radiological Science for Technologists by Stewart Carlyce Bushang, 9th Ed., Mosby Elsevier, 2008, p. 381.

101. CT number of water is

(a) Zero
(b) –1000
(c) + 1000
(d) 200–300

Ans. (a). Radiological Science for Technologists by Stewart Carlyce Bushang, 9th Ed., Mosby Elsevier, 2008, p. 304.

102. CT number of air is

(a) Zero
(b) –1000
(c) + 1000
(d) 200–300

Ans. (b). Radiological Science for Technologists by Stewart Carlyce Bushang, 9th Ed., Mosby Elsevier, 2008, p. 304.

103. CT number of bone is

(a) Zero
(b) –1000
(c) +1000
(d) 200–300

Ans. (c). Radiological Science for Technologists by Stewart Carlyce Bushang, 9th Ed., Mosby Elsevier, 2008, p. 304.

104. In CT reference material is

(a) Water
(b) Air
(c) Bone
(d) None of the above

Ans. (a). Radiological Science for Technologists by Stewart Carlyce Bushang, 9th Ed., Mosby Elsevier, 2008, p. 305.

105. Which of the following is not true for reduced mottle in CT scan

(a) Reduced when photons in every pixel is available
(b) Reduced by reducing slice thickness
(c) Reduced by increasing scan time
(d) Increased by increasing scan time

Ans. (b). Radiological Science for Technologists by Stewart Carlyce Bushang, 9th Ed., Mosby Elsevier, 2008, p. 369.

106. With narrowing of the window, each gray scale covers

(a) Larger CT number
(b) Less CT number
(c) No effect on CT number
(d) None of the above

Ans. (a). Radiological Science for Technologists by Stewart Carlyce Bushang, 9th Ed., Mosby Elsevier, 2008, p. 370.

107. Zooming of the CT image

(a) Increase the effect of noise
(b) Decrease the effect of noise
(c) No effect on noise
(d) All of the above

Ans. (a). *Radiological Science for Technologists by Stewart Carlyce Bushang, 9th Ed., Mosby Elsevier, 2008, p. 371.*

108. Which is not true of use of the high kV in CT scan

(a) Reduced patient dose
(b) Reduce the effect of beam hardening
(c) Reduces the efficiency of detectors and image contrast
(d) Reduces scatter

Ans. (d). *Radiological Science for Technologists by Stewart Carlyce Bushang, 9th Ed., Mosby Elsevier, 2008, p. 372.*

109. CT scan uses tube

(a) Rotating anode tube
(b) Stationary anode tube
(c) Gassy tube
(d) None of the above

Ans. (a). *Radiological Science for Technologists by Stewart Carlyce Bushang, 9th Ed., Mosby Elsevier, 2008, p. 372.*

110. Beam hardening in CT is increased by using

(a) Copper filter
(b) Aluminium filter
(c) Tin filter
(d) Lead filter

Ans. (a). *Radiological Science for Technologists by Stewart Carlyce Bushang, 9th Ed., Mosby Elsevier, 2008, p. 374.*

111. To minimize heel effect in CT scan

(a) X-ray tube long axis is perpendicular to CT slice
(b) X-ray tube long axis is parallel to CT slice
(c) X-ray tube long axis is oblique to CT slice
(d) X-ray tube long axis is angulated to CT slice

Ans. (a). *Radiological Science for Technologists by Stewart Carlyce Bushang, 9th Ed., Mosby Elsevier, 2008, p. 375.*

112. 1st generation CT scan uses

(a) Pencil beam of X-rays
(b) Narrow fan beam
(c) Broad fan beam
(d) Multiple X-ray beam

Ans. (a). *Radiological Science for Technologists by Stewart Carlyce Bushang, 9th Ed., Mosby Elsevier, 2008, p. 376.*

113. 2nd generation CT scan uses

(a) Pencil beam of X-rays
(b) Narrow fan beam
(c) Broad fan beam
(d) Multiple X-ray beams

Ans. (b). *Radiological Science for Technologists by Stewart Carlyce Bushang, 9th Ed., Mosby Elsevier, 2008, p. 376.*

114. 3rd and 4th generation CT scan uses

(a) Pencil beam of X-rays (b) Narrow fan beam
(c) Broad fan beam (d) Multiple X-ray beams

Ans. (c). *Radiological Science for Technologists by Stewart Carlyce Bushang, 9th Ed., Mosby Elsevier, 2008, p. 376.*

115. 5th generation CT scan uses

(a) Pencil beam of X-rays (b) Narrow fan beam
(c) Broad fan beam (d) Multiple X-ray beams

Ans. (d). *Radiological Science for Technologists by Stewart Carlyce Bushang, 9th Ed., Mosby Elsevier, 2008, p. 376.*

116. In CT scan the 1st generation is

(a) Translate-rotate type (b) Rotate-rotate type
(c) Stationary-rotate type (d) None of the above

Ans. (a). *Radiological Science for Technologists by Stewart Carlyce Bushang, 9th Ed., Mosby Elsevier, 2008, p. 377.*

117. In CT scan the 2nd generation is

(a) Translate-rotate type (b) Rotate-rotate type
(c) Stationary-rotate type (d) None of the above

Ans. (a). *Radiological Science for Technologists by Stewart Carlyce Bushang, 9th Ed., Mosby Elsevier, 2008, p. 377.*

118. In CT scan the 3rd generation is

(a) Translate-rotate type (b) Rotate-rotate type
(c) Stationary-rotate type (d) None of the above

Ans. (b). *Radiological Science for Technologists by Stewart Carlyce Bushang, 9th Ed., Mosby Elsevier, 2008, p. 377.*

119. In CT scan the 4th generation is

(a) Translate-rotate type (b) Rotate-rotate type
(c) Stationary-rotate type (d) None of the above

Ans. (c). *Radiological Science for Technologists by Stewart Carlyce Bushang, 9th Ed., Mosby Elsevier, 2008, p. 377.*

120. Sharp and high contrast boundaries artifact occur due to

(a) Patient movement (b) Aliasing
(c) Beam hardening (d) Metals in the body

Ans. (b). *Radiological Science for Technologists by Stewart Carlyce Bushang, 9th Ed., Mosby Elsevier, 2008, p. 389.*

121. Streak artifact in CT scan are due to

(a) Movement due to heart patient
(b) Aliasing
(c) Beam hardening
(d) Metals in the body

Ans. (a). *Radiological Science for Technologists by Stewart Carlyce Bushang, 9th Ed., Mosby Elsevier, 2008, p. 389.*

122. Cupping artifact in CT scan is due to

(a) Patient movement
(b) Aliasing
(c) Beam hardening
(d) Metals in the body

Ans. (c). *Radiological Science for Technologists by Stewart Carlyce Bushang, 9th Ed., Mosby Elsevier, 2008, p. 389.*

123. Star artifact in CT scan is due to

(a) Patient movement
(b) Aliasing
(c) Beam hardening
(d) Metals in the body

Ans. (d). *Radiological Science for Technologists by Stewart Carlyce Bushang, 9th Ed., Mosby Elsevier, 2008, p. 389.*

124. Spatial resolution in CT depends on

(a) High contrast objects
(b) Pixel size
(c) Noise
(d) All of the above

Ans. (d). *Radiological Science for Technologists by Stewart Carlyce Bushang, 9th Ed., Mosby Elsevier, 2008, p. 389.*

125. Resolution of CT image improves on

(a) Increase matrix and decrease pixel size
(b) Reducing field of view and immobilization of patient
(c) Decreasing size of focal spot
(d) All of the above

Ans. (d). *Radiological Science for Technologists by Stewart Carlyce Bushang, 9th Ed., Mosby Elsevier, 2008, p. 389.*

126. Anode heat storage capacity in multislice spiral CT is

(a) 2 MHU
(b) 4 MHU
(c) 6 MHU
(d) 8 MHU or more

Ans. (d). *Radiological Science for Technologists by Stewart Carlyce Bushang, 9th Ed., Mosby Elsevier, 2008, p. 373.*

127. Pixel size is

(a) FOV multiplied by matrix size
(b) FOV divided by matrix size

(c) FOV added by matrix size
(d) None of the above

Ans. (b). *Radiological Science for Technologists by Stewart Carlyce Bushang, 9th Ed., Mosby Elsevier, 2008, p. 389.*

128. Slice acquisition rate is

(a) Slices acquired per 360° divided by rotation time
(b) Slices acquired per 360° multiplied by rotation time
(c) Slices acquired per 360° added by rotation time
(d) None of the above

Ans. (a). *Radiological Science for Technologists by Stewart Carlyce Bushang, 9th Ed., Mosby Elsevier, 2008, p. 389.*

129. Pitch is

(a) Couch movement each 360° divided by slice thickness
(b) Couch movement each 360° multiplied by slice thickness
(c) Couch movement each 360° added by slice thickness
(d) None of the above

Ans. (a). *Textbook of Radiology for Residents & Technicians, 5th ed., S.K. Bhargava & Sumeet Bhargava, p. 381.*

130. Detectors used in modern CT scanners are

(a) Scintillation detectors (b) Gas detectors
(c) Either (a) or (b) (d) None of the above

Ans. (c). *Textbook of Radiology for Residents & Technicians, 5th ed., S.K. Bhargava & Sumeet Bhargava, p. 372–385.*

131. The first CT scanner was developed in the year

(a) 1905 (b) 1943
(c) 1972 (d) 1986

Ans. (c). *Textbook of Radiology for Residents & Technicians, 5th ed., S.K. Bhargava & Sumeet Bhargava, p. 372-407.*

132. The first CT scanner was developed by

(a) W.C. Roentgen (b) Paul Lauterberg
(c) Purcell and Bloch (d) Godfrey Hounsfield

Ans. (d). *Textbook of Radiology for Residents & Technicians, 5th ed., S.K. Bhargava & Sumeet Bhargava, p. 372-407.*

133. Who developed the mathematics used to reconstruct the CT images?

(a) Godfrey Hounsfield (b) Alan Cormack
(c) Paul Lauterberg (d) W.C. Roentgen

Ans. (b). *Textbook of Radiology for Residents & Technicians, 5th ed., S.K. Bhargava & Sumeet Bhargava, p. 372-407.*

134. Who is the father of computed tomography?

(a) Curie (b) Felix Bloch
(c) Godfrey Hounsfield (d) W.C. Roentgen

Ans. (c). *Textbook of Radiology for Residents & Technicians, 5th ed., S.K. Bhargava & Sumeet Bhargava, p. 372-407.*

135. The internal structure of body attenuates the X-ray beam according to their

(a) Size (b) Field of view
(c) Slice thickness (d) Atomic number

Ans. (d). *Textbook of Radiology for Residents & Technicians, 5th ed., S.K. Bhargava & Sumeet Bhargava, p. 372-407.*

136. How many detectors were used to measure transmitted beam in first generation CT scanner?

(a) 64 (b) 16
(c) 128 (d) 2

Ans. (d). *Textbook of Radiology for Residents & Technicians, 5th ed., S.K. Bhargava & Sumeet Bhargava, p. 372-407.*

137. First generation CT scanner was designed specifically for evaluation of

(a) Angiography (b) STN
(c) Brain (d) Stomach

Ans. (c). *Textbook of Radiology for Residents & Technicians, 5th ed., S.K. Bhargava & Sumeet Bhargava, p. 372-407.*

138. In first generation of CT scanner head was enclosed in

(a) Air (b) Water
(c) Chlorine (d) Methanol

Ans. (b). *Textbook of Radiology for Residents & Technicians, 5th ed., S.K. Bhargava & Sumeet Bhargava, p. 372-407.*

139. What is the meaning of 'EMI' in EMI CT scanner?

(a) Electric motion imaging
(b) Electromagnetic induction
(c) Electric musical instrumentation
(d) Easy magnetic imaging

Ans. (c). *Textbook of Radiology for Residents & Technicians, 5th ed., S.K. Bhargava & Sumeet Bhargava, p. 372-407.*

140. CT numbers were proportional to the

(a) Atomic number (b) Matrix size
(c) Linear attenuation coefficient (d) Energy of X-ray beam

Ans. ***(c).*** *Textbook of Radiology for Residents & Technicians, 5th ed., S.K. Bhargava & Sumeet Bhargava, p. 372-407.*

141. Each square in the image matrix is known as

(a) Pixel (b) Voxel
(c) Troxel (d) Squaxel

Ans. ***(a).*** *Textbook of Radiology for Residents & Technicians, 5th ed., S.K. Bhargava & Sumeet Bhargava, p. 372-407.*

142. In first generation of CT scanner, the detectors were made-up of

(a) Bismuth germenate (b) Sodium thiosulphate
(c) Phosphor (d) Sodium iodide

Ans. ***(d).*** *Textbook of Radiology for Residents & Technicians, 5th ed., S.K. Bhargava & Sumeet Bhargava, p. 372-407.*

143. Which of the following were used in first generation of CT scanner?

(a) Pencil beam (b) Narrow fan beam
(c) Fan beam (d) Wide fan beam

Ans. ***(a).*** *Textbook of Radiology for Residents & Technicians, 5th ed., S.K. Bhargava & Sumeet Bhargava, p. 372-407.*

144. In second generation of CT scanner, how many detectors were used?

(a) 2 (b) 30
(c) 79 (d) 64

Ans. ***(b).*** *Textbook of Radiology for Residents & Technicians, 5th ed., S.K. Bhargava & Sumeet Bhargava, p. 372-407.*

145. In second generation of CT scanner, the rotatory steps are around

(a) 1° (b) 15°
(c) 30° (d) 90°

Ans. ***(c).*** *Textbook of Radiology for Residents & Technicians, 5th ed., S.K. Bhargava & Sumeet Bhargava, p. 372-407.*

146. In second generation of CT scanner, _______ used.

(a) Rotate/translate, fan beam (b) Rotate/translate, pencil beam
(c) Rotate/rotate (d) Rotate/stationary

Ans. ***(a).*** *Textbook of Radiology for Residents & Technicians, 5th ed., S.K. Bhargava & Sumeet Bhargava, p. 372-407.*

147. Third generation of CT scanner was introduced in

(a) 1970 (b) 1972
(c) 1975 (d) 1979

Ans. (c). *Textbook of Radiology for Residents & Technicians, 5th ed., S.K. Bhargava & Sumeet Bhargava, p. 372-407.*

148. Third generation of CT scanner uses a _____ tube, _____ detector configuration.

(a) rotate/translate, pencil beam (b) translate/rotate, fan beam
(c) rotate, rotate (d) rotate, stationary

Ans. (c). *Textbook of Radiology for Residents & Technicians, 5th ed., S.K. Bhargava & Sumeet Bhargava, p. 372-407.*

149. How much time is taken by third generation CT scanner to produce an image?

(a) 0.25 msec (b) 5 sec
(c) less than 5 min (d) 1 min

Ans. (b). *Textbook of Radiology for Residents & Technicians, 5th ed., S.K. Bhargava & Sumeet Bhargava, p. 372-407.*

150. When third generation of CT scanner were recently introduced, then how many detectors were used in scanner?

(a) 288 (b) 30
(c) 600 (d) 912

Ans. (a). *Textbook of Radiology for Residents & Technicians, 5th ed., S.K. Bhargava & Sumeet Bhargava, p. 372-407.*

151. In fourth generation of CT scanner _____ used.

(a) Rotate/translate, narrow beam (b) Rotate/translate, fan beam
(c) Rotate/rotate, wide beam (d) Rotate/stationary

Ans. (d). *Textbook of Radiology for Residents & Technicians, 5th ed., S.K. Bhargava & Sumeet Bhargava, p. 372-407.*

152. How many detectors were used in fourth generation of CT scanner?

(a) 400 (b) Less than 900
(c) 1000-1800 (d) More than 2000

Ans. (d). *Textbook of Radiology for Residents & Technicians, 5th ed., S.K. Bhargava & Sumeet Bhargava, p. 372-407.*

153. Which of the following interaction occur when high energy X-ray photon are used in CT (around 120 kV_p)?

(a) Photoelectric (b) Compton scattering
(c) Coherent scattering (d) Pair production

Ans. (b). *Textbook of Radiology for Residents & Technicians, 5th ed., S.K. Bhargava & Sumeet Bhargava, p. 372-407.*

154. In currently available CT scanner, *k* has a value of

(a) 100 (b) 1000
(c) 10000 (d) 100000

Ans. (b). *Textbook of Radiology for Residents & Technicians, 5th ed., S.K. Bhargava & Sumeet Bhargava, p. 372-407.*

155. The range of CT number above and below the window level is called the

(a) Window level (b) Window width
(c) Window slice (d) All of the above

Ans. (b). *Textbook of Radiology for Residents & Technicians, 5th ed., S.K. Bhargava & Sumeet Bhargava, p. 372-407.*

156. In which generation of CT scanner ring artifact are produced?

(a) 1st generation (b) 2nd generation
(c) 3rd generation (d) 4th generation

Ans. (c). *Textbook of Radiology for Residents & Technicians, 5th ed., S.K. Bhargava & Sumeet Bhargava, p. 372-407.*

157. In multislice CT scanner, an anode heat storage capacity is around

(a) 1 MHU (b) 10^8 MHU
(c) $10^2 \times 8$ MHU (d) 8 MHU

Ans. (d). *Textbook of Radiology for Residents & Technicians, 5th ed., S.K. Bhargava & Sumeet Bhargava, p. 372-407.*

158. An anode cooling rate of multislice spiral CT is approximately

(a) 1 KHU/hr (b) 15 MHU/min
(c) 1 MHU/min (d) 8 MHU/min

Ans. (c). *Textbook of Radiology for Residents & Technicians, 5th ed., S.K. Bhargava & Sumeet Bhargava, p. 372-407.*

159. In CT scanner, the patient couch must be constructed of

(a) High atomic material (b) According to patient load
(c) Low atomic material (d) All of the above

Ans. (c). *Textbook of Radiology for Residents & Technicians, 5th ed., S.K. Bhargava & Sumeet Bhargava, p. 372-407.*

160. Which of the following materials is used to construct the patient couch?

(a) Plastic (b) Fibre
(c) Aluminium (d) Cardboard

Ans. (b). *Textbook of Radiology for Residents & Technicians, 5th ed., S.K. Bhargava & Sumeet Bhargava, p. 372-407.*

161. Spiral CT scanner was made possible by the use of

(a) Multiple row detector (b) Array processor
(c) Light weight of X-ray tube (d) Slip ring technology

Ans. (d). *Textbook of Radiology for Residents & Technicians, 5th ed., S.K. Bhargava & Sumeet Bhargava, p. 372-407.*

162. Slip rings allows to

(a) Rotate gantry (b) Rotate patient couch
(c) Reduce patient dose (d) None of the above

Ans. (a). *Textbook of Radiology for Residents & Technicians, 5th ed., S.K. Bhargava & Sumeet Bhargava, p. 372-407.*

163. Slip ring brushes are made-up of

(a) Tungsten (b) Cobalt
(c) Nickle (d) Silver graphite

Ans. (d). *Textbook of Radiology for Residents & Technicians, 5th ed., S.K. Bhargava & Sumeet Bhargava, p. 372-407.*

164. The numeric information contained in each pixel is called

(a) CT number (b) Intensity
(c) Attenuation coefficient (d) Density

Ans. (a). *Textbook of Radiology for Residents & Technicians, 5th ed., S.K. Bhargava & Sumeet Bhargava, p. 372-407.*

165. CT number for dense bone material is

(a) –1000 (b) 0
(c) 3000 (d) 25

Ans. (c). *Textbook of Radiology for Residents & Technicians, 5th ed., S.K. Bhargava & Sumeet Bhargava, p. 372-407.*

166. A CT number of –1000 corresponds to

(a) Bone (b) Lung
(c) Fat (d) Air

Ans. (d). *Textbook of Radiology for Residents & Technicians, 5th ed., S.K. Bhargava & Sumeet Bhargava, p. 372-407.*

167. A CT number of 0 indicates

(a) Air (b) Lung
(c) Water (d) Space

Ans. (c). *Textbook of Radiology for Residents & Technicians, 5th ed., S.K. Bhargava & Sumeet Bhargava, p. 372-407.*

168. MIP images are widely used in

(a) Angiography (b) Virtual colonoscopy

(c) Bone structure (d) All of the above

Ans. (a). *Textbook of Radiology for Residents & Technicians, 5th ed., S.K. Bhargava & Sumeet Bhargava, p. 372-407.*

169. SSD images are used in

(a) Bone imaging (b) Angiography
(c) CT fluoroscopy (d) CECT head

Ans. (a). *Textbook of Radiology for Residents & Technicians, 5th ed., S.K. Bhargava & Sumeet Bhargava, p. 372-407.*

170. Spatial frequency is expressed in

(a) LP/cm (b) LP/m
(c) LP/mm (d) LP/m^2

Ans. (a). *Textbook of Radiology for Residents & Technicians, 5th ed., S.K. Bhargava & Sumeet Bhargava, p. 372-407.*

171. Thickness of a CT slice is controlled by the

(a) Beam collimators (b) Exposure factor
(c) Target angle (d) Filament size

Ans. (a). *Textbook of Radiology for Residents & Technicians, 5th ed., S.K. Bhargava & Sumeet Bhargava, p. 372-407.*

172. Reconstruction of an image at any z-axis position is possible by

(a) Straight line method (b) Interpolation algorithm
(c) Back projection method (d) Analytical method

Ans. (b). *Textbook of Radiology for Residents & Technicians, 5th ed., S.K. Bhargava & Sumeet Bhargava, p. 372-407.*

173. Linear interpolation at 180° improves

(a) Resolution along x and y axis (b) Resolution along z axis
(c) Signal to noise ratio (d) Contrast

Ans. (b). *Textbook of Radiology for Residents & Technicians, 5th ed., S.K. Bhargava & Sumeet Bhargava, p. 372-407.*

174. The smaller detector size result in better

(a) Contrast resolution (b) Spatial resolution
(c) Image clarity (d) All of the above

Ans. (b). *Textbook of Radiology for Residents & Technicians, 5th ed., S.K. Bhargava & Sumeet Bhargava, p. 372-407.*

175. The principal advantage of multislice spiral CT is

(a) Increased patient dose (b) High cost
(c) Imaged large volume (d) All of the above

Ans. (c). *Textbook of Radiology for Residents & Technicians, 5th ed., S.K. Bhargava & Sumeet Bhargava, p. 372-407.*

176. CT number also known as

(a) HU
(b) MHU
(c) LAC
(d) TWF

Ans. (a). *Textbook of Radiology for Residents & Technicians, 5th ed., S.K. Bhargava & Sumeet Bhargava, p. 372-407.*

177. The major clinical application of MSCT is

(a) Angiographic studies
(b) Perfusion studies
(c) Virtual endoscope
(d) All of the above

Ans. (d). *Textbook of Radiology for Residents & Technicians, 5th ed., S.K. Bhargava & Sumeet Bhargava, p. 372-407.*

178. Spatial resolution of dual source MSCT is

(a) < 0.4 mm
(b) > 0.6 mm
(c) 1.2 mm
(d) 1 mm

Ans. (a). *Textbook of Radiology for Residents & Technicians, 5th ed., S.K. Bhargava & Sumeet Bhargava, p. 372-407.*

179. In dual source CT scanner, one tube operated at _____ and other tube operated at ____.

(a) 80 kV_p and 140 kV_p
(b) 30 kV_p and 100 kV_p
(c) 80 kV_p and 80 kV_p
(d) 100 kV_p and 100 kV_p

Ans. (a). *Textbook of Radiology for Residents & Technicians, 5th ed., S.K. Bhargava & Sumeet Bhargava, p. 372-407.*

180. Which of the following has a HU value of approximately –90?

(a) Fat
(b) Grey matter
(c) Water
(d) Lung

Ans. (a). *Textbook of Radiology for Residents & Technicians, 5th ed., S.K. Bhargava & Sumeet Bhargava, p. 372-407.*

181. The main advantage of helical CT over conventional CT is improved

(a) Spatial resolution
(b) Data acquisition rate
(c) Patient dose
(d) Image reconstruction time

Ans. (b). *Textbook of Radiology for Residents & Technicians, 5th ed., S.K. Bhargava & Sumeet Bhargava, p. 372-407.*

182. CT fluoroscopy minimizes radiation doses by using

(a) Filtration
(b) High tube current
(c) Lower collimator thickness
(d) Low tube current

Ans. (d). Textbook of Radiology for Residents & Technicians, 5th ed., S.K. Bhargava & Sumeet Bhargava, p. 372-407.

183. The difference in X-ray attenuation between white (40 HU) and grey matter (50 HU) is

(a) 0.1% (b) 1%
(c) 10% (d) 25%

Ans. (c). Textbook of Radiology for Residents & Technicians, 5th ed., S.K. Bhargava & Sumeet Bhargava, p. 372-407.

184. Which of the following is not a source of CT artifacts?

(a) Patient motion (b) Metal implants
(c) Beam hardening (d) Low tube current

Ans. (d). Textbook of Radiology for Residents & Technicians, 5th ed., S.K. Bhargava & Sumeet Bhargava, p. 372-407.

185. To reduce X-ray beam hardening effects, which types of filter are used?

(a) Copper (b) Nickle
(c) Cobalt (d) Cadmium

Ans. (a). Textbook of Radiology for Residents & Technicians, 5th ed., S.K. Bhargava & Sumeet Bhargava, p. 372-407.

186. The relation between patient and tube motion is known as

(a) Pitch (b) Spatial frequency
(c) Dose profile (d) HU

Ans. (a). Textbook of Radiology for Residents & Technicians, 5th ed., S.K. Bhargava & Sumeet Bhargava, p. 372-407.

187. Quantum mottle decreases as the number of photons

(a) Increases (b) Decreases
(c) No effect on quantum mottle (d) None of the above

Ans. (a). Textbook of Radiology for Residents & Technicians, 5th ed., S.K. Bhargava & Sumeet Bhargava, p. 372-407.

188. CT noise is reduced by

(a) Decreased scan time (b) Increased mAs
(c) Increased voxel size (d) Detector thickness

Ans. (c). Textbook of Radiology for Residents & Technicians, 5th ed., S.K. Bhargava & Sumeet Bhargava, p. 372-407.

189. The mathematical technique that involves the estimation of an unknown value from values on either side of it is known as

(a) Filtering (b) Interpolation
(c) Convolution (d) Summation

Ans. (b). *Textbook of Radiology for Residents & Technicians, 5th ed., S.K. Bhargava & Sumeet Bhargava, p. 372-407.*

190. What is the average linear attenuation coefficient for water?
(a) 0.0007 (b) 0.155
(c) 0.206 (d) 0.530

Ans. (c). *Textbook of Radiology for Residents & Technicians, 5th ed., S.K. Bhargava & Sumeet Bhargava, p. 372-407.*

191. Ring artifacts on the CT image are associated with which of the following tube detector relationships?
(a) Rotate-rotate (b) Rotate-stationary
(c) Translate-translate (d) Translate-rotate

Ans. (a). *Textbook of Radiology for Residents & Technicians, 5th ed., S.K. Bhargava & Sumeet Bhargava, p. 372-407.*

192. Which of the following increases the signal-to-noise ratio of a CT image?
(a) Decreased aperture size (b) Decreased mAs
(c) Increased aperture size (d) Increased filtration

Ans. (a). *Textbook of Radiology for Residents & Technicians, 5th ed., S.K. Bhargava & Sumeet Bhargava, p. 372-407.*

193. Which one of the following statements regarding collimation of the CT X-ray beam is false?
(a) Collimation of the X-ray beam occurs both before and after the beam passes through the patient.
(b) Collimation of the X-ray beam occurs in the Z-axis, thus controlling the thickness.
(c) Increases in collimation increases the intensity of the X-ray beam.
(d) Collimation of the CT X-ray beam is used to limit the detection of scatter radiation.

Ans. (c). *Textbook of Radiology for Residents & Technicians, 5th ed., S.K. Bhargava & Sumeet Bhargava, p. 372-407.*

194. The information included during the 3D reconstruction of a CT scan is controlled by
(a) Algorithm (b) Window setting
(c) Threshold setting (d) Grey scale map

Ans. (c). *Textbook of Radiology for Residents & Technicians, 5th ed., S.K. Bhargava & Sumeet Bhargava, p. 372-407.*

195. The device constructed to house the X-ray tube and data acquisition system for a CT scanner is termed as

(a) Central processing unit (b) Generator
(c) Gantry (d) Array processor

Ans. (c). *Textbook of Radiology for Residents & Technicians, 5th ed., S.K. Bhargava & Sumeet Bhargava, p. 372-407.*

196. The term voxel is the shortened form of the phrase

(a) Volume data acquisition (b) Volume data limitation
(c) Volume element (d) Voxel pixels

Ans. (d). *Textbook of Radiology for Residents & Technicians, 5th ed., S.K. Bhargava & Sumeet Bhargava, p. 372-407.*

197. CT image of a shoulder phantom shows streaking artifacts caused by

(a) Tube arching (b) Edge gradient
(c) Beam hardening (d) Photon starvation

Ans. (c). *Textbook of Radiology for Residents & Technicians, 5th ed., S.K. Bhargava & Sumeet Bhargava, p. 632-640.*

198. For imaging the heart, techniques have been developed to produce images by using data from just a fraction of the cardiac cycle. When there is least cardiac motion, this technique is called

(a) Electrocardiogram triggering (b) Cardiac cycle monitoring
(c) ECG data acquisition (d) Cardiac gating

Ans. (d). *Textbook of Radiology for Residents & Technicians, 5th ed., S.K. Bhargava & Sumeet Bhargava, p. 372-407.*

199. The computed tomography _________ was proposed to account for the dose from multiple scans in CT.

(a) Polypscan index (b) Exposure index
(c) Compound index (d) Dose index

Ans. (d). *Textbook of Radiology for Residents & Technicians, 5th ed., S.K. Bhargava & Sumeet Bhargava, p. 372-407.*

200. Slip ring technology allows

(a) The tube to rotate around the patient
(b) Increased resolution
(c) Increased contrast brightness
(d) The gantry to rotate around the patient

Ans. (c). *Textbook of Radiology for Residents & Technicians, 5th ed., S.K. Bhargava & Sumeet Bhargava, p. 372-407.*

201. Anode cooling rate of straton tube is

(a) 0.3–1 MHU
(b) 1–3 MHU
(c) 5–8 MHU
(d) 15–20 MHU

Ans. (c). *Textbook of Radiology for Residents & Technicians, 5th ed., S.K. Bhargava & Sumeet Bhargava, p. 372-407.*

202. In dual source CT, which of the following filters are used?

(a) Lead
(b) Tungsten
(c) Rhenium
(d) Tin

Ans. (d). *Textbook of Radiology for Residents & Technicians, 5th ed., S.K. Bhargava & Sumeet Bhargava, p. 372-407.*

ULTRASOUND

203. The ultrasound frequency used in the diagnosis is

(a) 20 kHz
(b) 40 kHz
(c) 60 kHz
(d) 1 MHz – 20 MHz

Ans. (d). *Textbook of Radiology for Residents & Technicians, 5th ed., S.K. Bhargava & Sumeet Bhargava, p. 343.*

204. On applying the electric field certain materials change

(a) Physical dimension
(b) Chemical dimension
(c) Both (a) and (b)
(d) None of these

Ans. (d). *Textbook of Radiology for Residents & Technicians, 5th ed., S.K. Bhargava & Sumeet Bhargava, p. 348.*

205. Piezoelectric material used in medical ultrasound

(a) Lead zirconate titanate
(b) Calcium tungstate
(c) Zinc cadmium sulphate
(d) None of these

Ans. (a). *Textbook of Radiology for Residents & Technicians, 5th ed., S.K. Bhargava & Sumeet Bhargava, p. 347.*

206. To sterilize the transducer, it should be

(a) Autoclaved
(b) Heated
(c) Cleaned with spirit
(d) None of the above

Ans. (c). *Textbook of Radiology for Residents & Technicians, 5th ed., S.K. Bhargava & Sumeet Bhargava, p. 348.*

207. Though he was not the first person to use sonography for medical purpose but who is generally known as the father of medical ultrasound

(a) John Wilde
(b) George Ludwid
(c) Ralph Joseph Holmes
(d) Geoff Stevenson

Ans. (a). Textbook of Radiology for Residents & Technicians, 5th ed., S.K. Bhargava & Sumeet Bhargava, p. 343-358.

208. While doing US scans you notice that the echoes at a depth of 4–6 cm appear relatively weak. The appropriate action to increase their brightness in image would be to adjust the

(a) Frequency (b) Focussing
(c) TGC (d) Beam intensity

Ans. (c). Textbook of Radiology for Residents & Technicians, 5th ed., S.K. Bhargava & Sumeet Bhargava, p. 343-358.

209. Piezoelectric effect is

(a) Application of electric field causes change in physical dimension
(b) Application of magnetic field causes change in physical dimension
(c) Application of either electric or magnetic field causes change in physical dimension
(d) None of the above

Ans. (a). Textbook of Radiology for Residents & Technicians, 5th ed., S.K. Bhargava & Sumeet Bhargava, p. 343-358.

210. Now-a-days, PE material is

(a) Lead zirconate titanate (b) Bismuth zirconate
(c) Phosphor (d) All of the above

Ans. (a). Textbook of Radiology for Residents & Technicians, 5th ed., S.K. Bhargava & Sumeet Bhargava, p. 343-358.

211. PE crystal is of

(a) 1 mm (b) 0.1 mm
(c) 0.3 mm (d) 0.5 mm

Ans. (d). Textbook of Radiology for Residents & Technicians, 5th ed., S.K. Bhargava & Sumeet Bhargava, p. 343-358.

212. Decreased sector angle will produce

(a) Low resolution (b) High resolution
(c) No relation with resolution (d) Large FOV

Ans. (b). Textbook of Radiology for Residents & Technicians, 5th ed., S.K. Bhargava & Sumeet Bhargava, p. 343-358.

213. Transrectal scanner best at which frequency?

(a) 5–7.5 (b) 3–5
(c) 3–7.5 (d) 8–12

Ans. (a). Textbook of Radiology for Residents & Technicians, 5th ed., S.K. Bhargava & Sumeet Bhargava, p. 343-358.

214. US produces which of the following biological effects?

(a) Heating (b) Cavitation
(c) Both of these (d) None of these

Ans. (c). Textbook of Radiology for Residents & Technicians, 5th ed., S.K. Bhargava & Sumeet Bhargava, p. 343-358.

215. Heating can cause biological effect at which intensity?

(a) 400 mW/cm^2 (b) 300 mW/cm^2
(c) Above 100 mW/cm^2 (d) None of these

Ans. (c). Textbook of Radiology for Residents & Technicians, 5th ed., S.K. Bhargava & Sumeet Bhargava, p. 359-371.

216. During systolic flow, what is the flow?

(a) Plug flow (b) Laminar flow
(c) Circular flow (d) None of the above

Ans. (a). Textbook of Radiology for Residents & Technicians, 5th ed., S.K. Bhargava & Sumeet Bhargava, p. 359-371.

217. Venous flow is normally which type of flow?

(a) Plug flow (b) Laminar flow
(c) Circular flow (d) None of the above

Ans. (b). Textbook of Radiology for Residents & Technicians, 5th ed., S.K. Bhargava & Sumeet Bhargava, p. 359-371.

218. In which of the following, Doppler has two piezoelectric elements with single head?

(a) C.W. Doppler
(b) Pulsed
(c) Duplex
(d) Doppler color flow imaging

Ans. (a). Textbook of Radiology for Residents & Technicians, 5th ed., S.K. Bhargava & Sumeet Bhargava, p. 359-371.

219. Unit of pulse repetition frequency is

(a) Per minute (b) msec
(c) mm/US (d) MHz

Ans. (a). Textbook of Radiology for Residents & Technicians, 5th ed., S.K. Bhargava & Sumeet Bhargava, p. 359-371.

220. The duty factor for continuous wave US is

(a) 10.0 (b) 1%
(c) 1.0 (d) 0.00001

Ans. (c). Textbook of Radiology for Residents & Technicians, 5th ed., S.K. Bhargava & Sumeet Bhargava, p. 359-371.

221. Which pair of intensities has the same value for continuous wave US?

(a) Spatial peak and spatial average.
(b) Temporal peak and spatial peak.
(c) Pulse average and temporal average.
(d) Spatial average and temporal average.

Ans. (c). *Textbook of Radiology for Residents & Technicians, 5th ed., S.K. Bhargava & Sumeet Bhargava, p. 359-371.*

222. Which of the following is best lateral resolution?

(a) 15 cm
(b) 6 cm
(c) 0.06 cm
(d) 2 cm

Ans. (c). *Textbook of Radiology for Residents & Technicians, 5th ed., S.K. Bhargava & Sumeet Bhargava, p. 343-358.*

223. What determines the frequency of a sound beam from a pulsed transducer?

(a) Voltage applied to PZT
(b) PZT thickness
(c) Frequency of the system
(d) PRF of the pulses

Ans. (b). *Textbook of Radiology for Residents & Technicians, 5th ed., S.K. Bhargava & Sumeet Bhargava, p. 359-371.*

224. What component of a transducer changes electrical to mechanical and mechanical back to electrical energy?

(a) PZT
(b) Scan converter
(c) Demodulator
(d) Receiver

Ans. (a). *Textbook of Radiology for Residents & Technicians, 5th ed., S.K. Bhargava & Sumeet Bhargava, p. 343-358.*

225. What has the greatest amount of attenuation?

(a) Bone
(b) Fat
(c) Water
(b) Muscle

Ans. (a). *Textbook of Radiology for Residents & Technicians, 5th ed., S.K. Bhargava & Sumeet Bhargava, p. 343-358.*

226. Azimuthal resolution is also known as

(a) Lateral resolution
(b) Range resolution
(c) Axial resolution
(d) None of the above

Ans. (a). *Textbook of Radiology for Residents & Technicians, 5th ed., S.K. Bhargava & Sumeet Bhargava, p. 343-358.*

227. Poiseuille's equation states that the volume rate of flow through a vessel is inversely proportional to

(a) Vessel radius
(b) Blood viscosity
(c) Blood density
(d) Pressure gradient

Ans. (b). *Textbook of Radiology for Residents & Technicians, 5th ed., S.K. Bhargava & Sumeet Bhargava, p. 359-371.*

228. Aliasing is a potential problem in PW Doppler because

(a) Of the use of high pulse repetition frequency.
(b) The Doppler signal is sampled rather than recorded continuously.
(c) Of dynamic focussing.
(d) Of perpendicular incidence.

Ans. (c). *Textbook of Radiology for Residents & Technicians, 5th ed., S.K. Bhargava & Sumeet Bhargava, p. 359-371.*

229. The transducer with more than one element is known as

(a) Multipurpose
(b) Annular
(c) Mechanical
(d) Array

Ans. (d). *Textbook of Radiology for Residents & Technicians, 5th ed., S.K. Bhargava & Sumeet Bhargava, p. 343-358.*

230. Doppler shift produces information about

(a) Location
(b) RBC motion
(c) Velocity
(d) None of the above

Ans. (c). *Textbook of Radiology for Residents & Technicians, 5th ed., S.K. Bhargava & Sumeet Bhargava, p. 343-358.*

231. The transducer _____ is equal to the ratio of the operating frequency to the frequency bandwidth.

(a) Frequency
(b) Q-factor
(c) Resolution
(d) Polarity

Ans. (b). *Textbook of Radiology for Residents & Technicians, 5th ed., S.K. Bhargava & Sumeet Bhargava, p. 343-358.*

232. Color Doppler frame rates are ______ gray scale rates.

(a) Equal to
(b) Less than
(c) More than
(d) Depends on color map

Ans. (b). *Textbook of Radiology for Residents & Technicians, 5th ed., S.K. Bhargava & Sumeet Bhargava, p. 343-358.*

233. For obese patient, which transducer is mostly preferred?

(a) High frequency
(b) Medium frequency
(c) Low frequency
(d) None of the above

Ans. (c). *Textbook of Radiology for Residents & Technicians, 5th ed., S.K. Bhargava & Sumeet Bhargava, p. 343-358.*

234. THI improved

(a) Resolution
(b) Artifacts
(c) Contrast
(d) Image noise

Ans. (a). *Textbook of Radiology for Residents & Technicians, 5th ed., S.K. Bhargava & Sumeet Bhargava, p. 343-358.*

235. Another name of sono-CT is

(a) Hybrid imaging
(b) THI
(c) Spatial compound imaging
(d) Elastography

Ans. (c). *Textbook of Radiology for Residents & Technicians, 5th ed., S.K. Bhargava & Sumeet Bhargava, p. 372-407.*

236. HIFU

(a) High Intensity Focussed Ultrasound
(b) Hypoechoic Intensity of Fusion Ultrasound
(c) Hyperechoic Intensity of Fusion Ultrasound
(d) High Information Fusion Ultrasound

Ans. (a). *Textbook of Radiology for Residents & Technicians, 5th ed., S.K. Bhargava & Sumeet Bhargava, p. 359-371.*

237. SMURF

(a) Spatial Modified Ultrasound Radiation Filament
(b) Spatially Modulated Ultrasound Radiation Force
(c) Shear Mode Ultrasound Radio-frequency
(d) None of the above

Ans. (b). *Textbook of Radiology for Residents & Technicians, 5th ed., S.K. Bhargava & Sumeet Bhargava, p. 359-371.*

238. EUS

(a) Elastography Ultrasound
(b) External Ultrasound
(c) Endoscopic Ultrasonography
(d) None of the above

Ans. (c). *Textbook of Radiology for Residents & Technicians, 5th ed., S.K. Bhargava & Sumeet Bhargava, p. 359-371.*

239. What would be the most likely result from increasing the transmit frequency of the Color Doppler?

(a) Improved sensitivity to slow flow
(b) Improved penetration for imaging flow in deep tissues
(c) Reduced flash artifact obscuring small vessel flow
(d) Reduced Color Doppler aliasing

Ans. (a). *Textbook of Radiology for Residents & Technicians, 5th ed., S.K. Bhargava & Sumeet Bhargava, p. 359-371.*

CT ARTIFACTS

240. Contrast media used during CT can result in

(a) Ring artifacts
(b) Beam hardening artifacts
(c) Partial volume artifacts
(d) Incomplete projection artifacts

Ans. (b). *Textbook of Radiology for Residents & Technicians, 5th ed., S.K.Bhargava, p. 632-640.*

241. Ring artifact is

(a) Motion artifact
(b) Scanner based artifact
(c) Physics based artifact
(d) Cupping artifact

Ans. (b). *Textbook of Radiology for Residents & Technicians, 5th ed., S.K. Bhargava & Sumeet Bhargava, p. 632-640.*

242. One of the following is not physics based artifact

(a) Cupping artifact
(b) Photon starvation
(c) Partial volume
(d) Incomplete projection

Ans. (d). *Textbook of Radiology for Residents & Technicians, 5th ed., S.K. Bhargava & Sumeet Bhargava, p. 632-640.*

243. Photon starvation artifact can be minimized by

(a) Automatic tube current modulation
(b) Slower rotation speed
(c) Quarter-detection shift technique
(d) Flying focal spot technique

Ans. (a). *Textbook of Radiology for Residents & Technicians, 5th ed., S.K. Bhargava & Sumeet Bhargava, p. 632-640.*

244. Metallic material can result in

(a) Beam hardening artifact
(b) Partial volume
(c) Aliasing artifact
(d) All of the above

Ans. (d). *Textbook of Radiology for Residents & Technicians, 5th ed., S.K.Bhargava, p. 632-640.*

245. Which of the following artifacts can not be avoided by the operator?

(a) Metallic material artifact
(b) Ring artifact
(c) Incomplete projection
(d) Beam hardening artifact

Ans. (b). *Textbook of Radiology for Residents & Technicians, 5th ed., S.K. Bhargava & Sumeet Bhargava, p. 632-640.*

246. Partial volume artifact can be avoided by

(a) Using as short scan time as possible
(b) Asking the patient to hold their breath
(c) Taking thin slice section
(d) None of the above

Ans. (c). *Textbook of Radiology for Residents & Technicians, 5th ed., S.K. Bhargava & Sumeet Bhargava, p. 632-640.*

247. Cone beam effect is seen in

(a) Single section scanning
(b) Multisection scanning
(c) Both of the above
(d) None of the above

Ans. (b). *Textbook of Radiology for Residents & Technicians, 5th ed., S.K. Bhargava & Sumeet Bhargava, p. 632-640.*

248. Under sampling artifact depends on

(a) Number of projection
(b) Patient positioning
(c) Scanner function
(d) Patient motion

Ans. (a). *Textbook of Radiology for Residents & Technicians, 5th ed., S.K. Bhargava & Sumeet Bhargava, p. 632-640.*

249. Cardiac gating is used for minimizing

(a) Motion artifact
(b) Ring artifact
(c) Beam hardening effect
(d) Photon starvation effect

Ans. (a). *Textbook of Radiology for Residents & Technicians, 5th ed., S.K. Bhargava & Sumeet Bhargava, p. 632-642.*

250. Beam hardening effect can be avoided

(a) By tilting the gantry
(b) By means of sedation
(c) By using as short scan time as possible
(d) None of the above

Ans. (a). *Textbook of Radiology for Residents & Technicians, 5th ed., S.K. Bhargava & Sumeet Bhargava, p. 632-642.*

251. Stair step artifacts are avoided

(a) By taking thin section
(b) By proper position
(c) By using position aid
(d) By tilting gantry

Ans. (a). *Textbook of Radiology for Residents & Technicians, 5th ed., S.K.Bhargava, p. 632-642.*

252. Bow-tie filter is used for minimizing

(a) Photon starvation
(b) Beam hardening effect
(c) Under sampling artifact
(d) All of the above

Ans. ***(b).*** *Textbook of Radiology for Residents & Technicians, 5th ed., S.K. Bhargava & Sumeet Bhargava, p. 632-642.*

253. Beam hardening software should be used to avoid

(a) Metal artifact
(b) Motion artifact
(c) Under sampling
(d) All above

Ans. ***(a).*** *Textbook of Radiology for Residents & Technicians, 5th ed., S.K.Bhargava, p. 632-642.*

254. Beam hardening artifact is due to

(a) Absorption of high energy photons
(b) Absorption of low energy photons
(c) Both (a) and (b)
(d) None

Ans. ***(b).*** *Textbook of Radiology for Residents & Technicians, 5th ed., S.K. Bhargava & Sumeet Bhargava, p. 632-642.*

255. Partial volume artifact results in following type of artifact

(a) Streaking
(b) Shading
(c) Ring
(d) Distortion artifact

Ans. ***(b).*** *Textbook of Radiology for Residents & Technicians, 5th ed., S.K. Bhargava & Sumeet Bhargava, p. 632-642.*

256. Multidimensional adaptive filtration technique is used for minimizing

(a) Photon starvation artifact
(b) Under sampling
(c) Ring artifact
(d) Zebra artifact

Ans. ***(a).*** *Textbook of Radiology for Residents & Technicians, 5th ed., S.K. Bhargava & Sumeet Bhargava, p. 632-642.*

257. View aliasing and ray aliasing effect occurs due to

(a) Incomplete projection
(b) Photon starvation
(c) Under sampling
(d) All of above

Ans. ***(c).*** *Textbook of Radiology for Residents & Technicians, 5th ed., S.K. Bhargava & Sumeet Bhargava, p. 632-642.*

258. View aliasing can be minimized by

(a) Increase number of projection
(b) Decrease number of projection
(c) Gantry angulations
(d) By taking thick sections

Ans. ***(a).*** *Textbook of Radiology for Residents & Technicians, 5th ed., S.K. Bhargava & Sumeet Bhargava, p. 632-642.*

259. If one of the detectors is out of calibration on a scanner, it gives rise to

(a) Ring artifact
(b) Stair step artifact
(c) Cone beam effect artifact
(d) Streaks and dark effect

Ans. (a). *Textbook of Radiology for Residents & Technicians, 5th ed., S.K. Bhargava & Sumeet Bhargava, p. 632-642.*

MR ARTIFACTS

260. The angle at which magic angle artifact occurs is

(a) 60
(b) 45
(c) 55
(d) 90

Ans. (c). *Textbook of Radiology for Residents & Technicians, 5th ed., S.K.Bhargava, p. 650-659.*

261. About chemical shift, false is

(a) Worst at lower fields strength
(b) Due to different resonant frequency of protons in fat and water
(c) Common in solid organs surrounded by fat
(d) Less with stronger gradients

Ans. (a). *Textbook of Radiology for Residents & Technicians, 5th ed., S.K. Bhargava & Sumeet Bhargava, p. 650-659.*

262. Chemical shift artifact reduced by

(a) Using fat suppression
(b) Increasing bandwidth
(c) Both (a) and (b)
(d) None

Ans. (c). *Textbook of Radiology for Residents & Technicians, 5th ed., S.K. Bhargava & Sumeet Bhargava, p. 650-659.*

263. Aliasing artifact, false is

(a) Decreasing by increasing FOV
(b) Decreased by using surface coil
(c) Occurs at initial slices of 3D acquisition.
(d) Occurs at end slices of 3D acquisition.

Ans. (c). *Textbook of Radiology for Residents & Technicians, 5th ed., S.K. Bhargava & Sumeet Bhargava, p. 650-659.*

264. Black line artifact occurs in

(a) Short TE
(b) Long TE
(c) In phase
(d) None of these

Ans. (a). *Textbook of Radiology for Residents & Technicians, 5th ed., S.K. Bhargava & Sumeet Bhargava, p. 650-659.*

265. Method to remove black line artifact includes

(a) In phase sequences (b) Long TE
(c) Fat suppression (d) All of the above

Ans. (d). *Textbook of Radiology for Residents & Technicians, 5th ed., S.K. Bhargava & Sumeet Bhargava, p. 650-659.*

266. Artifacts seen as bright and dark lines parallel to and next to borders of abrupt intensity change

(a) Gibbs artifact (b) Chemical shift artifacts
(c) Zipper artifact (d) Magic angle artifact

Ans. (a). *Textbook of Radiology for Residents & Technicians, 5th ed., S.K. Bhargava & Sumeet Bhargava, p. 650-659.*

267. One of the following is a useful artifact

(a) Chemical shift artifact (b) Gibbs artifact
(c) Zipper artifact (d) Magic angle artifact

Ans. (a). *Textbook of Radiology for Residents & Technicians, 5th ed., S.K. Bhargava & Sumeet Bhargava, p. 650-659.*

268. Artifacts caused due to radiofrequency waves entering the MR room

(a) Gibbs artifact (b) Zipper artifact
(c) Chemical artifact (d) Cross-talk artifact

Ans. (b). *Textbook of Radiology for Residents & Technicians, 5th ed., S.K. Bhargava & Sumeet Bhargava, p. 650-659.*

269. Artifact that occur from a multi-angle, multi-slice acquisition

(a) Slice overlap (b) Slice cross-talk
(c) Zipper artifact (d) Gibbs artifact

Ans. (a). *Textbook of Radiology for Residents & Technicians, 5th ed., S.K. Bhargava & Sumeet Bhargava, p. 650-659.*

270. Methods used to remove slice overlap artifact

(a) Avoiding steep change in angle between slice groups
(b) Using separate acquisition
(c) None of the above
(d) Both (a) and (b)

Ans. (d). *Textbook of Radiology for Residents & Technicians, 5th ed., S.K. Bhargava & Sumeet Bhargava, p. 650-659.*

271. Methods of removing magic angle artifact includes

(a) Repositioning of patient
(b) Increasing TE
(c) Comparing with T_2 or other sequences

(d) All of the above

Ans. (d). Textbook of Radiology for Residents & Technicians, 5th ed., S.K. Bhargava & Sumeet Bhargava, p. 650-659.

272. Artifact useful as mechanism of angiography
(a) Entry slice artifact (b) Gibbs artifact
(c) Zipper artifact (d) Susceptibility artifact

Ans. (a). Textbook of Radiology for Residents & Technicians, 5th ed., S.K. Bhargava & Sumeet Bhargava, p. 650-659.

273. True about susceptibility artifact
(a) Worse at higher field strength (b) Less with FSE
(c) None of the above (d) Both of the above

Ans. (d). Textbook of Radiology for Residents & Technicians, 5th ed., S.K. Bhargava & Sumeet Bhargava, p. 650-659.

274. Susceptibility artifacts reduced by
(a) Using smallest voxel size
(b) Using FSE
(c) Optimal positioning of patients with metallic implant
(d) All of the above

Ans. (d). Textbook of Radiology for Residents & Technicians, 5th ed., S.K. Bhargava & Sumeet Bhargava, p. 650-659.

275. Artifact that occur as band-like strips due to loss of data in K-space
(a) Gibbs artifact (b) Moire fringes
(c) Clipping artifact (d) Zebra artifact

Ans. (b). Textbook of Radiology for Residents & Technicians, 5th ed., S.K. Bhargava & Sumeet Bhargava, p. 650-659.

276. Artifact produced due to induced electric current in conductor due to varying magnetic fields
(a) Zipper artifact (b) Zebra artifact
(c) Moire fringes (d) Eddy current

Ans. (d). Textbook of Radiology for Residents & Technicians, 5th ed., S.K. Bhargava & Sumeet Bhargava, p. 650-659.

277. Artifact produced due to distortion of the linear magnetic field by metallic objects with ferromagnetic properties
(a) Zebra artifact (b) Zipper artifact
(c) Susceptibility artifact (d) Eddy artifact

Ans. (c). Textbook of Radiology for Residents & Technicians, 5th ed., S.K. Bhargava & Sumeet Bhargava, p. 650-659.

278. Partial voluming artifact reduced by using

(a) Small voxel (b) Large voxel
(c) None (d) Both (a) and (b)

Ans. (a). *Textbook of Radiology for Residents & Technicians, 5th ed., S.K. Bhargava & Sumeet Bhargava, p. 650-659.*

279. Artifacts produced due to decreased FOV as compared to the anatomical part being examined is

(a) Moire fringes (b) Aliasing artifact
(c) Gibbs artifact (d) Clipping artifact

Ans. (b). *Textbook of Radiology for Residents & Technicians, 5th ed., S.K. Bhargava & Sumeet Bhargava, p. 650-659.*

280. Static marks, which are black tree-like or circular marks on radiograph, are often caused by

(a) Film being bent when inserted in a cassette or holder
(b) Foreign material or dirt imbedded in screen
(c) Scratches on lead foil's screens
(d) Improper film handling techniques

Ans. (d). *Textbook of Radiology for Residents & Technicians, 5th ed., S.K. Bhargava & Sumeet Bhargava, p. 632-662.*

281. Water spots on films can be minimized by

(a) Rapid drying of wet film
(b) Immersing wet film for one or two minutes in a wetting agent solution
(c) By using a fresh fixer solution
(d) By cascading water during the rinse cycle

Ans. (d). *Textbook of Radiology for Residents & Technicians, 5th ed., S.K. Bhargava & Sumeet Bhargava, p. 632-662.*

282. Contrast media used during CT scan cause

(a) Partial volume artifacts
(b) Ring artifacts
(c) Beam hardening artifacts
(d) Incomplete projection artifacts

Ans. (c). *Textbook of Radiology for Residents & Technicians, 5th ed., S.K. Bhargava & Sumeet Bhargava, p. 632-662.*

283. Photon starvation artifacts can be minimized by

(a) Automatic tube current modulation
(b) Large FOV
(c) Flying focal spot technique
(d) Low mAs technique

Ans. (a). Textbook of Radiology for Residents & Technicians, 5th ed., S.K. Bhargava & Sumeet Bhargava, p. 632-662.

284. Which of the following is a useful artifact in imaging?

(a) Chemical shift artifacts
(b) Gibbs artifacts
(c) Zipper artifacts
(d) Ghost artifacts

Ans. (a). Textbook of Radiology for Residents & Technicians, 5th ed., S.K. Bhargava & Sumeet Bhargava, p. 632-662.

285. Artifacts produced due to decreased FOV as compared to the anatomical part being examined is

(a) Moire fringe artifact
(b) Aliasing artifact
(c) Gibbs artifact
(d) Clipping artifact

Ans. (b). Textbook of Radiology for Residents & Technicians, 5th ed., S.K. Bhargava & Sumeet Bhargava, p. 632-662.

286. When gas bubbles interact with US, which artifact is produced?

(a) Reverberation
(b) Comet tail
(c) Ring down
(d) Multipath

Ans. (c). Textbook of Radiology for Residents & Technicians, 5th ed., S.K. Bhargava & Sumeet Bhargava, p. 632-662.

287. Dirty shadowing is produced by

(a) Air
(b) Water
(c) Fat
(d) Fluid

Ans. (a). Textbook of Radiology for Residents & Technicians, 5th ed., S.K. Bhargava & Sumeet Bhargava, p. 632-662.

288. When gas bubbles interact with US, which artifact is produced?

(a) Reverberation
(b) Comet tail
(c) Ring down
(d) Multipath

Ans. (c). Textbook of Radiology for Residents & Technicians, 5th ed., S.K. Bhargava & Sumeet Bhargava, p. 632-662.

289. Dirty shadowing is produced by

(a) Air
(b) Water
(c) Fat
(d) Fluid

Ans. (a). Textbook of Radiology for Residents & Technicians, 5th ed., S.K. Bhargava & Sumeet Bhargava, p. 632-662.

290. Presence of the highly reflectors in the path of a US beam produces

(a) Reverberation artifacts
(b) Posterior enhancement
(c) Acoustic shadowing
(d) Speckle

Ans. ***(a)****. Textbook of Radiology for Residents & Technicians, 5th ed., S.K. Bhargava & Sumeet Bhargava, p. 632-662.*

291. Which of the following is not an attenuation artifact?

(a) Acoustic shadowing (b) Edge enhancement
(c) Speckle (d) Misregistration

Ans. ***(d)****. Textbook of Radiology for Residents & Technicians, 5th ed., S.K. Bhargava & Sumeet Bhargava, p. 632-662.*

292. Screen marks appear as a

(a) White on radiograph (b) Blue on radiograph
(c) Black on radiograph (d) Green on radiograph

Ans. ***(a)****. Textbook of Radiology for Residents & Technicians, 5th ed., S.K. Bhargava & Sumeet Bhargava, p. 632-662.*

293. Crimp marks appear/caused by

(a) Finger print (b) Finger nail pressure
(c) Film becomes cressed (d) All of the above

Ans. ***(d)****. Textbook of Radiology for Residents & Technicians, 5th ed., S.K. Bhargava & Sumeet Bhargava, p. 632-662.*

294. Generally, white pressure marks are produced when packet of film

(a) Kept in vertical position (b) Kept on boxes
(c) Box kept in wet place (d) All of the above

Ans. ***(b)****. Textbook of Radiology for Residents & Technicians, 5th ed., S.K. Bhargava & Sumeet Bhargava, p. 632-662.*

295. Static marks produced due to

(a) Wet surface (b) Static electric charges
(c) Rough development (d) Misalignment of screen

Ans. ***(b)****. Textbook of Radiology for Residents & Technicians, 5th ed., S.K. Bhargava & Sumeet Bhargava, p. 632-662.*

296. Handling the surface of a film with the finger before it has been processed may lead to formation of

(a) Chemical staining (b) Static marks
(c) Finger marks (d) Pressure marks

Ans. ***(c)****. Textbook of Radiology for Residents & Technicians, 5th ed., S.K. Bhargava & Sumeet Bhargava, p. 632-662.*

297. After some time (week or month) yellow or brown shades appear on the radiograph. This is due to

(a) Finger marks (b) Screen marks
(c) Chemical staining (d) Storage

Ans. (c). Textbook of Radiology for Residents & Technicians, 5th ed., S.K. Bhargava & Sumeet Bhargava, p. 632-662.

298. When an exposed cassette is re-exposed

(a) Magnification occurs (b) Artifact occurs
(c) Distortion occurs (d) All of the above

Ans. (b). Textbook of Radiology for Residents & Technicians, 5th ed., S.K. Bhargava & Sumeet Bhargava, p. 632-662.

299. Fogging is

(a) Loss of radiographic contrast (b) Loss of sharpness
(c) Loss of radiographic detail (d) All of the above

Ans. (d). Textbook of Radiology for Residents & Technicians, 5th ed., S.K. Bhargava & Sumeet Bhargava, p. 632-662.

300. Structure mottle is due to

(a) Excessive processing temperature
(b) Excessive exposure factor
(c) Excessive focus to film distance
(d) Excessive motion during exposure

Ans. (a). Textbook of Radiology for Residents & Technicians, 5th ed., S.K. Bhargava & Sumeet Bhargava, p. 632-662.

301. Quantum mottle is due to

(a) High speed rare earth intensifying screen with low mAs exposure
(b) Low speed rare earth intensifying screen with high mAs exposure
(c) High speed rare earth intensifying screen with high mAs exposure
(d) Low speed rare earth intensifying screen with low mAs exposure

Ans. (a). Textbook of Radiology for Residents & Technicians, 5th ed., S.K. Bhargava & Sumeet Bhargava, p. 632-662.

302. Fog is

(a) Unwanted film density which lower radiographic contrast
(b) Leakage of radiation in darkroom
(c) Increase in radiation dose
(d) All of the above

Ans. (a). Textbook of Radiology for Residents & Technicians, 5th ed., S.K. Bhargava & Sumeet Bhargava, p. 632-662.

303. Discoloration of film is

(a) Fog (b) Artifact
(c) Stain (d) None of the above

Ans. (c). Textbook of Radiology for Residents & Technicians, 5th ed., S.K. Bhargava & Sumeet Bhargava, p. 632-662.

304. Regular agitation can be removed by

(a) Finger marks
(b) Flow marks
(c) Static electric marks
(d) Abrasion marks

Ans. (b). *Textbook of Radiology for Residents & Technicians, 5th ed., S.K. Bhargava & Sumeet Bhargava, p. 632-662.*

305. Cupping artifact is type of

(a) Patient-based
(b) Physics-based
(c) Scanner-based
(d) Not recognised

Ans. (b). *Textbook of Radiology for Residents & Technicians, 5th ed., S.K. Bhargava & Sumeet Bhargava, p. 632-662.*

306. Zebra artifact is

(a) Patient-based
(b) Physics-based
(c) Scanner-based
(d) Helical and multisection artifact

Ans. (d). *Textbook of Radiology for Residents & Technicians, 5th ed., S.K. Bhargava & Sumeet Bhargava, p. 632-662.*

307. Photon starvation

(a) Insufficient photons reach the detector
(b) Sufficient photons reach the detector
(c) Number of photon increase when they reach the detector
(d) No photons reached to the detector

Ans. (a). *Textbook of Radiology for Residents & Technicians, 5th ed., S.K. Bhargava & Sumeet Bhargava, p. 632-662.*

308. The problem of photon starvation will be overcome by

(a) Increased tube current
(b) Increased kV_p
(c) Decreased the FOV
(d) Increased slice thickness

Ans. (a). *Textbook of Radiology for Residents & Technicians, 5th ed., S.K. Bhargava & Sumeet Bhargava, p. 632-662.*

309. In CT scanner 'ECG cardiac gating' is used

(a) Because it minimizes motion artifact
(b) Because it captures all the signals from heart
(c) To remove incomplete projection
(d) To check the heart valve function

Ans. (a). *Textbook of Radiology for Residents & Technicians, 5th ed., S.K. Bhargava & Sumeet Bhargava, p. 632-662.*

310. Histogram error produces

(a) Acquisition artifact
(b) Post-processing
(c) Display artifact
(d) None of the above

Ans. (b). Textbook of Radiology for Residents & Technicians, 5th ed., S.K. Bhargava & Sumeet Bhargava, p. 632-662.

311. In which generation of CT scanner 'ring artifact' is produce

(a) 1st generation
(b) 2nd generation
(c) 3rd generation
(d) 4th generation

Ans. (c). Textbook of Radiology for Residents & Technicians, 5th ed., S.K. Bhargava & Sumeet Bhargava, p. 632-662.

312. Which artifact is due to resonance of air bubble

(a) Reverberation
(b) Mirror image
(c) Ring down
(d) None of the above

Ans. (c). Textbook of Radiology for Residents & Technicians, 5th ed., S.K. Bhargava & Sumeet Bhargava, p. 632-662.

313. CT image of a shoulder phantom shows streaking artifacts caused by

(a) Tube arcing
(b) Edge gradient
(c) Beam hardening
(d) Photon starvation

Ans. (d). Textbook of Radiology for Residents & Technicians, 5th ed., S.K. Bhargava & Sumeet Bhargava, p. 632-662.

ULTRASOUND ARTIFACT

314. Weak off axis lobes associated with a single piezoelectric element is

(a) Grating lobe
(b) Side lobe
(c) Superficial lobe
(d) Deep lobe

Ans. (b). Textbook of Radiology for Residents & Technicians, 5th ed., S.K. Bhargava & Sumeet Bhargava, p. 660-662.

315. Which of the following are not attenuation artifacts?

(a) Acoustic shadowing
(b) Enhancement
(c) Speckle
(d) Misregistration

Ans. (d). Textbook of Radiology for Residents & Technicians, 5th ed., S.K. Bhargava & Sumeet Bhargava, p. 660-662.

316. Speed of the sound is

(a) 1340 m/s
(b) 1440 m/s
(c) 1540 m/s
(d) 1640 m/s

Ans. (c). *Textbook of Radiology for Residents & Technicians, 5th ed., S.K. Bhargava & Sumeet Bhargava, p. 660-662.*

317. Which of the following is not a type of resolution encountered in ultrasound?

(a) Axial (b) Elevational
(c) Lateral (d) Superficial

Ans. (d). *Textbook of Radiology for Residents & Technicians, 5th ed., S.K. Bhargava & Sumeet Bhargava, p. 660-662.*

318. Spatial pulse length is

(a) No. of cycles in pulse × the wavelength
(b) No. of the cycles in pulse/the wavelength
(c) No. of the cycles in pulse + the wavelength
(d) None of the above

Ans. (a). *Textbook of Radiology for Residents & Technicians, 5th ed., S.K. Bhargava & Sumeet Bhargava, p. 660-662.*

319. Which of the resolution is the best?

(a) Axial (b) Lateral
(c) Elevational (d) Horizontal

Ans. (a). *Textbook of Radiology for Residents & Technicians, 5th ed., S.K. Bhargava & Sumeet Bhargava, p. 660-662.*

320. Non-imaging plane is

(a) Axial (b) Lateral
(c) Elevational (d) Horizontal

Ans. (c). *Textbook of Radiology for Residents & Technicians, 5th ed., S.K. Bhargava & Sumeet Bhargava, p. 660-662.*

321. When gas bubble are bombarded with ultrasound, artifact produced is

(a) Reverberation
(b) Comet tail
(c) Ring down
(d) Multipath

Ans. (c). *Textbook of Radiology for Residents & Technicians, 5th ed., S.K. Bhargava & Sumeet Bhargava, p. 660-662.*

322. Clean shadowing is produced by

(a) Calcification (b) Air
(c) Fat (d) Water

Ans. (a). *Textbook of Radiology for Residents & Technicians, 5th ed., S.K. Bhargava & Sumeet Bhargava, p. 660-662.*

323. Dirty shadowing is produced by

(a) Calcification (b) Air
(c) Fat (d) Water

Ans. (b). Textbook of Radiology for Residents & Technicians, 5th ed., S.K. Bhargava & Sumeet Bhargava, p. 660-662.

324. Enhancement occurs deep to a _______ attenuating structure.

(a) Low (b) High
(c) Both (a) and (b) (d) None

Ans. (a). Textbook of Radiology for Residents & Technicians, 5th ed., S.K. Bhargava & Sumeet Bhargava, p. 660-662.

325. Presence of the reflectors in the path of a ultrasound beam produces

(a) Reverberation artifact
(b) Posterior enhancement
(c) Acoustic shadowing
(d) Speckle

Ans. (a). Textbook of Radiology for Residents & Technicians, 5th ed., S.K.Bhargava, p. 660-662.

326. Sin@ r/ sin @ I = c 2/c1 is

(a) Boyle's law (b) Newton's law
(c) Snell's law (d) Archimedes law

Ans. (c). Textbook of Radiology for Residents & Technicians, 5th ed., S.K. Bhargava & Sumeet Bhargava, p. 660-662.

327. If propagation velocity in the liasion coming in the path of a sound beam is less than 1540 m/s

(a) Reflector appears deep
(b) Reflector appears superficial
(c) Reflector appears at the same position
(d) None of these

Ans. (a). Textbook of Radiology for Residents & Technicians, 5th ed., S.K. Bhargava & Sumeet Bhargava, p. 660-662.

328. If propagation velocity in the liasion coming in the path of a sound beam is more than 1540 m/s

(a) Reflector appears deep
(b) Reflector appears superficial
(c) Reflector appears at the same position
(d) None of these

Ans. (b). Textbook of Radiology for Residents & Technicians, 5th ed., S.K. Bhargava & Sumeet Bhargava, p. 660-662.

CR AND DR SYSTEM

329. Digital luminescence radiography is another name for

(a) Computed tomography (b) Direct digital radiography
(c) Indirect digital radiography (d) CCD

Ans. (a). *Textbook of Radiology for Residents & Technicians, 5th ed., S.K. Bhargava & Sumeet Bhargava, p. 372.*

330. Image receptor in CR is

(a) Photomultiplier tube
(b) Silicone TFT
(c) Amorphous selenium
(d) Photostimulable phosphor

Ans. (d). *Textbook of Radiology for Residents & Technicians, 5th ed., S.K. Bhargava & Sumeet Bhargava, p. 579.*

331. Fading of latent image on photostimulable phosphor occurs by

(a) Fluorescence
(b) Photostimulable luminescence
(c) Phosphorescence
(d) Light exposure

Ans. (c). *Textbook of Radiology for Residents & Technicians, 5th ed., S.K. Bhargava & Sumeet Bhargava, p. 581.*

332. Which one of the following is not the desirable characteristic of photostimulable phosphor?

(a) Stimulation-absorption peak at a wavelength produced by common lasers.
(b) A stimulated emission peak readily absorbed by common photomultiplier tube input phosphors.
(c) Retention of the latent image without significant signal loss due to phosphorescence.
(d) Release of the latent image by fluorescence.

Ans. (d). *Textbook of Radiology for Residents & Technicians, 5th ed., S.K. Bhargava & Sumeet Bhargava, p. 581.*

333. Luminescence center/activator in PSP is

(a) GdO_2S_2 (b) BaFBr
(c) Eu (d) BaFI

Ans. (c). *Textbook of Radiology for Residents & Technicians, 5th ed., S.K. Bhargava & Sumeet Bhargava, p. 582.*

334. Percentage loss of latent image on PSP between 10 min to 8 hrs. is

(a) 75% (b) 50%

(c) 25% (d) 100%

Ans. (c). Textbook of Radiology for Residents & Technicians, 5th ed., S.K. Bhargava & Sumeet Bhargava, p. 581-582.

335. Energy of laser beams required to read latent image is of the order of

(a) 4 eV (b) 6 eV
(c) 5 eV (d) 2 eV

Ans. (d). Textbook of Radiology for Residents & Technicians, 5th ed., S.K. Bhargava & Sumeet Bhargava, p. 582.

336. Fast scan/scan direction is the direction of motion of

(a) Laser beam (b) Phosphor plate
(c) X-ray beam (d) Grid

Ans. (a). Textbook of Radiology for Residents & Technicians, 5th ed., S.K. Bhargava & Sumeet Bhargava, p. 641-650.

337. Slow scan/sub-scan direction is the direction of motion of

(a) Laser beam (b) Phosphor plate
(c) X-ray beam (d) Grid

Ans. (b). Textbook of Radiology for Residents & Technicians, 5th ed., S.K. Bhargava & Sumeet Bhargava, p. 580.

338. Light erasure of residual signal of PSP is a function of

(a) Size of the object
(b) Degree of the X-ray exposure
(c) Laser beam energy
(d) Size of the phosphor plate

Ans. (b). Textbook of Radiology for Residents & Technicians, 5th ed., S.K. Bhargava & Sumeet Bhargava, p. 581.

339. The pixel size in CR is

(a) 20–100 micrometer (b) 50–200 micrometer
(c) 100–200 micrometer (d) 200–1000 micrometer

Ans. (b). Textbook of Radiology for Residents & Technicians, 5th ed., S.K. Bhargava & Sumeet Bhargava, p. 580.

340. Characteristic curve of PSP is

(a) Linear wide latitude (b) Non-linear wide latitude
(c) Linear narrow latitude (d) Non-linear narrow latitude

Ans. (a). Textbook of Radiology for Residents & Technicians, 5th ed., S.K. Bhargava & Sumeet Bhargava, p. 580.

341. In PSP histogram, X and Y axis denotes respectively

(a) Pixel value and spectrum
(b) Exposure and time of exposure
(c) Pixel width and gray scale
(d) Pixel spectrum and pixel value

Ans. (a). *Textbook of Radiology for Residents & Technicians, 5th ed., S.K. Bhargava & Sumeet Bhargava, p. 582.*

342. Which of these is correctly matched for the exposure information by PSP manufacturer?

(a) Fuji – sensitivity no; Kodak – exposure index; Agfa – relative exposure value 1 gm
(b) Kodak – relative exposure value 1 gm; Fuji – exposure index; Agfa – sensitivity no.
(c) Fuji – relative exposure value 1 gm; Kodak – sensitivity no; Agfa – exposure index
(d) None of the above.

Ans. (a). *Textbook of Radiology for Residents & Technicians, 5th ed., S.K. Bhargava & Sumeet Bhargava, p. 582.*

343. Overexposure is difficult to detect in CR due to

(a) Post-processing
(b) Quantum mottle
(c) Poor image quality
(d) Plate read out by laser beam

Ans. (a). *Textbook of Radiology for Residents & Technicians, 5th ed., S.K. Bhargava & Sumeet Bhargava, p. 579.*

344. All of these increases spatial resolution in CR except

(a) Smaller plate
(b) Larger pixel size
(c) Thinner phosphor plate
(d) Reduced phosphorescence lag

Ans. (b). *Textbook of Radiology for Residents & Technicians, 5th ed., S.K. Bhargava & Sumeet Bhargava, p. 579.*

345. Contrast of digital image depends upon all except

(a) Number of bits per pixel
(b) Gain
(c) Contrast enhancement
(d) Pixel size

Ans. (d). *Textbook of Radiology for Residents & Technicians, 5th ed., S.K. Bhargava & Sumeet Bhargava, p. 583.*

346. Which of the following is not a disadvantage of laser print?

(a) High cost
(b) Cannot be transilluminated

(c) Reduction in size complicated direct measurement and comparison
(d) Single rendition

Ans. (b). *Textbook of Radiology for Residents & Technicians, 5th ed., S.K. Bhargava & Sumeet Bhargava, p. 581.*

347. First PSP device implemented in US by
(a) Phillips in 1983
(b) Kodak in 1975
(c) Fuji in 1960
(d) Agfa in 1990

Ans. (a). *Textbook of Radiology for Residents & Technicians, 5th ed., S.K.Bhargava, p. 581.*

348. Digital radiography differs from computed radiography in
(a) Reduced radiation exposure
(b) Digitalization of the image
(c) Combined image capture and read-out capability
(d) Reduced retakes

Ans. (c). *Textbook of Radiology for Residents & Technicians, 5th ed., S.K. Bhargava & Sumeet Bhargava, p. 580.*

349. Which of these is not direct DR system?
(a) Flat panel detector
(b) Charged couple device
(c) Slot scanning type
(d) Photon counting type

Ans. (b). *Textbook of Radiology for Residents & Technicians, 5th ed., S.K. Bhargava & Sumeet Bhargava, p. 580.*

350. The disadvantage of CsI over gadox is
(a) Better spatial resolution
(b) Fragile
(c) Efficient X-ray absorption
(d) Better quantum efficiency

Ans. (b). *Textbook of Radiology for Residents & Technicians, 5th ed., S.K. Bhargava & Sumeet Bhargava, p. 581.*

351. The maximum detector size available in FPD currently is
(a) 43 × 43 cm
(b) 43 × 36 cm
(c) 36 × 36 cm
(d) 36 × 43 cm

Ans. (d). *Textbook of Radiology for Residents & Technicians, 5th ed., S.K.Bhargava, p. 583.*

352. Newer software application available with CR & DR are all, except
(a) Tomosynthesis
(b) CAD
(c) Dual energy imaging
(d) Perfusion imaging

Ans. (d). *Textbook of Radiology for Residents & Technicians, 5th ed., S.K. Bhargava & Sumeet Bhargava, p. 585.*

353. Image readout of PSP has been reduced to

(a) 30 s (b) 45 s
(c) 10 s (d) 75 s

Ans. (c). *Textbook of Radiology for Residents & Technicians, 5th ed., S.K. Bhargava & Sumeet Bhargava, p. 581.*

354. First DR system appeared in

(a) 1983 (b) 1975
(c) 1990 (d) 2000

Ans. (c). *Textbook of Radiology for Residents & Technicians, 5th ed., S.K. Bhargava & Sumeet Bhargava, p. 582.*

355. First DR system was type of

(a) CCD slot scan type (b) Flat panel type
(c) Photon counting type (d) Photostimulable type

Ans. (a). *Textbook of Radiology for Residents & Technicians, 5th ed., S.K. Bhargava,, p. 478.*

356. Following are used in direct DR, except

(a) Amorphous selenium (b) Lead iodide
(c) Mercury iodide (d) Barium fluorohalide

Ans. (d). *Textbook of Radiology for Residents & Technicians, 5th ed., S.K. Bhargava & Sumeet Bhargava, p. 584.*

357. Thalium doped cesium iodide is a

(a) Photoscintillator (b) Photoconductor
(c) Photostimulable phosphor (d) Protective layer

Ans. (a). *Textbook of Radiology for Residents & Technicians, 5th ed., S.K. Bhargava & Sumeet Bhargava, p. 585.*

358. Gadolinium oxysulphide is a

(a) Structured photoscintillator
(b) Unstructured photoscintillator
(c) Photostimulable phosphor
(d) Activator

Ans. (b). *Textbook of Radiology for Residents & Technicians, 5th ed., S.K. Bhargava & Sumeet Bhargava, p. 586.*

359. In digital radiography, spatial resolution is determined by all, except

(a) Pixel size (b) Matrix size
(c) Type of detector (d) mAs

Ans. (a). *Textbook of Radiology for Residents & Technicians, 5th ed., S.K. Bhargava & Sumeet Bhargava, p. 478-479.*

360. Bit depth is

(a) Size of pixel
(b) Size of matrix
(c) Number of pixels/unit length
(d) Number of shades/pixel

Ans. (d). *Textbook of Radiology for Residents & Technicians, 5th ed., S.K. Bhargava & Sumeet Bhargava, p. 478-480.*

361. Minimum bit depth for gray scale and color scale are

(a) 4 & 2
(b) 8 & 2
(c) 8 & 24
(d) 2 & 8

Ans. (d). *Textbook of Radiology for Residents & Technicians, 5th ed., S.K. Bhargava & Sumeet Bhargava, p. 478-480.*

362. Conduction layer of phosphor plate is used to

(a) Protect phosphor layer
(b) Prevents light from erasing data
(c) Prevents problem due to static charge and increases image sharpness
(d) Improves X-ray to photon conversion

Ans. (c). *Textbook of Radiology for Residents & Technicians, 5th ed., S.K. Bhargava & Sumeet Bhargava, p. 580.*

363. Photon counting type DR is used in

(a) OPG
(b) Extremities
(c) Tomography
(d) Mammography

Ans. (d). *Textbook of Radiology for Residents & Technicians, 5th ed., S.K. Bhargava & Sumeet Bhargava, p. 584.*

364. DICOM is

(a) Digital Imaging and Computation in Medicine
(b) Digital Imaging and Communication in Mammography
(c) Diagnostic Imaging and Communication in Musculoskeletal Imaging
(d) Diagnostic Imaging and Communication in Medicine

Ans. (a). *Textbook of Radiology for Residents & Technicians, 5th ed., S.K. Bhargava & Sumeet Bhargava, p. 584.*

365. Smallest complete sample of an image is

(a) Detector
(b) Pixel
(c) Bit
(d) Byte

Ans. (b). *Textbook of Radiology for Residents & Technicians, 5th ed., S.K. Bhargava & Sumeet Bhargava, p. 476.*

366. Size of pixel in DR is

(a) 100–200 microns
(b) 10–20 microns.
(c) 500–600 microns
(d) 45–50 microns

Ans. (a). *Textbook of Radiology for Residents & Technicians, 5th ed., S.K. Bhargava & Sumeet Bhargava, p. 476-477.*

367. Basic unit of binary coded information is

(a) Bit
(b) Byte
(c) Kilobyte
(d) Megabyte

Ans. (b). *Textbook of Radiology for Residents & Technicians, 5th ed., S.K. Bhargava & Sumeet Bhargava, p. 476.*

368. Greater bits per pixel has got the advantage of

(a) Greater tones of gray/pixel
(b) Reduced resolution
(c) Larger field size
(d) Improved resolution

Ans. (c). *Textbook of Radiology for Residents & Technicians, 5th ed., S.K. Bhargava & Sumeet Bhargava, p. 479.*

369. An artifact is

(a) Unnecessary clinical feature in an image
(b) Useful but less important clinical feature in an image
(c) Feature which masks important clinical information in an image
(d) Annotation used in an image

Ans. (c). *Textbook of Radiology for Residents & Technicians, 5th ed., S.K. Bhargava & Sumeet Bhargava, p. 479.*

370. Grid use is not required with

(a) CR
(b) Conventional film screen
(c) Slot scan DR
(d) Structured phosphor plate

Ans. (c). *Textbook of Radiology for Residents & Technicians, 5th ed., S.K. Bhargava & Sumeet Bhargava, p. 583.*

371. Histogram errors can occur due to all, except

(a) Improper collimation
(b) Improper exposure
(c) Improper shield placement
(d) Single image per plate

Ans. (d). *Textbook of Radiology for Residents & Technicians, 5th ed., S.K. Bhargava & Sumeet Bhargava, p. 584.*

372. Halo effect occurs due to

(a) Inaccurate edge identification
(b) Inaccurate collimation edges
(c) Inaccurate edge enhancement
(d) Overlapping of edges of multiple images per plate

Ans. (a). *Textbook of Radiology for Residents & Technicians, 5th ed., S.K. Bhargava & Sumeet Bhargava, p. 641.*

373. For multiple images per plate following are required except

(a) Overlap of edges
(b) Appropriate radiographic technique of each view
(c) Clear boundaries between image and plate edge
(d) Symmetrical division of the plate

Ans. (a). *Textbook of Radiology for Residents & Technicians, 5th ed., S.K. Bhargava & Sumeet Bhargava, p. 584.*

374. Ghost images occur due to

(a) Faulty laser beam head
(b) Faulty CR plate
(c) Faulty detector element
(d) Improper light erasure of CR plate

Ans. (d). *Textbook of Radiology for Residents & Technicians, 5th ed., S.K. Bhargava & Sumeet Bhargava, p. 643.*

375. Differentiation of CR reader artifact from dirt are

(a) Reader artifacts are shorter in length
(b) Reader artifacts extends along entire plate
(c) Reader artifacts are sharp
(d) Reader artifacts are curved

Ans. (b). *Textbook of Radiology for Residents & Technicians, 5th ed., S.K. Bhargava & Sumeet Bhargava, p. 643.*

376. Grid frequency of CR grid is

(a) 100 lines/inch (b) 103 lines/inch
(c) 105 lines/inch (d) 33 lines/inch

Ans. (b). *Textbook of Radiology for Residents & Technicians, 5th ed., S.K. Bhargava & Sumeet Bhargava, p. 648.*

377. Artifacts due to mismatch of grid frequency and laser frequency are all except

(a) Aliasing artifact
(b) Moire artifact
(c) Quantum mottle
(d) Beam pattern

Ans. (c). *Textbook of Radiology for Residents & Technicians, 5th ed., S.K. Bhargava & Sumeet Bhargava, p. 648.*

378. Tendency of technologists for overexposure in DR is known as

(a) Exposure creep (b) Quantum sink
(c) Quantum mottle (d) Exposure failure

Ans. (a). *Textbook of Radiology for Residents & Technicians, 5th ed., S.K. Bhargava & Sumeet Bhargava, p. 641.*

379. Sedation in children during MRI is important as

(a) Create noise (b) Takes long time to scan
(c) Both (a) and (b) (d) None

Ans. (c). *A Guide to Radiological Procedures, Chapman, 4th ed., Chapman, p. 9.*

380. Children who are at high risk from sedation

(a) With airway obstruction or respiratory failure
(b) With raised intracranial pressure
(c) With severe renal or hepatic failure
(d) All of the above

Ans. (d). *A Guide to Radiological Procedures, Chapman, 4th ed., Chapman, p. 8.*

381. Double head gamma camera has advantage of

(a) Able to image two sites simultaneously
(b) Imaging time reduced to half
(c) Both (a) and (b)
(d) None

Ans. (c). *A Guide to Radiological Procedures, Chapman, 4th ed., Chapman, p. 15.*

382. Recent double headed gamma camera has

(a) Transmission line sources for measured attenuation correction.
(b) Coinicidence imaging system for PET
(c) Both (a) and (b)
(d) None

Ans. (c). *A Guide to Radiological Procedures, Chapman, 4th ed., Chapman, p. 15.*

383. Potential hazard in MRI are due to

(a) Magnetic field
(b) Auditory effect due to noise
(c) Claustrophobia
(d) All above

Ans. (d). *A Guide to Radiological Procedures, Chapman, 4th ed., Chapman, p. 18.*

384. Magnetic field in MRI

(a) Static field (b) Gradient field
(c) Radiofrequency field (d) Any of the above

Ans. (d). *A Guide to Radiological Procedures, Chapman, 4th ed., Chapman, p. 18.*

385. Which is true for static magnetic field in MRI
(a) No deleterious physiological effect
(b) Effect on ferromagnetic material
(c) Effect on electric field
(d) All of the above

Ans. (d). *A Guide to Radiological Procedures, Chapman, 4th ed., Chapman, p. 20.*

386. The noise arising in MRI during scanning depends on
(a) Strength of the magnetic field
(b) Pulse sequences
(c) Design
(d) All of the above

Ans. (d). *A Guide to Radiological Procedures, Chapman, 4th ed., Chapman, p. 21.*

387. For pelvic ultrasound, urinary bladder should be
(a) Empty
(b) Partially filled
(c) About 2/3rd filled
(d) Filled to full of its capacity

Ans. (d). *A Guide to Radiological Procedures, Chapman, 4th ed., Chapman, p. 24.*

388. PACS
(a) Pocket Adopter Computer System
(b) Picture Archiving and Computer System
(c) Picture Archiving and Communication System
(d) Printing And Copying System

Ans. (c). *Textbook of Radiology for Residents & Technicians, 5th ed., S.K. Bhargava & Sumeet Bhargava, p. 591-593.*

389. Interaction between the PACS and the imaging modalities are made possible by the development of the
(a) RIS
(b) HIS
(c) DICOM
(d) HL-7

Ans. (c). *Textbook of Radiology for Residents & Technicians, 5th ed., S.K. Bhargava & Sumeet Bhargava, p. 591-593.*

390. RAID
(a) Rapid Absorb Image Doses
(b) Rapid Acquisition Image Doses
(c) Random Array of In-expensive Doses
(d) None of the above

Ans. (c). *Textbook of Radiology for Residents & Technicians, 5th ed., S.K. Bhargava & Sumeet Bhargava, p. 591-593.*

391. ASP

(a) Analog Service Provider
(b) Application Service Provider
(c) Automatic Service Provider
(d) None of the above

Ans. (b). *Textbook of Radiology for Residents & Technicians, 5th ed., S.K. Bhargava & Sumeet Bhargava, p. 591-593.*

392. _______ resolutions are required for CT, MRI, USG and DR.

(a) 1 K (b) 2 K
(c) 5 K (d) 10 K

Ans. (a). *Textbook of Radiology for Residents & Technicians, 5th ed., S.K. Bhargava & Sumeet Bhargava, p. 474-480.*

393. What are the main component of PACS?

(a) Digitization (b) Memory
(c) Network (d) All of the above

Ans. (d). *Textbook of Radiology for Residents & Technicians, 5th ed., S.K. Bhargava & Sumeet Bhargava, p. 591-593.*

394. Local Area Network (LAN) are devices connected by

(a) Cable (b) Router
(c) Telecommunication devices (d) Ring

Ans. (a). *Textbook of Radiology for Residents & Technicians, 5th ed., S.K. Bhargava & Sumeet Bhargava, p. 591-593.*

395. Wide Area Network (WAN) devices are connected by

(a) Cable (b) Router
(c) Telecommunication devices (d) Ring

Ans. (c). *Textbook of Radiology for Residents & Technicians, 5th ed., S.K. Bhargava & Sumeet Bhargava, p. 591-593.*

396. The first 'film less' radiology department appeared in the

(a) 1980 (b) 1972
(c) 1990 (d) 1985

Ans. (c). *Textbook of Radiology for Residents & Technicians, 5th ed., S.K. Bhargava & Sumeet Bhargava, p. 591-593.*

397. Luminescence centre/activator in PSP is

(a) GdO_2S_2 (b) BaFBr
(c) Eu (d) BaFI

Ans. (b). *Textbook of Radiology for Residents & Technicians, 5th ed., S.K. Bhargava & Sumeet Bhargava, p. 578-586.*

398. Energy of laser beams required to read latent image is of the order of

(a) 4 eV
(b) 6 eV
(c) 5 eV
(d) 2 eV

Ans. (d). *Textbook of Radiology for Residents & Technicians, 5th ed., S.K. Bhargava & Sumeet Bhargava, p. 578-586.*

399. Characteristic curve of PSP is

(a) Linear wide latitude
(b) Non-linear wide latitude
(c) Linear narrow latitude
(d) Non-linear narrow latitude

Ans. (a). *Textbook of Radiology for Residents & Technicians, 5th ed., S.K. Bhargava & Sumeet Bhargava, p. 591-593.*

400. Over-exposure is difficult to detect in CR due to

(a) Post-processing
(b) Quantum mottle
(c) Poor image quality
(d) Plate readout by laser beam

Ans. (a). *Textbook of Radiology for Residents & Technicians, 5th ed., S.K. Bhargava & Sumeet Bhargava, p. 576-586.*

401. First PSP device implemented in US by

(a) Philips in 1983
(b) Kodak in 1975
(c) Fuji in 1960
(d) Agfa in 1990

Ans. (a). *Textbook of Radiology for Residents & Technicians, 5th ed., S.K. Bhargava & Sumeet Bhargava, p. 576-586.*

402. Digital radiography differs from computed radiography in

(a) Reduced radiation exposure
(b) Digitization of image
(c) Combined image capture and readout capability
(d) Reduced retakes

Ans. (c). *Textbook of Radiology for Residents & Technicians, 5th ed., S.K. Bhargava & Sumeet Bhargava, p. 576-586.*

403. Which of these is not a direct DR system

(a) Flat panel detector
(b) Charged coupled device
(c) Slot scanning type
(d) Photon counting type

Ans. (b). *Textbook of Radiology for Residents & Technicians, 5th ed., S.K. Bhargava & Sumeet Bhargava, p. 474-480.*

404. First DR systems appeared in

(a) 1983
(b) 1975
(c) 1990
(d) 2000

Ans. (c). *Textbook of Radiology for Residents & Technicians, 5th ed., S.K. Bhargava & Sumeet Bhargava, p. 474-480.*

405. First DR system was of

(a) CCD type
(b) FPD type
(c) Photon counting type
(d) PSP type

Ans. (a). *Textbook of Radiology for Residents & Technicians, 5th ed., S.K. Bhargava & Sumeet Bhargava, p. 474-480.*

406. In digital radiography, spatial resolution is determined by all except

(a) Pixel size
(b) Matrix size
(c) Type of detector
(d) mAs

Ans. (a). *Textbook of Radiology for Residents & Technicians, 5th ed., S.K. Bhargava & Sumeet Bhargava, p. 474-480 and 578-586.*

407. Size of pixel in DR is

(a) 100–200 microns
(b) 10–40 microns
(c) 500–800 microns
(d) 1000–1200 microns

Ans. (a). *Textbook of Radiology for Residents & Technicians, 5th ed., S.K. Bhargava & Sumeet Bhargava, p. 578-586.*

408. Basic unit of binary coded information is

(a) Bit
(b) Byte
(c) Kilobyte
(d) Megabyte

Ans. (b). *Textbook of Radiology for Residents & Technicians, 5th ed., S.K. Bhargava & Sumeet Bhargava, p. 578-586.*

409. Halo effect occurs due to

(a) Inaccurate edge identification
(b) Inaccurate collimation edges
(c) Inaccurate edge enhancement
(d) Overlapping of edges of multiple images per plate

Ans. (c). *Textbook of Radiology for Residents & Technicians, 5th ed., S.K. Bhargava & Sumeet Bhargava, p. 578-586.*

410. Ghost images occur due to

(a) Faulty laser beam head
(b) Faulty CR plate
(c) Faulty detector element
(d) Improper light eraser of CR plate

Ans. (d). *Textbook of Radiology for Residents & Technicians, 5th ed., S.K. Bhargava & Sumeet Bhargava, p. 578-586.*

411. Grid frequency of CR grid is

(a) 80 lines/inch
(b) 103 lines/inch
(c) 140 lines/inch
(d) 33 lines/inch

Ans. (b). Textbook of Radiology for Residents & Technicians, 5th ed., S.K. Bhargava & Sumeet Bhargava, p. 578-586.

412. For comparable image mottle, which has the highest patient dose?

(a) Screen film
(b) Photostimulable phosphor
(c) Direct flat panel detector
(d) Digital photospot

Ans. (b). Textbook of Radiology for Residents & Technicians, 5th ed., S.K. Bhargava & Sumeet Bhargava, p. 578-586.

413. The matrix size in a DSA image is typically

(a) 128 × 128
(b) 512 × 512
(c) 256 × 256
(d) 1024 × 1024

Ans. (d). Textbook of Radiology for Residents & Technicians, 5th ed., S.K. Bhargava & Sumeet Bhargava, p. 611-621.

414. DSA image acquisition normally do not make use of

(a) High voltages
(b) Low noise TV system
(c) 2 LP/mm resolution
(d) 2 micro Gy/frame

Ans. (a). Textbook of Radiology for Residents & Technicians, 5th ed., S.K. Bhargava & Sumeet Bhargava, p. 611-621.

415. The most important component affecting spatial resolution in DSA is the

(a) Focal spot size
(b) Image intensifier input phosphor thickness
(c) Image intensifier output phosphor thickness
(d) Digitization matrix

Ans. (d). Textbook of Radiology for Residents & Technicians, 5th ed., S.K. Bhargava & Sumeet Bhargava, p. 611-621.

416. How many bits are present in 1 byte?

(a) Eight
(b) Sixteen
(c) One
(d) Nine

Ans. (a). Textbook of Radiology for Residents & Technicians, 5th ed., S.K. Bhargava & Sumeet Bhargava, p. 611-621.

417. A limiting resolution of digital imaging is approximately

(a) 1 LP/mm
(b) 10 LP/mm
(c) 5 LP/mm
(d) 0.05 LP/mm

Ans. (c). Textbook of Radiology for Residents & Technicians, 5th ed., S.K. Bhargava & Sumeet Bhargava, p. 578-586.

418. Which is the most common photoconductor used in digital radiography?

(a) Gadolinium oxysulphide (b) Cesium iodide
(c) Barium fluorohalide (d) Selenium

Ans. (d). *Textbook of Radiology for Residents & Technicians, 5th ed., S.K. Bhargava & Sumeet Bhargava, p. 578-586.*

419. The limiting spatial resolution is also known as
(a) Aliasing (b) Nyquist frequency
(c) Aperture (d) Contrast to noise ratio

Ans. (b). *Textbook of Radiology for Residents & Technicians, 5th ed., S.K. Bhargava & Sumeet Bhargava, p. 578-586.*

420. In CR system, at room temperature, the image should, however, be readable up to _____ after exposure.
(a) 4 hr (b) 24 hr
(c) 12 hr (d) 8 hr

Ans. (d). *Textbook of Radiology for Residents & Technicians, 5th ed., S.K. Bhargava & Sumeet Bhargava, p. 578-586.*

421. In which technique, detector system remains stationary while X-ray tube moves in an arc during multiple low dose exposures given from various angles?
(a) Dual energy imaging (b) Automatic image stitching
(c) Mobile DR (d) Tomosynthesis

Ans. (d). *Textbook of Radiology for Residents & Technicians, 5th ed., S.K. Bhargava & Sumeet Bhargava, p. 622-625.*

422. Dual energy imaging is very useful in
(a) Chest radiography (b) Head radiography
(c) Hip radiography (d) Joint radiography

Ans. (a). *Textbook of Radiology for Residents & Technicians, 5th ed., S.K. Bhargava & Sumeet Bhargava, p. 372-407.*

423. Digital mammography biopsy system makes use of
(a) Fiberoptic coupled (b) Large screen with TFT
(c) Small screen with TFT (d) None of the above

Ans. (a). *Textbook of Radiology for Residents & Technicians, 5th ed., S.K. Bhargava & Sumeet Bhargava, p. 259-326.*

424. Dual energy subtraction technique uses
(a) Low energy (b) High energy
(c) Medium energy (d) Both (a) and (b)

Ans. (d). *Textbook of Radiology for Residents & Technicians, 5th ed., S.K. Bhargava & Sumeet Bhargava, p. 474-480.*

425. Alternative to conventional image intensifier

(a) Use optical coupling (b) Use 2D array detectors
(c) Use 3D array detectors (d) All of the above

Ans. (a). Textbook of Radiology for Residents & Technicians, 5th ed., S.K. Bhargava & Sumeet Bhargava, p. 434-480.

RECENT ADVANCES

426. Film screen radiography is preferred due to

(a) Familiar with higher comfort level and confidence
(b) Cheaper as compare to digital
(c) Easy to pinpoint the cause of poor quality of the film
(d) All of the above

Ans. (d). Textbook of Radiology for Residents & Technicians, 5th ed., S.K. Bhargava & Sumeet Bhargava, p. 578.

427. Limitation of film screen mammography are

(a) Limited exposure latitude, less detail and contrast.
(b) Artifacts more common due to chemical processing.
(c) True magnification not possible.
(d) All of the above

Ans. (d). Textbook of Radiology for Residents & Technicians, 5th ed., S.K. Bhargava & Sumeet Bhargava, p. 298.

428. Film screen mammography has following limitation

(a) Film quality deteriorates with time
(b) Repeat X-ray hence more radiation
(c) All aspects like acquisition, display and storage not separable
(d) All of the above

Ans. (d). Textbook of Radiology for Residents & Technicians, 5th ed., S.K. Bhargava & Sumeet Bhargava, p. 298.

429. Advantages of digital radiography is

(a) Better contrast as images can be manipulated
(b) Quick display, storage, and retrieval
(c) Decrease repeat rate
(d) All of the above

Ans. (d). Textbook of Radiology for Residents & Technicians, 5th ed., S.K. Bhargava,p. 583.

430. In CR the photostimulable phosphor is made-up of

(a) Europiam-activated barium fluorohalide (Ba Fx Ev^{2+})
(b) Calcium tungstate activated in silver

(c) Zn Cd sulphide
(d) None of these

Ans. (a). *Textbook of Radiology for Residents & Technicians, 5th ed., S.K. Bhargava & Sumeet Bhargava, p. 580.*

431. The advantages of CR system are
(a) More latitude, better quality, and thus less repetition
(b) Consistant image density and contrast
(c) Simultaneous availability of Images at different places
(d) All of the above

Ans. (d). *Textbook of Radiology for Residents & Technicians, 5th ed., S.K. Bhargava & Sumeet Bhargava, p. 581.*

432. Limitation of digital radiography systems are
(a) High cost of the equipment
(b) Image enhancement not proper
(c) Radiation dose and film density relation no longer valid
(d) All of the above

Ans. (d). *Textbook of Radiology for Residents & Technicians, 5th ed., S.K. Bhargava & Sumeet Bhargava, p. 582.*

433. Digital image storage has advantages of
(a) Rapid storage and retrieval
(b) Less physical storage
(c) Ability to copy and duplicate without loss of quality
(d) All of the above

Ans. (d). *Textbook of Radiology for Residents & Technicians, 5th ed., S.K. Bhargava & Sumeet Bhargava, p. 582.*

434. The advantages of the digital image storage are
(a) Good communication and networking
(b) Display and adjust of the optimum contrast
(c) Both (a) and (b)
(d) None of these

Ans. (c). *Textbook of Radiology for Residents & Technicians, 5th ed., S.K. Bhargava & Sumeet Bhargava, p. 583.*

435. Advantages of digital radiography system is
(a) Quality control of the images are good so less repetition
(b) Work flow increased, thus saving time and labour
(c) Radiation dose is less
(d) All of the above

Ans. (d). *Textbook of Radiology for Residents & Technicians, 5th ed., S.K. Bhargava & Sumeet Bhargava, p. 582.*

436. The digital radiography system has following advantages
- (a) Preset available for various anatomical studies including optimized post processing e.g. chest and spine
- (b) Various selectors for filters, focal spots etc. are available
- (c) Motion blur eliminated because of short exposure time
- (d) All of the above

Ans. (d). *Textbook of Radiology for Residents & Technicians, 5th ed., S.K. Bhargava & Sumeet Bhargava, p. 582.*

437. Diagnostic radiography system has following disadvantages
- (a) Fragile detectors so handle carefully
- (b) High initial cost
- (c) Some radiographic views not possible as detectors can not be placed in all places
- (d) All of the above

Ans. (d). *Textbook of Radiology for Residents & Technicians, 5th ed., S.K. Bhargava & Sumeet Bhargava, p. 582.*

438. 100% of fill factor is available in
- (a) Direct X-ray conversion type of Flat Panel Detector (FPD)
- (b) Indirect X-ray conversion type of Flat Panel Detector (FPD)
- (c) Both (a) and (b)
- (c) None of these

Ans. (a). *Textbook of Radiology for Residents & Technicians, 5th ed., S.K. Bhargava & Sumeet Bhargava, p. 583.*

439. Amorphous selenium substance is used in detector in
- (a) Flat Panel Detector (FPD) based system (direct X-ray conversion type)
- (b) Flat Panel Detector (FPD) based system (indirect X-ray conversion type)
- (c) Both (a) and (b)
- (d) None of these

Ans. (a). *Textbook of Radiology for Residents & Technicians, 5th ed., S.K. Bhargava & Sumeet Bhargava, p. 583.*

440. Thallium doped cesium iodide or gadolinium oxysulphide are used as phosphores in
- (a) Flat Panel Detector (FPD) based system (Direct X-ray conversion type)
- (b) Flat Panel Detector (FPD) based system (Indirect X-ray conversion type)
- (c) Photon counting type D.R. system
- (d) None of these

Ans. (b). Textbook of Radiology for Residents & Technicians, 5th ed., S.K. Bhargava & Sumeet Bhargava, p. 585.

441. Dual energy imaging is possible with

(a) DR system
(b) CR system
(c) None of these
(d) Both (a) and (b)

Ans. (a). Textbook of Radiology for Residents & Technicians, 5th ed., S.K. Bhargava & Sumeet Bhargava, p. 584.

442. Tomosynthesis is possible with

(a) D.R. system
(b) C.R. system
(c) None of these
(d) Both (a) and (b)

Ans. (a). Textbook of Radiology for Residents & Technicians, 5th ed., S.K. Bhargava & Sumeet Bhargava, p. 584.

443. Maximum Digital Quantum Efficiency (DQE) is available with detectors made-up of

(a) Brusidium chloride or barium fluorohalides doped with europium
(b) Thallium doped cesium iodide
(c) Amorphous selenium
(d) None of the above

Ans. (a). Textbook of Radiology for Residents & Technicians, 5th ed., S.K. Bhargava & Sumeet Bhargava, p. 380.

444. Attenuation i.e. reduction in intensity of X-ray beam (reducing the number of photons) is due to

(a) Absorption
(b) Compression
(c) Scattering
(d) None

Ans. (a). Textbook of Radiology for Residents & Technicians, 5th ed., S.K. Bhargava & Sumeet Bhargava, p. 589-590.

445. Attenuation is effected by

(a) Radiation energy i.e. electron per gram of matter
(b) Density of the matter
(c) Atomic number of the matter
(d) All of the above

Ans. (a). Textbook of Radiology for Residents & Technicians, 5th ed., S.K. Bhargava & Sumeet Bhargava, p. 589-590.

446. Elastography in ultrasound machine observes the principle of

(a) Relaxation properties of the tissue
(b) Atomic number of the tissue
(c) Both (a) and (b)
(d) None of these

Ans. (a). *Textbook of Radiology for Residents & Technicians, 5th ed., S.K. Bhargava & Sumeet Bhargava, p. 594.*

447. In radiofrequency ablation, the requirement is
(a) Tissue temperature rises above 113°F (50°C)
(b) Time required is less than 10–15 mts.
(c) Size of the tissue 2–3 cm.
(d) All of the above

Ans. (d). *Textbook of Radiology for Residents & Technicians, 5th ed., S.K. Bhargava & Sumeet Bhargava, p. 603-610.*

448. Radiofrequency Ablation (RFA) can be performed by
(a) Percutaneous approach (b) Laparoscopic approach
(c) Open approach (d) All of the above

Ans. (d). *Textbook of Radiology for Residents & Technicians, 5th ed., S.K. Bhargava & Sumeet Bhargava, p. 603-610.*

449. Benefits of the RFA are
(a) Decreased cost and morbidity
(b) Possibility of the performing the procedure in outpatient.
(c) Treating patient not considered fit for surgery, due to age, comfort or extent of the disease
(d) All of the above

Ans. (d). *Textbook of Radiology for Residents & Technicians, 5th ed., S.K. Bhargava & Sumeet Bhargava, p. 603-610.*

450. RFA not useful in patients with
(a) Bile duct or major vessel invasion
(b) Extra hepatic disease
(c) Child with cirrhosis or active infection
(d) All of the above

Ans. (d). *Textbook of Radiology for Residents & Technicians, 5th ed., S.K. Bhargava & Sumeet Bhargava, p. 603-610.*

451. RFA not indicated when
(a) Tumor occupy more than 40% of the volume of the liver
(b) Lesion larger than 5 cm
(c) Metastatic tumor more than 3 cm or more than 3 in number
(d) All of the above

Ans. (d). *Textbook of Radiology for Residents & Technicians, 5th ed., S.K. Bhargava & Sumeet Bhargava, p. 603-610.*

452. Angiography is a procedure
(a) Utilizes the use of catheter to enter the vessel

(b) Contrast to inject to make the artery/vein visible
(c) Visualization of vessels to diagnose blockage and other vessel problem
(d) All of the above

Ans. (d). *Textbook of Radiology for Residents & Technicians, 5th ed., S.K. Bhargava & Sumeet Bhargava, p. 611.*

453. Digital image intensifiers and flat panel detectors technology technique is utilized in interventional radiology as it provide

(a) Film less environment
(b) Has capability to store images easily in PACS and picture achieving
(c) Increase image quality and reduce radiation dose to the patient.
(d) All of the above

Ans. (d). *Textbook of Radiology for Residents & Technicians, 5th ed., S.K. Bhargava & Sumeet Bhargava, p. 612.*

454. The fixed flat panel detector system in fluoroscopy during interventional radiology has advantages over conventional image intensifier

(a) Less radiation
(b) Approximately 40% more coverage with larger field of view
(c) Dynamic range is 5–10 times greater
(d) All of the above

Ans. (d). *Textbook of Radiology for Residents & Technicians, 5th ed., S.K. Bhargava & Sumeet Bhargava, p. 612.*

455. The advantages of fixed flat panel detector system in fluoroscopy over conventional image intensifier are

(a) Better and improved visualization of vasculature
(b) Contrast agent utilization reduced by approx. 30%
(c) Both (a) and (b)
(d) None of these

Ans. (c). *Textbook of Radiology for Residents & Technicians, 5th ed., S.K. Bhargava & Sumeet Bhargava, p. 283.*

456. Digital tomosynthesis utilizes restructuring of multiple Tomographic images from the data acquired during

(a) Isocenteric Rotational (IR) motion of the gantry
(b) Linear motion of the tube
(c) Both (a) and (b)
(d) None of these

Ans. (a). *Textbook of Radiology for Residents & Technicians, 5th ed., S.K. Bhargava & Sumeet Bhargava, p. 584.*

457. Digital tomosynthesis has advantage

(a) Study time is short so less radiation
(b) Acquired digitalized image can be enhanced through manipulation of window and display
(c) The technique can be applied for dynamic study
(d) All of the Above

Ans. (d). *Textbook of Radiology for Residents & Technicians, 5th ed., S.K. Bhargava & Sumeet Bhargava, p. 584.*

458. Limitation of digital tomography are

(a) Limited field of view
(b) Low spatial and contrast resolution
(c) Geometric magnification and pin-cushion distortion
(d) All of the above

Ans. (d). *Textbook of Radiology for Residents & Technicians, 5th ed., S.K. Bhargava & Sumeet Bhargava, p. 584.*

459. Disadvantages of the PET are

(a) No anatomical detail
(b) Large number of false positive and false negative results
(c) Difficult to differentiate lesions from areas of normal physiological uptake
(d) All of the above

Ans. (d). *Textbook of Radiology for Residents & Technicians, 5th ed., S.K. Bhargava & Sumeet Bhargava, p. 626.*

460. The advantages of the PET-CT are

(a) Increase both sensitivity and specificity
(b) Minimal/Subtle disease/equivocal CT images can be detected.
(c) Hybrid scanner utilizes more accurate tumor
(d) All of the above

Ans. (d). *Textbook of Radiology for Residents & Technicians, 5th ed., S.K. Bhargava & Sumeet Bhargava, p. 626.*

461. PET-CT has following disadvantages

(a) More ionizing radiation
(b) Focal physiological uptake from large or small bowel malignancy
(c) Residual tumor from post-therapy chances immediately after surgery or radiotherapy
(d) All of the above

Ans. (d). *Textbook of Radiology for Residents & Technicians, 5th ed., S.K. Bhargava & Sumeet Bhargava, p. 626.*

462. PET-MRI has advantages
(a) Almost no radiation
(b) Specific molecular, enzymes and gene suppression
(c) High sensitivity
(d) All of the above

Ans. (d). *Textbook of Radiology for Residents & Technicians, 5th ed., S.K. Bhargava & Sumeet Bhargava, p. 629.*

463. In condenser discharge mobile equipment, does kV_p has following changes during exposure
(a) Increases
(b) Decreases
(c) No change
(d) Fluctuate

Ans. (b). *Textbook of Radiology for Residents & Technicians, 5th ed., S.K. Bhargava & Sumeet Bhargava, p. 118.*

464. Which of the following equipment shows decrease in kV_p during actual length of exposure?
(a) Fixed X-ray units
(b) Battery operated mobile units
(c) Condenser discharge mobile equipments
(d) CT scan equipments

Ans. (c). *Textbook of Radiology for Residents & Technicians, 5th ed., S.K. Bhargava & Sumeet Bhargava, p. 118.*

465. Capacitor discharge mobile X-rays equipment has
(a) Light weight
(b) Large size
(c) High kVp
(d) High mAs

Ans. (a). *Textbook of Radiology for Residents & Technicians, 5th ed., S.K. Bhargava & Sumeet Bhargava, p. 111.*

466. Full form of PACS is
(a) Picture and Associated Communication Set-up
(b) Picture Archiving and Communicating Systems
(c) Poster and Sign Set-up
(d) Processing and Cutting System

Ans. (b). *Textbook of Radiology for Residents & Technicians, 5th ed., S.K. Bhargava & Sumeet Bhargava, p. 591-593.*

467. The benefits of the PACS include
(a) Security of the image storage
(b) Elimination of the film stores
(c) Better availability of the images
(d) All of the above

Ans. (d). Textbook of Radiology for Residents & Technicians, 5th ed., S.K. Bhargava & Sumeet Bhargava, p. 591-593.

468. The standard used in PACS is

(a) Analog (b) DICOM
(c) Windows (d) Office

Ans. (b). Textbook of Radiology for Residents & Technicians, 5th ed., S.K. Bhargava & Sumeet Bhargava, p. 591-593.

469. The PACS workflow manager from the archieve can

(a) Send the image (b) Retrieve the image
(c) Both of the above (d) None of the above

Ans. (c). Textbook of Radiology for Residents & Technicians, 5th ed., S.K. Bhargava & Sumeet Bhargava, p. 591-593.

470. Service class user functions required on imaging modalities are

(a) Modality push (b) Modality pull
(c) Print service (d) All of the above

Ans. (d). Textbook of Radiology for Residents & Technicians, 5th ed., S.K.Bhargava, p. 591-593.

MAMMOGRAPHY

471. The target in mammography is made of

(a) Tungsten (b) Molybdenum
(c) Copper (d) Aluminium

Ans. (b). Textbook of Radiology for Residents & Technicians, 5th ed., S.K. Bhargava & Sumeet Bhargava, p. 297.

472. The filter used in mammography can be

(a) Molybdenum (b) Rhodium
(c) Any of the above (d) None of the above

Ans. (c). Textbook of Radiology for Residents & Technicians, 5th ed., S.K. Bhargava & Sumeet Bhargava, p. 295.

473. The energy level of X-rays used in mammography is

(a) Low energy (b) High energy
(c) Very high energy (d) None of the above

Ans. (a). Textbook of Radiology for Residents & Technicians, 5th ed., S.K. Bhargava & Sumeet Bhargava, p. 295.

474. Films used in mammography are

(a) Single emulsion (b) Double emulsion

(c) Triple emulsion
(d) None of the above

Ans. (a). Textbook of Radiology for Residents & Technicians, 5th ed., S.K. Bhargava & Sumeet Bhargava, p. 172.

475. The screens used in mammography are made of

(a) Calcium tungstate
(b) Iron oxide
(c) Silver halide
(d) Rare earth screen

Ans. (d). Textbook of Radiology for Residents & Technicians, 5th ed., S.K. Bhargava & Sumeet Bhargava, p. 172.

476. Focal spot size for mammography is

(a) 0.5–1 mm
(b) 1–2 mm
(c) 2–3 mm
(d) 0.1–0.4 mm

Ans. (d). Textbook of Radiology for Residents & Technicians, 5th ed., S.K. Bhargava & Sumeet Bhargava, p. 297.

477. Operating potential in mammography are in the range of

(a) 100–200 Kv
(b) 50–100 Kv
(c) 10–20 Kv
(d) 24–35 Kv

Ans. (d). Textbook of Radiology for Residents & Technicians, 5th ed., S.K. Bhargava & Sumeet Bhargava, p. 297.

478. By compression, the dose to the breast tissue is

(a) Reduced
(b) Increased
(c) No change
(d) Initially increases then decreases

Ans. (a). Textbook of Radiology for Residents & Technicians, 5th ed., S.K. Bhargava & Sumeet Bhargava, p. 297.

479. Exposure times for mammography when compared to conventional radiography are

(a) Same
(b) Shorter
(c) Longer
(d) Any of the above

Ans. (c). Textbook of Radiology for Residents & Technicians, 5th ed., S.K. Bhargava & Sumeet Bhargava, p. 297.

480. The average absorbed dose to the glandular tissue per film in mammography is

(a) 5–10 mGy
(b) 1.5–3 mGy
(c) 10–15 mGy
(d) 15–20 mGy

Ans. (b). Textbook of Radiology for Residents & Technicians, 5th ed., S.K.Bhargava, p. 297.

481. The following are true of mammographic equipment

(a) The focal spot size is fixed. (False)
(b) The size of the air can be altered. (True)
(c) Target is made-up of aluminium. (False)
(d) Grids are not used in mammography. (False)
(e) The X-ray tube is made-up from glass. (True)

482. Regarding the film-screen combinations used in mammography

(a) Double emulsion film is used to improve resolution. (False)
(b) A single screen is used. (True)
(c) A vacuum is applied to ensure good film/grid contact. (False)
(d) Films with high gamma are used. (True)
(e) Films with wide exposure latitude are used to detect as much pathology as possible. (False)

483. Regarding compression in mammography

(a) Compression is mandatory in all patients having mammography. (False)
(b) Compression reduces object-film distance. (True)
(c) Compression results in good immobilization of the breast. (True)
(d) Compression is necessary as mammography is a relatively short exposure. (False)
(e) Compression increases geometrical unsharpness. (False)

484. Concerning mammography

(a) The dose is so low that there is no risk of breast cancer. (False)
(b) The mean dose to the average breast should be less than 2.5 mGy. per exposure. (True)
(c) K-edge filters are used. (True)
(d) A molybdenum filter cannot be used when a molybdenum target is used. (False)
(e) A molybdenum filter can not be used when rhodium target is used. (True)

485. Concerning mammography

(a) The anode heel effect is harmful. (False)
(b) An automated exposure control is utilized in mammography. (True)
(c) A molybdenum target with a molybdenum filter is typically used to image large breasts. (False)
(d) Typical resolution in film/screen mammography is between 15–20 line pairs/mm. (True)
(e) A tungsten target with a rhodium filter is used to image small breasts. (False)

486. Concerning mammographic equipment

(a) Source image distance is 75 cm. (True)

(b) Window is made of beryllium. (True)
(c) Fast screens are used in mammography. (False)
(d) Operating potential in mammography is 25–35 kV. (True)
(e) Focal spot size in mammography is 1–2 mm. (False)

487. Concerning radiation dose in mammography

(a) The radiation dose is quoted in terms of the effective dose. (False)
(b) The radiation dose is measured in mGy. (False)
(c) The glandular tissue in the breast is the most sensitive to radiation. (True)
(d) Radiation dose is reduced by compression. (True)
(e) Radiation dose in mammography is lower than chest X-ray. (False)

488. Which tissue is most sensitive to cancer by radiation?

(a) Fibrous tissue (b) Glandular tissue
(c) Adipose tissue (d) Connective tissue

Ans. (b). *Textbook of Radiology for Residents & Technicians, 5th ed., S.K. Bhargava & Sumeet Bhargava, p. 259-326.*

489. Low kV_P is used in mammography to maximize the

(a) Compton scattering (b) Photoelectric absorption
(c) Coherent (d) Both (a) and (b)

Ans. (b). *Textbook of Radiology for Residents & Technicians, 5th ed., S.K. Bhargava & Sumeet Bhargava, p. 259-326.*

490. X-ray mammography requires a

(a) Low kV_p, low mAs (b) Low kV_p, high mAs
(c) High kV_p, low mAs (d) High kV_p, high mAs

Ans. (b). *Textbook of Radiology for Residents & Technicians, 5th ed., S.K. Bhargava & Sumeet Bhargava, p. 259-326.*

491. The X-rays most useful for enhancing differential absorption in breast tissue and for maximizing radiographic contrast are those in the range of

(a) 17 to 25 keV (b) 17 to 35 kV_p
(c) 20 to 40 kV_p (d) 15 to 60 keV

Ans. (a). *Textbook of Radiology for Residents & Technicians, 5th ed., S.K. Bhargava & Sumeet Bhargava, p. 259-326.*

492. Molybdenum has an atomic number of

(a) 74 (b) 89
(c) 42 (d) 37

Ans. (c). *Textbook of Radiology for Residents & Technicians, 5th ed., S.K. Bhargava & Sumeet Bhargava, p. 259-326.*

493. Imaging of micro-calcification requires

(a) Dual focal spots
(b) Large focal spots
(c) Small focal spots
(d) Both (b) and (c)

Ans. (c). *Textbook of Radiology for Residents & Technicians, 5th ed., S.K. Bhargava & Sumeet Bhargava, p. 259-326.*

494. In mammography unit, the positioning of the cathode is usually preferred towards

(a) The nipple side
(b) Near the chest wall
(c) Between nipple and chest wall
(d) Both (a) and (b)

Ans. (b). *Textbook of Radiology for Residents & Technicians, 5th ed., S.K. Bhargava & Sumeet Bhargava, p. 259-326.*

495. Image quality is improved with

(a) High kV_p technique
(b) Low mAs technique
(c) Compression
(d) Both (a) and (b)

Ans. (c). *Textbook of Radiology for Residents & Technicians, 5th ed., S.K. Bhargava & Sumeet Bhargava, p. 259-326.*

496. Compression improves

(a) Spatial resolution
(b) Vontrast resolution
(c) Reduces patient dose
(d) All of the above

Ans. (d). *Textbook of Radiology for Residents & Technicians, 5th ed., S.K. Bhargava & Sumeet Bhargava, p. 259-326.*

497. Most common grid ratios preferred in mammography are

(a) 12 : 1 to 14 : 1
(b) 4 : 1 to 5 : 1
(c) 8 : 1 to 12 : 1
(d) 6 : 1 to 9 : 1

Ans. (b). *Textbook of Radiology for Residents & Technicians, 5th ed., S.K. Bhargava & Sumeet Bhargava, p. 259-326.*

498. Grid frequencies for the moving grid are typical of

(a) 40 lines/cm
(b) 25 lines/m
(c) 90 lines/cm
(d) 72 lines/mm

Ans. (a). *Textbook of Radiology for Residents & Technicians, 5th ed., S.K. Bhargava & Sumeet Bhargava, p. 259-326.*

499. In mammography unit, shorter object-to-image receptor distance (OID) results in

(a) Reduced radiation dose
(b) Improved contrast resolution
(c) Improved spatial resolution

(d) Reduced motion blur

Ans. (c). *Textbook of Radiology for Residents & Technicians, 5th ed., S.K. Bhargava & Sumeet Bhargava, p. 259-326.*

500. AEC

(a) Automatic Enhancement Controller
(b) Automatic Exposure Control
(c) Applied Exposure Centre
(d) None of the above

Ans. (b). *Textbook of Radiology for Residents & Technicians, 5th ed., S.K. Bhargava & Sumeet Bhargava, p. 259-326.*

501. AEC are positioned

(a) Front to the image receptor
(b) Behind the image receptor
(c) Behind the patient body
(d) Front to the patient body

Ans. (b). *Textbook of Radiology for Residents & Technicians, 5th ed., S.K. Bhargava & Sumeet Bhargava, p. 259-326.*

502. The purpose of magnification mammography is to investigate

(a) Microcalcification
(b) Macrocalcification
(c) Malignancy
(d) Retromammary adipose tissue

Ans. (a). *Textbook of Radiology for Residents & Technicians, 5th ed., S.K. Bhargava & Sumeet Bhargava, p. 259-326.*

503. ________ X-ray tube window is used to minimize C-ray beam attenuation.

(a) Aluminium
(b) Lead
(c) Molybdenum
(d) Beryllium

Ans. (d). *Textbook of Radiology for Residents & Technicians, 5th ed., S.K. Bhargava & Sumeet Bhargava, p. 259-326.*

504. Grids are commonly used to

(a) Minimize patient dose
(b) Maximize image quality
(c) To achieve small focal spot
(d) Both (a) and (b)

Ans. (b). *Textbook of Radiology for Residents & Technicians, 5th ed., S.K. Bhargava & Sumeet Bhargava, p. 259-326.*

505. Optical film densities in mammography are between

(a) 15 to 20
(b) 0.05 to 0.2
(c) 3 to 8
(d) 1.5 to 2.0

Ans. (d). *Textbook of Radiology for Residents & Technicians, 5th ed., S.K. Bhargava & Sumeet Bhargava, p. 259-326.*

506. Compression is achieved by using

(a) Translucent paddles
(b) Translucent binder
(c) Nylon cloth
(d) Both (b) and (c)

Ans. (a). *Textbook of Radiology for Residents & Technicians, 5th ed., S.K. Bhargava & Sumeet Bhargava, p. 259-326.*

507. A typical source to image distance in mammography is

(a) 100 cm
(b) 180 cm
(c) 65 cm
(d) 40 cm

Ans. (c). *Textbook of Radiology for Residents & Technicians, 5th ed., S.K. Bhargava & Sumeet Bhargava, p. 259-326.*

508. In breast, most sensitive tissue to cancer by radiation is

(a) Adipose tissue
(b) Glandular tissue
(c) Fibrous tissue
(d) Nervous tissue

Ans. (b). *Textbook of Radiology for Residents & Technicians, 5th ed., S.K. Bhargava & Sumeet Bhargava, p. 259-326.*

509. Film used in mammography are

(a) Single emulsion
(b) Double emulsion
(c) Duplicating film
(d) Without emulsion

Ans. (a). *Textbook of Radiology for Residents & Technicians, 5th ed., S.K. Bhargava & Sumeet Bhargava, p. 259-326.*

510. The screens used in mammography are made of

(a) Calcium tungstate
(b) Iron oxide
(c) Silver halide
(d) Rare earth screen

Ans. (d). *Textbook of Radiology for Residents & Technicians, 5th ed., S.K. Bhargava & Sumeet Bhargava, p. 259-326.*

511. Focal spot size in mammography is

(a) 1–5 mm
(b) 0.1–0.5 mm
(c) 1–3 mm
(d) 0.5–1 mm

Ans. (a). *Textbook of Radiology for Residents & Technicians, 5th ed., S.K. Bhargava & Sumeet Bhargava, p. 259-326.*

512. The spatial resolution for digital mammography is

(a) 20 LP/mm
(b) 5-10 LP/mm
(c) 0.1-0.5 LP/mm
(d) 10-15 LP/mm

Ans. (b). *Textbook of Radiology for Residents & Technicians, 5th ed., S.K. Bhargava & Sumeet Bhargava, p. 259-326.*

513. Digital mammogram can be processed using _________ software.

(a) Computer-aided diagnosis (CAD)
(b) Computed mammogram processor (CMP)
(c) Computed data acquisition (CDA)
(d) None of the above

Ans. (a). *Textbook of Radiology for Residents & Technicians, 5th ed., S.K. Bhargava & Sumeet Bhargava, p. 259-326.*

514. ________ resolution and ______ frequency transducer are used for ultrasound imaging of the breast.

(a) High, high
(b) High, low
(c) Low, high
(d) Low, low

Ans. (a). *Textbook of Radiology for Residents & Technicians, 5th ed., S.K. Bhargava & Sumeet Bhargava, p. 259-326.*

515. The low voltage used in screen/film mammography reduces

(a) Subject contrast
(b) Dose
(c) Microcalcification visibility
(d) Scatter

Ans. (d). *Textbook of Radiology for Residents & Technicians, 5th ed., S.K. Bhargava & Sumeet Bhargava, p. 259-326.*

516. Which radionuclide does PET breast imaging use?

(a) $Technetium^{99m}$
(b) $Fluorine^{18}$
(c) $Iodine^{131}$
(d) Gadopentetate

Ans. (b). *Textbook of Radiology for Residents & Technicians, 5th ed., S.K. Bhargava & Sumeet Bhargava, p. 259-326.*

517. Xeroradiography was invented by

(a) W.C. Roentgen
(b) Chester F. Carlsan
(c) I. Carlton
(d) Micheal Henry

Ans. (b). *Textbook of Radiology for Residents & Technicians, 5th ed., S.K. Bhargava & Sumeet Bhargava, p. 259-326.*

518. In which year xeroradiography was invented?

(a) 1985
(b) 1895
(c) 1937
(d) 1974

Ans. (c). *Textbook of Radiology for Residents & Technicians, 5th ed., S.K. Bhargava & Sumeet Bhargava, p. 259-326.*

519. Xeroradiographic plate is exposed to

(a) X-rays
(b) Gamma rays
(c) Infrared rays
(d) Ultraviolet rays

Ans. (a). *Textbook of Radiology for Residents & Technicians, 5th ed., S.K. Bhargava & Sumeet Bhargava, p. 259-326.*

520. Xeroradiography utilizes a __________ target X-ray tube.

(a) Molybdenum
(b) Rhodium
(c) Tungsten
(d) None of these

Ans. (c). *Textbook of Radiology for Residents & Technicians, 5th ed., S.K. Bhargava & Sumeet Bhargava, p. 259-326.*

521. Which form of Se is used in the xeroradiography?

(a) Crystalline Se
(b) Liquid Se
(c) Amorphous Se
(d) Pure Se

Ans. (c). *Textbook of Radiology for Residents & Technicians, 5th ed., S.K. Bhargava & Sumeet Bhargava, p. 259-326.*

522. In a xeroradiographic plate, the outer surface of the Se layer behaves like

(a) An insulator
(b) A capacitor
(c) A dielectric
(d) None of the above

Ans. (b). *Textbook of Radiology for Residents & Technicians, 5th ed., S.K. Bhargava & Sumeet Bhargava, p. 259-326.*

523. The remaining charge pattern on the plate is called the

(a) Latent image
(b) Visible image
(c) Electrostatic latent image
(d) Invisible image

Ans. (c). *Textbook of Radiology for Residents & Technicians, 5th ed., S.K. Bhargava & Sumeet Bhargava, p. 259-326.*

524. Why liquid toner xeroradiography system was introduced?

(a) To reduced scan time
(b) To reduced patient dose
(c) To improve resolution
(d) To reduced artifacts

Ans. (b). *Textbook of Radiology for Residents & Technicians, 5th ed., S.K. Bhargava & Sumeet Bhargava, p. 259-326.*

525. Liquid toner xeroradiography system was introduced in the year

(a) 1895
(b) 1939
(c) 1985
(d) 1999

Ans. (c). *Textbook of Radiology for Residents & Technicians, 5th ed., S.K. Bhargava & Sumeet Bhargava, p. 259-326.*

CHAPTER

5

Radiographic Positioning

1. In PA projection of hand, it is

(a) Pronated (b) Supinated
(c) Everted (d) Flexed

Ans. (a). *Clark's Positioning, p. 59.*

2. In which view of wrist joint the fracture of scaphoid is well demonstrated?

(a) PA (b) Lateral
(c) PA with ulnar deviation (d) PA with radial deviation

Ans. (c). *Refer to p. 50 of Clark's or Eisenberg, p. 60.*

3. The forearm should not be X-rayed in PA position because

(a) It involves rotation of radius (b) It involves rotation of ulna
(c) It involves rotation of elbow (d) Radius and ulna lies parallel

Ans. (a). *Refer to p. 59 of Clark's.*

4 The first carpometacarpal joint of thumb can best visualized in

(a) AP view of hand (b) PA view of thumb
(c) AP view of thumb (d) Lateral view of thumb

Ans. (c). Refer to p. 48 of Clark's or Eisenberg, p. 46.

5. In the lateral view of elbow joint it is not advisable to keep the

(a) Arm and forearm in the same place
(b) Elbow flexed
(c) Elbow extended
(d) Epicondyle superimposed

Ans. (c). *Refer to p. 61 of Clark's or Eisenberg, p. 67.*

6. In order to demonstrate the anterior and posterior displacement in fracture of metacarpal bones the most useful view would be

(a) PA view of hand
(b) PA view of wrist with ulna deviation
(c) Lateral view of hand
(d) Lateral view of wrist joint

Ans. (c). *Refer to p. 45 of Clark's or Eisenberg, p. 49.*

7. The bicipital groove of humerus can be demonstrated in

(a) Axial view of shoulder (b) Tangential projection
(c) PA view of shoulder (d) Lateral view

Ans. (b). *Refer to p. 73 of Clark's or Eisenberg, p. 87.*

8. For the lateral view of scapula the patient is placed in erect position, facing vertical grid cassette and the patient is adjusted obliquely so that

(a) Scapula is parallel to cassette
(b) Scapula is parallel to perpendicular
(c) Plane of scapula is separated from the thorax
(d) Plane of scapula is within thorax

Ans. (b). *Refer to Eisenberg, p. 92.*

9. The medial malleolus is the part of

(a) Tibia (b) Fibula
(c) Calcaneum (d) Talus

Ans. (a). *Refer to Eisenberg, p. 119.*

10. To demonstrate the structural status of longitudinal arch of the foot which view is taken?

(a) Lateral position weight bearing
(b) Lateral position without weight bearing
(c) Mediolateral oblique
(d) Dorsoplantar projection

Ans. (a). *Refer to Eisenberg, p. 110.*

11. In axial view of calcaneum the cassette is kept under the ankle in planto-dorsal position and the tube is angled

(a) 20° towards head (b) 40° towards head
(c) 20° towards feet (d) 40° towards feet

Ans. (b). *Refer to p. 119 of Clark's or Eisenberg, p. 112.*

12. In order to better visualize joint space in AP view of knee joint the tube is angled 5 to 7 degree

(a) Cranially (b) Caudally
(c) Towards medial side (d) Towards lateral side

Ans. (a). *Refer to p. 126 of Clark's or Eisenberg, p. 121.*

13. To demonstrate joint space in lateral view of the knee joint, it is advisable to keep the knee

(a) Flexed to 90° (b) Flexed to 20° to 30°
(c) Extended fully (d) In oblique position

Ans. (b). *Refer to p. 127 of Clark's or Eisenberg, p. 126.*

14. The ileum, ischium and pubic are the parts of

(a) Small intestine (b) Hip bone
(c) Femur (d) Humerus

Ans. (b). *Refer to p. 145 of Clark's or Eisenberg, p. 142.*

15. The palpable bony prominence which is a landmark for localizing the hip joint for correct AP positioning is

(a) Anterior superior iliac spine (b) Sciatic notch
(c) Iliac spine (d) Obturator foramen

Ans. (a). *Refer to p. 145 of Clark's or Eisenberg, p. 142.*

16. The grid is not necessary in making a radiograph of

(a) Lateral pelvis (b) AP lumbar spine
(c) Lateral cervical spine (d) AP view of pelvis

Ans. (c). *Refer to p. 169 of Clark's or Eisenberg, p. 170.*

17. The vertebral column normally consist of _______ small irregular bones called vertebrae.

(a) 12 (b) 5
(c) 33 (d) 7

Ans. (c). *Refer to General Human Anatomy B.D. Chaurasia.*

18. In order to demonstrate atlas and axis in AP projection the patient is asked to

(a) Breath normally (b) Close the mouth
(c) Open the mouth (d) Move the head side-to-side

Ans. (c). *Refer to p. 171 of Clark's or Eisenberg, p. 169.*

19. The patient is asked to take some purgative one day before the examination of LS spine in order to

(a) Clear the bowel (b) To absorb the gases
(c) Both of the above (d) None of the above

Ans. (a). *Refer to Eisenberg, p. 186.*

20. For AP view of coccyx the central ray is directed

(a) 25° towards head | (b) 10° towards head
(c) 25° towards feet | (d) 10° towards feet

***Ans. (d).** Refer to p. 192 of Clark's or Eisenberg, p. 201.*

21. Manubrium is the _______ of the sternum.

(a) Middle part | (b) Upper part
(c) Lower part | (d) Body

***Ans. (b).** Refer to General Anatomy of B.D. Chaurasia.*

22. Interlobar effusion of the chest can be demonstrated in

(a) Lordotic projection | (b) Recumbent position
(c) PA view | (d) AP view

***Ans. (a).** Refer to p. 213 of Clark's or Eisenberg, p. 29.*

23. When the patient lies in lateral recumbent position the cassette is placed behind the patient and the horizontal beam is used. This projection is termed as

(a) Lateral decubitus | (b) Dorsal decubitus
(c) Ventral decubitus | (d) Axial view

***Ans. (a).** Refer to Eisenberg, p. 34.*

24. The specialized radiological examination of lungs and bronchial tree using an opaque contrast medium is called as

(a) Bronchoscopy | (b) Bronchography
(c) Cystography | (d) Urography

***Ans. (b).** A Guide to Radiological Procedures, Chapman, 4th ed., p. 190.*

25. The contrast medium used in bronchography examination is

(a) Urografin | (b) Dianosil
(c) Barium sulphate | (d) Osbil

***Ans. (b).** A Guide to Radiological Procedures, Chapman, 4th ed., p. 190.*

26. To decrease the magnification of the heart in PA view of chest, the film focal distance is kept at

(a) 40 inches | (b) 60 inches
(c) 72 inches | (d) 36 inches

***Ans. (c).** Refer to p. 26 of Eisenberg.*

27. Radiological examination of salivary glands and its ducts by means of contrast medium is termed as

(a) Ductography | (b) Sialography

(c) Sinography (d) Cholelithiasis

Ans. (b). *A Guide to Radiological Procedures, Chapman, 4th ed., p. 329.*

28. Percutaneous transhepatic cholangiography is performed using needles known as

(a) Fiber optic endoscopy needles
(b) Chiba needles
(c) Drip infusion needles
(d) Butterfly set of nec dles used for IVP

Ans. (b). *A Guide to Radiological Procedures, Chapman, 4th ed., p. 109.*

29. In a craniocaudal view of breast the following should be in profile

(a) Inferior margin of breast
(b) Nipple of breast to be radiographed
(c) Nipple of breast of opposite side
(d) Lactiferous tubules

Ans. (b). *Refer to p. 450 of Clark's or Eisenberg, p. 326.*

30. To demonstrate position for towns in AP projection the central ray is directed

(a) 25°–30° caudally (b) 25°–30° cranially
(c) 30°–45° caudally (d) 25°-30° cranially

Ans. (a). *Refer to p. 243 of Clark's or Eisenberg, p. 274.*

31. To demonstrate position for Caldwell in PA projection the central ray is directed

(a) 15° caudally (b) 25° caudally
(c) 25° cranially (d) 30° cranially

Ans. (a). *Refer to Eisenberg, p. 277.*

32. Stenver projection view basically done for

(a) Base of skull
(b) Petrous portion of temporal bone
(c) Oblique view of mandible
(d) Orbit

Ans. (b). *Refer to p. 254 of Clark's or Eisenberg, p. 318.*

33. Schuller projection view basically done for

(a) Petrous portion
(b) Mastoid portion of temporal bone
(c) Mandible
(d) EAM

Ans. (b). *Refer to Eisenberg, p. 320.*

34. Fetogram done for
(a) To detect suspected fetal abnormalities
(b) Abdominal preparation
(c) Lung cavity
(d) Obstruction in intestine

***Ans. (a).** Refer to Eisenberg, p. 338.*

35. Lauenstein's projection view basically done for
(a) Pelvis
(b) SI joint
(c) Hip joint & upper third of femur
(d) Chest region

***Ans. (c).** Refer to Eisenberg, p. 277.*

36. For cranium Caldwell projection, the central ray is
(a) 15° cranially
(b) 30° caudally
(c) 15° caudally
(d) 30° laterally

***Ans. (c).** Refer to Eisenberg, p. 277.*

37. In cranium SMV projection the central ray must be perpendicular to
(a) Infra orbital line
(b) Infra orbitomeatal line
(c) Supra orbital line
(d) Supra orbitomeatal line

***Ans. (b).** Refer to Eisenberg, p. 280.*

38. In orbit PA axial projection the central ray is at a
(a) 0°–40° caudal
(b) 15°–30° caudal
(c) 20°–25° caudal
(d) 0°–25° caudal

***Ans. (c).** Refer to p. 267 of Clark's or Eisenberg, p. 293.*

39. Parieto-orbital oblique projection also known as
(a) Judet projection
(b) Lauenstein's projection
(c) Waters projection
(d) Rhese projection

***Ans. (c).** Refer to Eisenberg, p. 296.*

40. Parieto-orbital oblique projection basically done for
(a) Head of femur
(b) Hip joint
(c) Paranasal sinuses
(d) Optic foramen

***Ans. (d).** Refer to Eisenberg, p. 296.*

41. In reverse Towne (PA) projection the central ray is at a
(a) 30° cephalic
(b) 30° cranially
(c) Can give both (a) and (b) projections

(d) 15° cephalic

Ans. (b). Refer to Clark's, p. 245.

42. In mandible (AP), oblique projection procedure may require a short subject tube distance upto _______ to blur the superimposed part distal from the film while the part of the mandible to be radiographed remain sharply outlined.

(a) 75 cm
(b) 65 cm
(c) 50 cm
(d) 100 cm

Ans. (a). Refer to Eisenberg, p. 308.

43. In these mandible projection (AP oblique)

(a) Grid should be used
(b) Non-bucky exposure
(c) No need to use grid
(d) Both (b) & (c)

Ans. (d). Refer to Eisenberg, p. 308.

44. In hand anterior oblique, the hand is _______ with the finger extended.

(a) Internally rotated 30°
(b) Externally rotated with 30°
(c) Internally rotated 45°
(d) Externally rotated with 45°

Ans. (d). Refer to Eisenberg, p. 51.

45. In hand anterior oblique, the vertical central ray is centered over the _______.

(a) Head of 5th metacarpal
(b) Head of 3rd metacarpal
(c) Head of 2nd metacarpal
(d) Head of 1st metacarpal

Ans. (b). Refer to Eisenberg, p. 51.

46. Bilateral hand posterior oblique projection is also called _______.

(a) Rhese projection
(b) Frog projection
(c) Ball catcher projection
(d) Stenver's view

Ans. (c). Refer to Clark's, p. 44.

47. In hand posterior oblique, both the hands are _______.

(a) Externally rotated with 30°
(b) Internally rotated with 45°
(c) Externally rotated with 45°
(d) Internally rotated with 30°

Ans. (b). Refer to Clark's, p. 44.

48. Hand lateral is used in addition to the routine posteroanterior projection to locate a _______.

(a) Foreign body
(b) Fracture
(c) Dislocation
(d) All of the above

Ans. (d). Refer to Clark's, p. 45.

49. Which one of the following is best view to demonstrate scaphoid bone _______.

(a) Ulnar deviation (b) Posterior oblique
(c) Lateral (d) All of the above

Ans. (a). *Refer to p. 50 of Clark's or Eisenberg, p. 60.*

50. Number of carpal bone present in hand

(a) 7 bone (b) 8 bone
(c) 14 bone (d) 33 bone

Ans. (b). *Refer to General Anatomy of B.D. Chaurasia.*

51. In carpal tunnel projection the image should demonstrate _______.

(a) Pisiform and the hook of hemate
(b) Tubercle of scaphoid & trapezium
(c) A concavity
(d) All of the above

Ans. (d). *Refer to Clark's p. 54 or Eisenberg, p. 62.*

52. In wrist PA projection the vertical central ray is centered at _______.

(a) Between 2nd and 3rd carpal
(b) Between 2nd and 3rd metacarpal
(c) Between radius and styloid process
(d) None of these

Ans. (c). *Refer to Clark's, p. 56.*

53. The carpal bones arranged in proximal row are named as _______.

(a) Scaphoid lunate
(b) Triquetral and pisiform
(c) Trapezium, trapezoid, capitate and hamate
(d) Both (a) & (b)

Ans. (d). *Refer to Clark's, p. 56.*

54. There are _______ phalanges in hand.

(a) 14 (b) 8
(c) 15 (d) 33

Ans. (a). *Refer to General Anatomy of B.D. Chaurasia.*

55. The palm of the hand is formed by the

(a) Carpal bone (b) Metacarpal bone
(c) Phalanges (d) Both (b) & (c)

Ans. (d). *Refer to General Anatomy of B.D. Chaurasia.*

56. The bicipital groove of humerus can be demonstrated in

(a) Axial view of shoulder (b) Tangenital projection
(c) PA view of shoulder (d) Lateral view of shoulder

Ans. ***(b).*** *Refer to Eisenberg, p. 87.*

57. Iliac crest is used as landmark in making a radiograph of

(a) AP view of hip (b) Neck of femur
(c) Plain KUB (d) Plain abdomen

Ans. ***(c).*** *Refer to Eisenberg, p. 254.*

58. DPT stands for

(a) Digital pantomography
(b) Dental panoramic-tomography
(c) Di-pantomography
(d) None of these

Ans. ***(b).*** *Refer to Clark's, p. 318.*

59. Dental radiography consist

(a) Intra-oral radiography (b) Extra-oral radiography
(c) Both (a) and (b) (d) None of these

Ans. ***(c).*** *Refer to Clark's, p. 286.*

60. Bitewing radiography is used for

(a) Demonstrates the crown of teeth
(b) Alveolar crest bone of the premolar & molar region
(c) Roots of the tooth
(d) Both (a) and (b)

Ans. ***(d).*** *Refer to Clark's, p. 280.*

61. Cephalometry technique used in

(a) Orthodontic (b) Orthomatic
(c) Implant treatment (d) All of these

Ans. ***(d).*** *Refer to Clark's, p-325.*

62. In the AP axial projection (Towne's method) of the skull, with the central ray directed 30 degrees caudal to the OML and passing midway between the external auditory meatus, which of the following is best demonstrated

(a) Frontal bone (b) Sella turcica
(c) Occipital bone (d) Basal foramina

Ans. ***(c).*** *Refer to Eisenberg, p. 274 or Clark's, p. 243.*

63. Which view is best demonstrate the radiographic examination of the sternum?

(a) PA
(b) AP
(c) Lateral
(d) LAO or RAO

Ans. (c). *Refer to Eisenberg, p. 152 or Clark's, p. 228.*

64. Xero-radiography is used in _______ cancer detection.

(a) Stomach
(b) Breast
(c) Colonic
(d) Pancreatic

Ans. (b). *Textbook of Radiology for Residents & Technicians, 5th ed., S.K.Bhargava, p. 288.*

65. Patella is a _______.

(a) Flat bone
(b) Long bone
(c) Irregular bone
(d) Sesamoid bone

Ans. (d). *General Human Anatomy of B.D. Chaurasia.*

66. The main constituent of bone is _______.

(a) Calcium and phosphate
(b) Magnesium
(c) Carbonate
(d) Iron

Ans. (a). *Human Anatomy of B.D. Chaurasia.*

67. Which of the following is false about mammography?

(a) It uses soft radiation
(b) It has molybdenum filter
(c) It requires higher KVP
(d) It is done to evaluate breast diseases

Ans. (c). *Refer to Eisenberg, p. 323 or Clark's, p. 435.*

68. Most common view used during chest X-ray

(a) AP view
(b) Supine AP view
(c) PA view (erect)
(d) Lateral view

Ans. (c). *Refer to Eisenberg, p. 26.*

69. Skyline view is used for

(a) Talus
(b) Scapula
(c) Patella
(d) Hip joint

Ans. (c). *Refer to Eisenberg, p. 128.*

70. Stryker's view is done for

(a) Shoulder
(b) Knee
(c) Ankle
(d) Hip

Ans. (a). *Refer to Clark's, p. 90.*

71. Lordotic view of chest is done for

(a) Lordosis of thoracic vertebrae

(b) Apices of lung
(c) Lower part of lung
(d) Thyroid gland

Ans. (b). *Refer to Eisenberg, p. 29.*

72. Radiographic examination of invertogram basically done for
(a) Vertebral column (b) Cardiac shadow
(c) Costophrenic angle of lung (d) Suspected anal atresia

Ans. (d). *Textbook of Radiology for Residents & Technicians, 5th ed., S.K. Bhargava & Sumeet Bhargava, p. 206.*

73. Series of X-rays in acute abdomen needed are
(a) Abdomen AP supine
(b) Abdomen AP erects
(c) Lateral decubitus
(d) Chest PA view including upper abdomen
(e) All of these

Ans. (e). *Textbook of Radiology for Residents & Technicians, 5th ed., S.K. Bhargava & Sumeet Bhargava, p. 211.*

74. Lateral decubitus view demonstrate
(a) On the affected sides to demonstrate fluid in pleural cavity
(b) On the non-affected side to demonstrate the air in pleural cavity
(c) Both (a) and (b)
(d) None of these

Ans. (c). *Refer to Clark's, p. 34.*

75. In sternum anterior oblique projection, why the patient is rotated to either side because
(a) Radiographic factor become less
(b) To avoid superposition of sternum over thoracic vertebrae
(c) Both (a) and (b)
(d) None of these

Ans. (b). *Refer to Eisenberg, p. 154 or Clark's, p. 226.*

76. In case of transthoracic lateral view of shoulder, if the patient is unable to lower the affected shoulder while elevating the opposite extremity, so what we can do to prevent super-imposition of the shoulders
(a) Central ray should be at a 90 degree
(b) Central ray should be at a 10 to 25 degree caudal angulation
(c) Central ray should be at a 10 to 25 degree cranially angulation
(d) Both (b) and (c)

Ans. (b). *Refer to Eisenberg, p. 77.*

77. Where is the central ray location for an PA oblique hand projection?

(a) Parallel to the third MCP joint
(b) Parallel to the third PIP joint
(c) Perpendicular to the third MCP joint
(d) Parallel to the third DIP joint

Ans. (c). Refer to Eisenberg, p. 51.

78. Where is the CR location for all lateral hand projections?

(a) Perpendicular to the third MCP joint
(b) Parallel to the second PIP joint
(c) Perpendicular to the second MCP joint
(d) Parallel to the third DIP joint

Ans. (c). Refer to Eisenberg, p. 53 or Clark's, p. 45.

79. What is the proper position for an AP forearm projection?

(a) Hand supinated
(b) Hand pronated
(c) Elbow at 90 degree
(d) Both (a) and (c)

Ans. (a). Refer to Clark's, p. 59.

80. Which projection shows the radial head free of superimposition?

(a) AP elbow
(b) Medial oblique elbow
(c) Lateral oblique elbow
(d) AP forearm

Ans. (c). Refer to Eisenberg, p. 69.

81. To do a medial oblique projection of the elbow

(a) Pronate the hand
(b) Place the hand in a neutral position
(c) Supinate the hand
(d) Bend the elbow 45 degrees

Ans. (d). Refer to Eisenberg, p. 68.

82. Which projection shows the coronoid process free of superimposition?

(a) AP elbow
(b) Medial oblique elbow
(c) Lateral oblique elbow
(d) AP forearm

Ans. (b). Refer to Eisenberg, p. 68.

83. The hand should be pronated for an

(a) AP elbow
(b) AP forearm
(c) Internal oblique elbow
(d) None of the above

Ans. (c). Refer to Eisenberg, p. 68.

84. Which structure is not included on a AP shoulder projection?

(a) Coronoid process
(b) Acromion process
(c) Lesser tubercle
(d) Glenoid fossa

Ans. (a). Refer to Eisenberg, p. 78.

85. The central ray location for an AP humerus is

(a) 1.5 inch below the shoulder joint
(b) Just below the greater trochanter
(c) Perpendicular to elbow joint
(d) None of these

Ans. (a). Refer to Eisenberg, p. 75.

86. Which view of the shoulder shows the greater tubercle in profile?

(a) External rotation
(b) Internal rotation
(c) Neutral
(d) Transthoracic

Ans. (a). Refer to Eisenberg, p. 83.

87. The Lawrence method is also known as

(a) Transthoracic lateral
(b) Inferosuperior axial projection
(c) Both (a) and (b)
(d) None of the above

Ans. (a). Refer to Eisenberg, p. 77.

88. The waters method is also known as a _______ projection.

(a) Parietocanthial
(b) Parietomental
(c) Parietoglabellar
(d) Parietonasal

Ans. (a). Refer to Eisenberg, p. 286.

89. Which is true about the lateral facial bone position?

(a) Central ray 2 inches above External Auditory Meatus (EAM)
(b) IOML parallel with axis of the image receptor
(c) Interpupillary line parallel with image receptor
(d) All of the above

Ans. (a). Refer to Eisenberg, p. 278.

90. Which of the following is not a cranial bone?

(a) Vomer
(b) Frontal
(c) Ethmoid
(d) Sphenoid

Ans. (a). Refer to Human Anatomy of B.D. Chaurasia.

91. Which skull shape is known by a 40 degrees angle of the petrous pyramids?

(a) Mesocephalic
(b) Bradycephalic
(c) Brachycephalic
(d) Dolichocephalic

Ans. (d). Refer to Eisenberg, p. 314.

92. The central ray enters 2 inches superior to the EAM for which position?

(a) Lateral skull
(b) Caldwell method
(c) Towne's method
(d) AP view

Ans. (a). *Refer to Eisenberg, p. 278.*

93. The central ray location for a Towne's method is

(a) 1.5 inches above glabella
(b) 2 inches above glabella
(c) 2.5 inches below glabella
(d) 2 inches below glabella

Ans. (b). *Refer to Eisenberg, p. 274.*

94. The occipital bone is best demonstrated with what skull positions?

(a) Towne's (AP) projection
(b) PA projection
(c) SMV
(d) Lateral

Ans. (a). *Refer to Eisenberg, p. 274.*

95. Which view of the nasal bone shows the bony nasal septum?

(a) Lateral projection
(b) AP projection
(c) Water's projection
(d) Oblique projection

Ans. (c). *Refer to Eisenberg, p. 300.*

96. Zygomatic arches best demonstrated in which view?

(a) Towne's projection
(b) SMV projection
(c) Oblique tangential projection
(d) All of the above

Ans. (d). *Refer to Eisenberg, p. 302–304.*

97. In case of cervical vertebral injured patient (trauma patient)

(a) Lateral horizontal beam used
(b) Lateral vertical beam used
(c) Both (a) and (b)
(d) None of the above

Ans. (a). *Refer to Clark's, p. 467.*

98. Where is central ray location for an urinary bladder projection?

(a) Lower border 2 cm below the pubic symphysis
(b) Lower border 5 cm below the P. symphysis
(c) Lower border 2 inches above the P. symphysis
(d) Lower border 5 inches above the P. symphysis

Ans. (b). *Refer to Clark's, p. 347.*

99. Which bone is the focus in the PA ulnar deviation projection of the wrists?

(a) Lunate
(b) Scaphoid
(c) Pisiform
(d) Capitate

Ans. ***(b).*** *Refer to Clark's, p. 347.*

100. Aspirated foreign bodies in older children and adults are most likely to lodge in the

(a) Right main bronchus
(b) Left main bronchus
(c) Esophagus
(d) Proximal stomach

Ans. ***(a).*** *Refer to Human Anatomy of B.D. Chaurasia.*

101. Which of the following position is obtained with the patient lying prone recumbent on the radiographic table, and the central ray directed horizontally to the iliac crest?

(a) Ventral decubitus position
(b) Dorsal decubitus position
(c) Left lateral decubitus position
(d) Right lateral decubitus position

Ans. ***(a).*** *Refer to Eisenberg, p. 15.*

102. The left sacroiliac joint is positioned perpendicular to the Incident Ray (IR) when the patient is positioned in a

(a) Left lateral position
(b) 25 degree to 30 degree LAO position
(c) 25 degree to 30 degree LPO position
(d) 30 degree to 40 degree LPO position

Ans. ***(b).*** *Refer to Eisenberg, p. 195.*

103. Which projection of the foot will best demonstrate the longitudinal arch?

(a) Mediolateral
(b) Lateromedial
(c) Lateral weight-bearing
(d) 30 degree medial oblique

Ans. ***(c).*** *Refer to Eisenberg, p. 110.*

104. Hallux view basically done for

(a) Wrist
(b) Metacarpal
(c) Patella
(d) Toe

Ans. ***(d).*** *Refer to Clark's, p. 113.*

105. Which of the following is not a structure found in the mediastinum?

(a) Oesophagus
(b) Trachea
(c) Thyroid gland
(d) Thymus gland

Ans. ***(c).*** *Textbook of Radiology for Residents & Technicians, 5th ed., S.K. Bhargava & Sumeet Bhargava, p. 209-258.*

106. What is the centering point for an average RAO stomach?

(a) Cardiac antrum
(b) Duodenal bulb
(c) Umbilicus
(d) Greater curvature

Ans. (b). *Textbook of Radiology for Residents & Technicians, 5th ed., S.K. Bhargava & Sumeet Bhargava, p. 209-258.*

107. What position of the elbow best demonstrates the olecranon process?

(a) AP
(b) Lateral
(c) Axial
(d) Oblique

Ans. (b). *Textbook of Radiology for Residents & Technicians, 5th ed., S.K. Bhargava & Sumeet Bhargava, p. 209-258.*

108. Which of the following structures are best demonstrated with a lateral oblique projection of the elbow?

(a) Radial head
(b) Capitellum
(c) Olecranon process
(d) Trochlea

Ans. (a). *Textbook of Radiology for Residents & Technicians, 5th ed., S.K. Bhargava & Sumeet Bhargava, p. 209-258.*

109. Which of the following is more desirable when positioning the breast?

(a) Compressing to demonstrate as much of posterior breast as possible.
(b) Compressing to profile the nipple.
(c) Avoiding compression.
(d) Medial side of the breast as for frame the cassette.

Ans. (a). *Textbook of Radiology for Residents & Technicians, 5th ed., S.K. Bhargava & Sumeet Bhargava, p. 298.*

110. When taking an AP cervical open mouth X-ray image, what is the tube tilt and distance?

(a) No tube tilt at 40 inches
(b) 15° tube tilt towards the head at a distance of 40 inches
(c) 15° tube tilt towards the floor at a distance of 40 inches
(d) 15° tube tilt towards the head at a distance of 72 inches

Ans. (b). *Textbook of Radiology for Residents & Technicians, 5th ed., S.K. Bhargava & Sumeet Bhargava, p. 209-258.*

111. When taking an AP lumbar X-ray image, where should the CR be focussed?

(a) 1″ above the iliac crest
(b) 1″–2″ below the iliac crest

(c) At the belly button
(d) Halfway between ASIS and PSIS

Ans. (b). Textbook of Radiology for Residents & Technicians, 5th ed., S.K. Bhargava & Sumeet Bhargava, p. 209-258.

112. Which of the lumbar and sacral X-ray views involves a tube tilt of 15°.
(a) AP lumbopelvic and lateral lumbar
(b) AP pelvis and l5-S1 spot
(c) l5-S1 spot AP
(d) Oblique lumbar spine

Ans. (b). Textbook of Radiology for Residents & Technicians, 5th ed., S.K. Bhargava & Sumeet Bhargava, p. 209-258.

113. When taking a 'swimmer's view' image, where should the CR be pointed and what should the tube tilt be?
(a) Through C7 prominence and 15° tube tilt towards the head
(b) Through C7 prominence and no tube tilt
(c) Through C7 prominence and 15° tube tilt towards the floor
(d) Through the inferior edge of the scapula and a 15° tube tilt towards the floor

Ans. (b). Textbook of Radiology for Residents & Technicians, 5th ed., S.K. Bhargava & Sumeet Bhargava, p. 209-258.

114. How must the patient arm be positioned for a good AP projection of the scapula?
(a) Adducted
(b) Abducted
(c) Internally rotated
(d) Externally rotated

Ans. (b). Textbook of Radiology for Residents & Technicians, 5th ed., S.K. Bhargava & Sumeet Bhargava, p. 209-258.

115. The transthoracic projection of the proximal humerus is also known as the _____ position.
(a) Jacobi
(b) Transaxillary
(c) Scobery
(d) Lawrence

Ans. (d). Textbook of Radiology for Residents & Technicians, 5th ed., S.K. Bhargava & Sumeet Bhargava, p. 209-258.

116. What are the proper breathing instruction for an AP abdomen?
(a) Full inspiration
(b) Rapid breathing
(c) Shallow breathing
(d) Full exhalation

Ans. (d). Textbook of Radiology for Residents & Technicians, 5th ed., S.K. Bhargava & Sumeet Bhargava, p. 209-258.

117. How many degrees of angulation are there between the orbito-meatal line and infraorbitomeatal line?

(a) 5° (b) 8°
(c) 12° (d) 7°

Ans. (d). Textbook of Radiology for Residents & Technicians, 5th ed., S.K. Bhargava & Sumeet Bhargava, p. 209-258.

118. Which of the following would best demonstrate fluid in the right pleural cavity?

(a) Left lateral decubitus (b) Right lateral decubitus
(c) Ventral decubitus (d) Dorsal decubitus

Ans. (b). Textbook of Radiology for Residents & Technicians, 5th ed., S.K. Bhargava & Sumeet Bhargava, p. 209-258.

119. Which of the following would best demonstrate the free air in the right pleural cavity?

(a) Left lateral decubitus (b) Right lateral decubitus
(c) Erect (d) Supine

Ans. (a). Textbook of Radiology for Residents & Technicians, 5th ed., S.K. Bhargava & Sumeet Bhargava, p. 209-258.

120. Another name for the seventh cervical vertebra is

(a) Atlas (b) Axis
(c) Dense (d) Vertebra prominens

Ans. (d). Textbook of Radiology for Residents & Technicians, 5th ed., S.K. Bhargava & Sumeet Bhargava, p. 209-258.

121. Which of the following are demonstrated in the oblique position of the cervical spine?

(a) Intervertebral foramina (b) Apophyseal joints
(c) Intervertebral joints (d) All of the above

Ans. (a). Textbook of Radiology for Residents & Technicians, 5th ed., S.K. Bhargava & Sumeet Bhargava, p. 209-258.

122. Aspirated foreign bodies in older children and adults are most likely to lodge in the

(a) Right main bronchus (b) Left main bronchus
(c) Oesophagus (d) G-junction

Ans. (a). Textbook of Radiology for Residents & Technicians, 5th ed., S.K. Bhargava & Sumeet Bhargava, p. 209-258.

123. Which of the following projection will best demonstrate the carpal scaphoid?

(a) Lateral
(b) Ulnar deviation
(c) Radial deviation
(d) Carpal tunnel

Ans. (c). *Textbook of Radiology for Residents & Technicians, 5th ed., S.K. Bhargava & Sumeet Bhargava, p. 209-258.*

124. Which of the following positions will best demonstrate sub-acromial dislocation?

(a) Tangential
(b) AP axial
(c) Transthoracic lateral
(d) PA oblique scapula

Ans. (d). *Textbook of Radiology for Residents & Technicians, 5th ed., S.K. Bhargava & Sumeet Bhargava, p. 209-258.*

125. Which projection will best demonstrate the sinus tarsi, cuboid and tuberosity of the fifth metatarsal?

(a) Lateral oblique foot
(b) Medial oblique foot
(c) Lateral foot
(d) All of the above

Ans. (b). *Textbook of Radiology for Residents & Technicians, 5th ed., S.K. Bhargava & Sumeet Bhargava, p. 209-258.*

126. The patient's chin should be elevated during chest radiography to

(a) Avoid superimposition on the apices.
(b) Keep midsagittal plane parallel.
(c) To reduce patient motion.
(d) To reduce patient dose.

Ans. (a). *Textbook of Radiology for Residents & Technicians, 5th ed., S.K. Bhargava & Sumeet Bhargava, p. 209-258.*

127. The plane that passes vertically through the body dividing it into anterior and posterior halves, is termed the

(a) Median saggital plane
(b) Midcoronal plane
(c) Sagittal plane
(d) Transverse plane

Ans. (b). *Textbook of Radiology for Residents & Technicians, 5th ed., S.K. Bhargava & Sumeet Bhargava, p. 209-258.*

128. The ileocecal valve is normally located in which of the following body regions?

(a) Left iliac fossa
(b) Right iliac fossa
(c) Right lumbar region
(d) Left hypochondrium

Ans. (b). *Textbook of Radiology for Residents & Technicians, 5th ed., S.K. Bhargava & Sumeet Bhargava, p. 209-258.*

129. Which of the following skull positions will demonstrate the cranial base, sphenoidal sinuses, atlas and odontoid process?

(a) AP axial (b) Towne's
(c) Submentovertical (d) Lateral

Ans. (c). *Textbook of Radiology for Residents & Technicians, 5th ed., S.K. Bhargava & Sumeet Bhargava, p. 209-258.*

130. The Water's method is also known as a ______ projection.

(a) Parietoacanthial (b) Parietomental
(c) Parietoglabella (d) Parietonasal

Ans. (a). *Textbook of Radiology for Residents & Technicians, 5th ed., S.K. Bhargava & Sumeet Bhargava, p. 209-258.*

131. Which view of the shoulder shows the greater tubercle in profile?

(a) External rotation (b) Internal rotation
(c) Neutral (d) Transthoracic

Ans. (a). *Textbook of Radiology for Residents & Technicians, 5th ed., S.K. Bhargava & Sumeet Bhargava, p. 209-258.*

132. The posterior aspect of the hand is against the leg for which view of the shoulder?

(a) External rotation (b) Internal rotation
(c) Neutral (d) Transthoracic

Ans. (b). *Textbook of Radiology for Residents & Technicians, 5th ed., S.K. Bhargava & Sumeet Bhargava, p. 209-258.*

133. The large end of the clavicle is the _____ end.

(a) Lateral (b) Medial
(c) Acromial (d) None of the above

Ans. (b). *Textbook of Radiology for Residents & Technicians, 5th ed., S.K. Bhargava & Sumeet Bhargava, p. 209-258.*

134. The _____ is the smallest wrist bone.

(a) Lunate (b) Hamate
(c) Pisiform (d) Scaphoid

Ans. (c). *Textbook of Radiology for Residents & Technicians, 5th ed., S.K. Bhargava & Sumeet Bhargava, p. 209-258.*

135. The wrist is made-up of ___ bones.

(a) 6 (b) 22
(c) 8 (d) 10

Ans. (c). *Textbook of Radiology for Residents & Technicians, 5th ed., S.K. Bhargava & Sumeet Bhargava, p. 209-258.*

136. The best projection to demonstrate the maxillary sinuses is the _____ method.

(a) Caldwell (b) Towne's
(c) Water's (d) SMV

Ans. (c). *Textbook of Radiology for Residents & Technicians, 5th ed., S.K. Bhargava & Sumeet Bhargava, p. 209-258.*

137. The best projection to demonstrate the frontal sinuses is the ______ method.

(a) Caldwell (b) Towne's
(c) Water's (d) SMV

Ans. (a). *Textbook of Radiology for Residents & Technicians, 5th ed., S.K. Bhargava & Sumeet Bhargava, p. 209-258.*

138. The bicipital groove of humerus can be demonstrated in

(a) Axial view of shoulder (b) Tangenital projection
(c) PA view of shoulder (d) Lateral view

Ans. (b). *Textbook of Radiology for Residents & Technicians, 5th ed., S.K. Bhargava & Sumeet Bhargava, p. 209-258.*

139. The vertebral column normally consists of_________small irregular bones called vertebrae.

(a) 12 (b) 5
(c) 33 (d) 7

Ans. (c). *Textbook of Radiology for Residents & Technicians, 5th ed., S.K. Bhargava & Sumeet Bhargava, p. 209-258.*

140. In order to demonstrate atlas and axis in AP projection, the patient is asked to

(a) Breathe normally (b) Close the mouth
(c) Open the mouth (d) Move the head side-to-side

Ans. (c). *Textbook of Radiology for Residents & Technicians, 5th ed., S.K. Bhargava & Sumeet Bhargava, p. 209-258.*

141. Interlobar effusion of the chest can be demonstrated in

(a) Lordotic projection (b) Recumbent position
(c) PA view (d) AP view

Ans. (a). *Textbook of Radiology for Residents & Technicians, 5th ed., S.K. Bhargava & Sumeet Bhargava, p. 209-258.*

142. When the patient lies in lateral recumbent position, the cassette is placed behind the patient and the horizontal beam is used. This projection is termed as

(a) Lateral decubitus (b) Dorsal decubitus
(c) Ventral decubitus (d) Axial view

Ans. (a). *Textbook of Radiology for Residents & Technicians, 5th ed., S.K. Bhargava & Sumeet Bhargava, p. 209-258.*

143. The contrast medium used in bronchography examination is

(a) Urografin
(b) Dianosil
(c) Barium sulphate
(d) Osbil

Ans. (b). *Textbook of Radiology for Residents & Technicians, 5th ed., S.K. Bhargava & Sumeet Bhargava, p. 209-258.*

144. Radiological examination of salivary glands and its ducts by means of contrast medium is termed as

(a) Ductography
(b) Sialography
(c) Sinography
(d) Cholelithiasis

Ans. (b). *Textbook of Radiology for Residents & Technicians, 5th ed., S.K. Bhargava & Sumeet Bhargava, p. 259-326.*

145. Percutaneous transhepatic cholangiography is performed using needles known as

(a) Fiberoptic endoscopy needles
(b) Chiba needles
(c) Drip infusion needles
(d) Butterfly set of needle used for IVP

Ans. (b). *Textbook of Radiology for Residents & Technicians, 5th ed., S.K. Bhargava & Sumeet Bhargava, p. 259-326.*

146. To demonstrate position for Towne's in AP projection, the central ray is directed

(a) 25°–30° caudally
(b) 25°–30° cranially
(c) 30°–45° caudally
(d) 30°–45° cranially

Ans. (a). *Textbook of Radiology for Residents & Technicians, 5th ed., S.K. Bhargava & Sumeet Bhargava, p. 209-258.*

147. To demonstrate position for Caldwell in PA projection the central ray is directed

(a) 15° caudally
(b) 25° caudally
(c) 25° cranially
(d) 30° cranially

Ans. (a). *Textbook of Radiology for Residents & Technicians, 5th ed., S.K. Bhargava & Sumeet Bhargava, p. 209-258.*

148. Fetogram done

(a) To detect suspected fetal abnormalities.
(b) For abdominal preparation.
(c) To detect lung cavity.
(d) To detect obstruction in intestine.

Ans. (a). *Textbook of Radiology for Residents & Technicians, 5th ed., S.K. Bhargava & Sumeet Bhargava, p. 259-326.*

149. Lauenstein's projection view is basically done for

(a) Pelvis
(b) SI joint
(c) Hip joint and upper-third of femur
(d) Chest region

Ans. (c). *Textbook of Radiology for Residents & Technicians, 5th ed., S.K. Bhargava & Sumeet Bhargava, p. 209-258.*

150. In reverse Towne's (PA) projection the central ray at

(a) 30° cephalic
(b) 30° cranially
(c) Can give both (a) and (b) projections
(d) 15° cephalic

Ans. (b). *Textbook of Radiology for Residents & Technicians, 5th ed., S.K. Bhargava & Sumeet Bhargava, p. 209-258.*

151. Bilateral hand posterior oblique projection is also called_______.

(a) Rhese projection
(b) Frog projection
(c) Ball catcher projection
(d) Stenver's view

Ans. (c). *Textbook of Radiology for Residents & Technicians, 5th ed., S.K. Bhargava & Sumeet Bhargava, p. 209-258.*

152. The bicipital groove of humerus can be demonstrated in

(a) Axial view of shoulder
(b) Tangential projection
(c) PA view of shoulder
(d) Lateral view of shoulder

Ans. (b). *Textbook of Radiology for Residents & Technicians, 5th ed., S.K. Bhargava & Sumeet Bhargava, p. 209-258.*

153. Iliac crest is used as landmark in making a radiograph of

(a) AP view of hip
(b) Neck of femur
(c) Plain KUB
(d) Plain abdomen

Ans. (c). *Textbook of Radiology for Residents & Technicians, 5th ed., S.K. Bhargava & Sumeet Bhargava, p. 209-258.*

154. Where is CR location for an urinary bladder projection?

(a) Lower border 2 cm below the pubic symphysis
(b) Lower border 5 cm below the pubic symphysis
(c) Lower border 2 inches above the pubic symphysis
(d) Lower border 5 inches above the pubic symphysis

Ans. (b). *Textbook of Radiology for Residents & Technicians, 5th ed., S.K. Bhargava & Sumeet Bhargava, p. 209-258.*

155. Which of the following is not a cranial bone?

(a) Vomer
(b) Frontal
(c) Ethamoid
(d) Sphenoid

Ans. (a). *Textbook of Radiology for Residents & Technicians, 5th ed., S.K. Bhargava & Sumeet Bhargava, p. 209-258.*

156. Skyline view is used for

(a) Talus
(b) Scapula
(c) Patella
(d) Hip joint

Ans. (c). *Textbook of Radiology for Residents & Technicians, 5th ed., S.K. Bhargava & Sumeet Bhargava, p. 209-258.*

157. Stryker's view is done for

(a) Shoulder
(b) Knee
(c) Ankle
(d) Hip

Ans. (a). *Textbook of Radiology for Residents & Technicians, 5th ed., S.K. Bhargava & Sumeet Bhargava, p. 209-258.*

CHAPTER

6

Hospital Practice, Patient Care & Radiation Protection

HOSPITAL AND PATIENT CARE

1. Radiographer has got the following responsibilities

(a) Clinical responsibilities (b) Ethical responsibilities
(c) Legal responsibilities (d) All above

Ans. (d). *Textbook of Radiology for Residents & Technicians, 5th ed., S.K. Bhargava & Sumeet Bhargava, p. 188.*

2. The radiographer should provide the following

(a) Should be cheerful, sympathetic and understandable
(b) Must show good confidence in patient care
(c) Check the requisition form properly and try to minimize the radiation dose to the patient
(d) All above

Ans. (d). *Textbook of Radiology for Residents & Technicians, 5th ed., S.K. Bhargava & Sumeet Bhargava, p. 188.*

3. Legal responsibilities of the radiographer are

(a) Not to disclose any information about the patient
(b) Always have a female attendant at the time of female patient
(c) Always have emergency drugs
(d) All above

Ans. (d). *Textbook of Radiology for Residents & Technicians, 5th ed., S.K. Bhargava & Sumeet Bhargava, p. 189.*

4. Purpose of the preparing the patient for abdominal, spine, IVP etc. is to

(a) Prevention of the gas
(b) Removal of the fecal matter

(c) Both
(d) None

Ans. ***(c).*** *Textbook of Radiology for Residents & Technicians, 5th ed., S.K. Bhargava & Sumeet Bhargava, p. 259.*

5. Radiation dose to the staff is more during mobile/bedside radiography
(a) Patient require support during radiography
(b) Radiographer has to stand close to the source of the exposure.
(c) Difficulty in limiting the beam strictly
(d) All above

Ans. ***(d).*** *Textbook of Radiology for Residents & Technicians, 5th ed., S.K. Bhargava & Sumeet Bhargava, p. 192.*

6. To use the mobile equipment in OT, it is advisable
(a) To enclose the tube head and image intensifier in a sterile linen/polythene cover
(b) To keep some mobile equipment permanent in OT
(c) Radiographer must wear like the theater staff required for sterilization
(d) All above

Ans. ***(d).*** *Textbook of Radiology for Residents & Technicians, 5th ed., S.K. Bhargava & Sumeet Bhargava, p. 192.*

7. Protective measures to be taken during radiography are
(a) Use of the fast imaging system consistent with adequate radiographic detail
(b) Use of the gonadal shield of similar lead
(c) Proper limitation of the area to be covered by X-ray beam
(d) All above

Ans. ***(d).*** *Textbook of Radiology for Residents & Technicians, 5th ed., S.K. Bhargava & Sumeet Bhargava, p. 192.*

8. Lead apron should be
(a) Keep clean (no stain of contrast agent)
(b) Periodically check fluoroscopically for any crack/defect
(c) Should not be left hanging partially over the edge of the chair-seat/doubled up on the shelf
(d) All above

Ans. ***(d).*** *Textbook of Radiology for Residents & Technicians, 5th ed., S.K. Bhargava & Sumeet Bhargava, p. 192 & 154.*

9. Natural environmental radiation contribute annual dose of

(a) 3 millisievert (b) 10 millisievert
(c) 20 millisievert (d) 40 millisievert

Ans. (a). *Radiological Science for Technologists by Stewart Carlyce Bushang, 9th Ed., Mosby Elsevier, 2008, p. 5.*

10. Man-made radiation results an annual dose of

(a) 60 millirem (0.6 mSv) (b) 100 millirem
(c) 200 millirem (d) 300 millirem

Ans. (a). *Radiological Science for Technologists by Stewart Carlyce Bushang, 9th Ed., Mosby Elsevier, 2008, p. 6.*

11. Diagnostic X-rays contribute an annual dose of

(a) 39 m rad (b) 56 m rad
(c) 225 m rad (d) 325 m rad

Ans. (a). *Radiological Science for Technologists by Stewart Carlyce Bushang, 9th Ed., Mosby Elsevier, 2008, p. 7.*

12. Sir Wilhelm Conrad Roentgen discovered X-rays on

(a) 8th November, 1895 (b) 28th August, 1895
(c) 8th November, 1825 (d) 8th November, 1795

Ans. (a). *Radiological Science for Technologists by Stewart Carlyce Bushang, 9th Ed., Mosby Elsevier, 2008, p. 6.*

13. Due to discovery of X-rays, Roentgen received the Noble Prize in

(a) 1901 (b) 1908
(c) 1921 (d) 1897

Ans. (a). *Radiological Science for Technologists by Stewart Carlyce Bushang, 9th Ed., Mosby Elsevier, 2008, p. 6.*

14. Stochastic effects of radiation are dose related and related to

(a) Early effects of radiation (b) Threshold dose
(c) Chromosomal aberration (d) Hematological changes

Ans. (b). *Radiological Science for Technologists by Stewart Carlyce Bushang, 9th Ed., Mosby Elsevier, 2008, p.*

15. Non-stochastic effects of radiation are related to

(a) Dose of the patient
(b) Have hematological effect
(c) Predominantly GIT symptoms
(d) All above

Ans. (d). *Textbook of Radiology for Residents & Technicians, 5th ed., S.K. Bhargava & Sumeet Bhargava, p. 149.*

16. The Annual occupational dose equivalent to the lens of the Eye as per NCRP recommendation

(a) 1 msv
(b) 25 msv
(c) 50 msv
(d) 150 msv

Ans. (d). *Textbook of Radiology for Residents & Technicians, 5th ed., S.K. Bhargava & Sumeet Bhargava, p. 150.*

17. The Annual occupational dose equivalent to the skin and extremities are (as per NCRP recommendation)

(a) 1 msv
(b) 50 msv
(c) 150 msv
(d) 500 msv

Ans. (d). *Textbook of Radiology for Residents & Technicians, 5th ed., S.K. Bhargava & Sumeet Bhargava, p. 150.*

18. The intensity of an X-ray photons affected each time, it scatters

(a) Intensity increases 4 times
(b) Intensity decreases 4 times
(c) Intensity increases 1000 times
(d) Intensity decreases 1000 times

Ans. (d). *Radiological Science for Technologists by Stewart Carlyce Bushang, 9th Ed., Mosby Elsevier, 2008, p. 309.*

19. If an exposure rate of an individual standing 2.0 metres from a source of radiation is 15 R/min, what will be the dose received after 2 mts. at a distance of 5 metres from the source

(a) 1.2 R
(b) 2.4 R
(c) 4.8 R
(d) 9.6 R

Ans. (c). *Radiological Science for Technologists by Stewart Carlyce Bushang, 9th Ed., Mosby Elsevier, 2008, p. 311.*

20. All the following statements regarding mobile radiographic equipments are true, except

(a) The exposure cord must permit the operator to stand at least 4 feet from the patient-ray tube and useful beam
(b) Expose switches must be the; "dead man" type
(c) Lead apron must be worn by radiographer during exposure
(d) The radiographer must explain to the person present in the area about radiation effect

Ans. (a). *Radiological Science for Technologists by Stewart Carlyce Bushang, 9th Ed., Mosby Elsevier, 2008, p. 391. (Correct is -6 Feet).*

21. If the exposure rate to a body standing 5 feet from radiation source is 10 mR/mts., what will be the dose to that body at a distance of 8 feet from the source?

(a) 25.6 mR/mts (b) 16.0 mR/mts
(c) 6.25 mR/mts (d) 3.9 mR/mts

Ans. (d). *Radiological Science for Technologists by Stewart Carlyce Bushang, 9th Ed., Mosby Elsevier, 2008, p. 311.*

22. Among the following, which of the intensifying screen phosphor material will have high patient dose

(a) Calcium tungstate (b) Gadolinium
(c) Lanthanum (d) Yttrium

Ans. (a). *Textbook of Radiology for Residents & Technicians, 5th ed., S.K. Bhargava & Sumeet Bhargava, p. 184.*

23. Which of the following devices does not help in reduction of the patient dose?

(a) Grid (b) Collimator
(c) Gonad shield (d) Reduce thickness of part

Ans. (a). *Textbook of Radiology for Residents & Technicians, 5th ed., S.K. Bhargava & Sumeet Bhargava, p. 200.*

24. Which of the following is (are) important for patient protection during fluoroscopic procedures

(a) Intermittent fluoroscopy (b) Fluoroscopic field side
(c) Patient-to-table distance (d) All above

Ans. (d). *Textbook of Radiology for Residents & Technicians, 5th ed., S.K. Bhargava & Sumeet Bhargava, p. 283.*

25. Thermoluminence dosimeter utilizes which of the following crystals

(a) Silver bromide (b) Sodium sulphite
(c) Lithium fluoride (d) Aluminium oxide

Ans. (c). *Textbook of Radiology for Residents & Technicians, 5th ed., S.K. Bhargava & Sumeet Bhargava, p. 538.*

26. In radiation protection, the product of absorbed dose and the correct modifying factor (RADX QF) is used to determine

(a) Roentgen (c/kg) (b) REM (sv)
(c) RAD (Gy) (d) Radiation quality

Ans. (b). *Textbook of Radiology for Residents & Technicians, 5th ed., S.K. Bhargava & Sumeet Bhargava, p. 601.*

27. Which is the safest investigation in terms of radiation dose in pregnant women

(a) X-rays (b) CT
(c) Ultrasound (d) PET-CT

Ans. (c). Textbook of Radiology for Residents & Technicians, 5th ed., S.K. Bhargava. p. 343.

28. Which of the following is (are) possible long term somatic effects of radiation exposure?

(a) Nausea and vomiting (b) Carcinogenesis
(c) Leukemia (d) Inborn defects

Ans. (a). Textbook of Radiology for Residents & Technicians, 5th ed., S.K. Bhargava. p. 150.

29. Which of the crystals used in optically stimulated luminance dosimeter

(a) Gadolinium (b) Calcium tungstate
(c) Lithium fluoride (d) Aluminium oxide

Ans. (d). Textbook of Radiology for Residents & Technicians, 5th ed., S.K. Bhargava & Sumeet Bhargava, p. 599-602.

30. The unit of measurement used to express occupational exposure is the

(a) Roentgen (c/kg) (b) RAD (Gy)
(c) REM (sv) (d) RBE

Ans. (b). Textbook of Radiology for Residents & Technicians, 5th ed., S.K. Bhargava & Sumeet Bhargava, p. 150.

31. The leakage radiation from the X-ray tube (when the tube is operated at maximum potential) must not exceed

(a) 10 mR/hr (b) 100 mR/hr
(c) 10 mR/mt (d) 100 mR/mt

Ans. (b). Textbook of Radiology for Residents & Technicians, 5th ed., S.K. Bhargava & Sumeet Bhargava, p. 151.

32. In the production of Bremsstrahlung radiation, the incident electron

(a) Ejects an inner shell electron
(b) Ejects an outer shell tungsten electron
(c) Is deflected, with resulting energy loss
(d) Is deflected with resulting energy increase

Ans. (c). Textbook of Radiology for Residents & Technicians, 5th ed., S.K. Bhargava & Sumeet Bhargava, p. 117.

33. Diagnostic X-ray radiation may be currently described as

(a) Low energy, low LET (b) Low energy, high LET
(c) High energy, low LET (d) High energy, high LET

Ans. (a). *Textbook of Radiology for Residents & Technicians, 5th ed., S.K. Bhargava & Sumeet Bhargava, p. 103.*

34. Which of the following shielding is required for secondary radiation barrier

(a) 1/4″ lead (b) 1/8″ lead
(c) 1/16″ lead (d) 1/32″ lead

Ans. (d). *Textbook of Radiology for Residents & Technicians, 5th ed., S.K. Bhargava & Sumeet Bhargava, p. 155.*

35. Aluminium filtration has its greatest effect on

(a) Long wavelength radiation (b) Short wavelength radiation
(c) Low MA factor (d) High MA factor

Ans. (a). *Textbook of Radiology for Residents & Technicians, 5th ed., S.K. Bhargava & Sumeet Bhargava, p. 167.*

36. The amount of time that X-ray are being produced and directed towards a particular wall is referred to as

(a) Workload (b) Use factor
(c) Occupancy factor (d) Controlling factor

Ans. (b). *Textbook of Radiology for Residents & Technicians, 5th ed., S.K. Bhargava & Sumeet Bhargava, p. 146.*

37. The most common and useful determination of thickness of protective barrier is

(a) Controlling factor (b) Workload
(c) Use factor (d) Occupancy factor

Ans. (c). *Textbook of Radiology for Residents & Technicians, 5th ed., S.K. Bhargava & Sumeet Bhargava, p. 152.*

38. The patient dose increases as

(a) FOV (field of view) increases
(b) FOV decreases
(c) FSS (focal spot size) increases
(d) FSS decreases

Ans. (b). *Textbook of Radiology for Residents & Technicians, 5th ed., S.K. Bhargava & Sumeet Bhargava, p. 152.*

39. The automatic exposure device that is located immediately under the X-ray table is the

(a) Photocathode
(b) Scintillation counter
(c) Ionization chamber
(d) Photomultiplier

Ans. (c). *Textbook of Radiology for Residents & Technicians, 5th ed., S.K. Bhargava & Sumeet Bhargava, p. 600.*

40. Filters used in radiographic X-ray tubes are generally composed of

(a) Aluminium
(b) Copper
(c) Tin
(d) Lead

Ans. (a). *Textbook of Radiology for Residents & Technicians, 5th ed., S.K. Bhargava & Sumeet Bhargava, p. 162.*

41. The thickness of Al-filter used in radiographic X-ray tube above 100 kVp

(a) 0.5 mm aluminium equivalent
(b) 1.0 mm aluminium equivalent
(c) 2.0 mm aluminium equivalent
(d) 2.5 mm aluminium equivalent

Ans. (d). *Textbook of Radiology for Residents & Technicians, 5th ed., S.K. Bhargava & Sumeet Bhargava, p. 120.*

42. The use of the following will function to reduce patient dose, except

(a) Collimation
(b) High kVp, low mAs factors
(c) Grid
(d) Fast intensifying screen

Ans. (c). *Textbook of Radiology for Residents & Technicians, 5th ed., S.K. Bhargava & Sumeet Bhargava, p. 152.*

43. Which of the following dose radiation hazard problem to personnel (radiographer)

(a) The photoelectric effect
(b) Compton effect
(c) Classical effect
(d) Pair production

Ans. (b). *Textbook of Radiology for Residents & Technicians, 5th ed., S.K. Bhargava & Sumeet Bhargava, p. 160.*

44. Which of the following personnel monitoring devices used in diagnostic radiography is considered to be the most sensitive and accurate

(a) TLD
(b) Film badge
(c) Pocket dosimeter
(d) OSL (optically stimulated luminance/light)

Ans. (d). *Textbook of Radiology for Residents & Technicians, 5th ed., S.K. Bhargava & Sumeet Bhargava, p. 145.*

45. What quantity of radiation exposure to the reproductive organs is required to cause temporary sterility?

(a) 100 rad (b) 200 rad
(c) 300 rad (d) 400 rad

Ans. (b). *Textbook of Radiology for Residents & Technicians, 5th ed., S.K. Bhargava & Sumeet Bhargava, p. 150.*

46. How much protection is provided from a 75 KVP X-ray beam when using 0.50 mm lead equivalent apron

(a) 51% (b) 66%
(c) 88% (d) 99%

Ans. (c). *Textbook of Radiology for Residents & Technicians, 5th ed., S.K. Bhargava & Sumeet Bhargava, p. 154.*

47. With the use of the rare earth (fast) intensifying screens, the patient dose is reduced because of

(a) Use of lower MAS
(b) Use of higher MAS
(c) Use of lower KVP
(d) No shielding required

Ans. (a). *Textbook of Radiology for Residents & Technicians, 5th ed., S.K. Bhargava & Sumeet Bhargava, p. 184.*

48. Which of the following monitoring device work on the principle of releasing electrons by interaction of photons with air?

(a) Pocket dosimeter
(b) Optically Stimulated Luminance (OSL)
(c) Film badge
(d) Thermoluminescent Dosimeter (TLD)

Ans. (d). *Textbook of Radiology for Residents & Technicians, 5th ed., S.K. Bhargava & Sumeet Bhargava, p. 148 & 538.*

49. Which of the following is responsible to completely implement the AERB radiation guidelines?

(a) Chief Technologist (b) Chief Radiologist
(c) Medical Superintendent (d) Radiation Safety Officer

Ans. (d). *Textbook of Radiology for Residents & Technicians, 5th ed., S.K. Bhargava & Sumeet Bhargava, p. 139.*

50. Most of the patient dose is contributed due to

(a) Classical scatter (b) Compton scatter
(c) Thompson scatter (d) Photoelectric effect

Ans. (d). *Textbook of Radiology for Residents & Technicians, 5th ed., S.K. Bhargava & Sumeet Bhargava, p. 161.*

51. Radiation exposure to patient can be reduced by

(a) Low mAs factor
(b) Collimation beam
(c) Shielding
(d) All above

Ans. (d). *Textbook of Radiology for Residents & Technicians, 5th ed., S.K. Bhargava & Sumeet Bhargava, p. 146.*

52. The primary function of the filtration is to reduce

(a) Image noise
(b) Scattered radiation
(c) Radiation/technologist dose
(d) To minimize the soft low energy photons – thus reducing patient skin dose

Ans. (d). *Textbook of Radiology for Residents & Technicians, 5th ed., S.K. Bhargava & Sumeet Bhargava, p. 166.*

53. The function of lead apron is to protect the personnel from

(a) Natural radiation
(b) Remnant radiation
(c) Primary beam
(d) Scattered radiation

Ans. (d). *Textbook of Radiology for Residents & Technicians, 5th ed., S.K. Bhargava & Sumeet Bhargava, p. 148.*

54. Which of the following factors contribute to radiation damage to biological tissues?

(a) Size of the irradiated area
(b) Absorbed dose
(c) Radiation quality
(d) All above

Ans. (d). *Textbook of Radiology for Residents & Technicians, 5th ed., S.K. Bhargava & Sumeet Bhargava, p. 147.*

55. Immediate reading can be obtained by the following personal monitoring devices

(a) Pocket dosimeter
(b) TLD
(c) Film badge
(d) Lithium fluoride chips

Ans. (a). *Textbook of Radiology for Residents & Technicians, 5th ed., S.K. Bhargava & Sumeet Bhargava, p. 600.*

56. Radiation that deviates in other direction while passing through the part is termed as

(a) Scattered radiation
(b) Secondary radiation
(c) Leakage radiation
(d) Remnant radiation

Ans. (a). *Textbook of Radiology for Residents & Technicians, 5th ed., S.K. Bhargava & Sumeet Bhargava, p. 163.*

57. Radiation that emerges from the leaded tube housing in directions other than that of useful beam is termed as

(a) Scattered radiation
(b) Secondary radiation
(c) Leakage radiation
(d) Remnant radiation

Ans. (c). *Textbook of Radiology for Residents & Technicians, 5th ed., S.K. Bhargava & Sumeet Bhargava, p. 163.*

58. The permissible limit of leakage radiation is

(a) Less than 0.1 R/Hr at 1 metre from the tube
(b) Less than 0.2 R/Hr at 1 metre from the tube
(c) Less than 0.3 R/Hr at 1 metre from the tube
(d) Less than 0.14 R/Hr at 1 metre from the tube

Ans. (a). *Textbook of Radiology for Residents & Technicians, 5th ed., S.K. Bhargava & Sumeet Bhargava, p. 147.*

59. The radiation that emerges from the patient to form the radiographic image is termed as

(a) Scattered radiation
(b) Remnant radiation
(c) Leakage radiation
(d) Secondary radiation

Ans. (b). *Textbook of Radiology for Residents & Technicians, 5th ed., S.K. Bhargava & Sumeet Bhargava, p. 163.*

60. During mobile radiography, the minimum distance between patient and X-ray tube during exposure is

(a) At least 1 feet
(b) At least 2 feet
(c) At least 4 feet
(d) At least 6 feet

Ans. (d). *Textbook of Radiology for Residents & Technicians, 5th ed., S.K. Bhargava & Sumeet Bhargava, p. 147.*

61. Which of the following are considered as mechanical waves?

(a) X-rays
(b) Gamma rays
(c) Beta rays
(d) Ultrasound waves

Ans. (d). *Textbook of Radiology for Residents & Technicians, 5th ed., S.K. Bhargava & Sumeet Bhargava, p. 108.*

62. Which of the following are considered as electromagnetic waves?

(a) X-rays
(b) Ultrasound
(c) Magnetic
(d) Beta

Ans. (a). *Textbook of Radiology for Residents & Technicians, 5th ed., S.K. Bhargava & Sumeet Bhargava, p. 108.*

63. The unit of exposure in diagnostic X-ray tube is

(a) RAD
(b) REM
(c) Roentgen
(d) Becquerel

Ans. (c). *Textbook of Radiology for Residents & Technicians, 5th ed., S.K. Bhargava & Sumeet Bhargava, p. 193.*

64. The use of copper and aluminium filters in film badge is
(a) To support the film contained within
(b) To eliminate harmful X-rays
(c) To measure radiation quantity
(d) To prevent exposure by Alpha particles

Ans. (c). *Textbook of Radiology for Residents & Technicians, 5th ed., S.K. Bhargava & Sumeet Bhargava, p. 140.*

65. Which of the following interaction is responsible for radiographic contrast and contribute significantly to patient dose?
(a) Pair production
(b) Compton scatter
(c) Coherent scatter
(d) Photoelectric effect

Ans. (d). *Textbook of Radiology for Residents & Technicians, 5th ed., S.K. Bhargava & Sumeet Bhargava, p. 160.*

66. Which of the following occurs at very high energy level, at least 1.02 MeV?
(a) Photoelectric effect
(b) Coherent effect
(c) Compton effect
(d) Pair production

Ans. (d). *Textbook of Radiology for Residents & Technicians, 5th ed., S.K. Bhargava & Sumeet Bhargava, p. 160.*

67. In which of the following, no energy is absorbed by the part and all merges as scattered photons
(a) Photoelectric effect
(b) Coherent effect
(c) Compton effect
(d) Pair production

Ans. (b). *Textbook of Radiology for Residents & Technicians, 5th ed., S.K. Bhargava & Sumeet Bhargava, p. 160.*

68. In which of the following a relatively high energy incident photon uses part of its energy to eject an outer shell electron and in doing so changes its direction is scattered. The energy retained by the scattered photon depends on the angle formed by the ejected electron and scattered photon. The greater the angle of deflection, the less is the retained energy. It is also responsible for the scatter radiation reaching the film in the form of fog?
(a) Photoelectric effect
(b) Coherent effect
(c) Compton effect
(d) Pair production

Ans. (c). *Textbook of Radiology for Residents & Technicians, 5th ed., S.K. Bhargava & Sumeet Bhargava, p. 160.*

69. In which of the following, a relatively low energy photons uses all its energy to eject an inner shell electron, leaving a vacancy? An electron from the shell above drops down to fill the vacancy

and in doing so gives up a characteristic ray, contribute to the patient dose

(a) Photoelectric effect (b) Coherent effect
(c) Compton effect (d) Pair production

Ans. (a). *Textbook of Radiology for Residents & Technicians, 5th ed., S.K. Bhargava & Sumeet Bhargava, p. 159.*

70. Relationship between LET and RBE

(a) As LET increases, RBE increases
(b) As LET increases, RBE decreases
(c) As LET decreases, RBE increases
(d) There is no relationship between LET and RBE

Ans. (a). *Textbook of Radiology for Residents & Technicians, 5th ed., S.K. Bhargava & Sumeet Bhargava, p. 156.*

71. An increase of 1.0 mm added aluminium filtration of X-ray beam should have the following

(a) Increase average energy of the beam
(b) Increase patient skin dose
(c) Increase MR output

Ans. (a). *Textbook of Radiology for Residents & Technicians, 5th ed., S.K. Bhargava & Sumeet Bhargava, p. 166-168.*

72. Which of the adult tissue is sensitive to radiation exposure?

(a) Muscle tissue (b) Nerve tissue
(c) Epithelial tissue (d) None

Ans. (c). *Textbook of Radiology for Residents & Technicians, 5th ed., S.K. Bhargava & Sumeet Bhargava, p. 147-157.*

73. Which of the following is correct regarding care of the protective leaded apparel?

(a) Lead aprons should be fluoroscoped yearly to check for cracks
(b) Lead gloves should be fluoroscoped yearly to check for cracks
(c) Lead aprons should be hung on appropriate racks when not in use
(d) All of the above

Ans. (d). *Textbook of Radiology for Residents & Technicians, 5th ed., S.K. Bhargava & Sumeet Bhargava, p. 155.*

74. The TLD/film badge be worn

(a) Under the lead apron at collar level
(b) Outside the lead apron at collar level
(c) Under the lead apron at waist level
(d) Over the lead apron at waist level

Ans. (a). Textbook of Radiology for Residents & Technicians, 5th ed., S.K. Bhargava & Sumeet Bhargava, p. 145.

75. The 10 days rule is applicable to

(a) The first 10 days following the cessation of menstruation
(b) The first 10 days following the onset of menstruation
(c) The 10 days preceding the onset of menstruation
(d) About 14 days before menstruation

Ans. (b). Textbook of Radiology for Residents & Technicians, 5th ed., S.K. Bhargava & Sumeet Bhargava, p. 147-157.

76. Which of the following are considered most radiosensitive

(a) Lymphocytes (b) Ova
(c) Neurons (d) Myocytes

Ans. (a). Textbook of Radiology for Residents & Technicians, 5th ed., S.K. Bhargava & Sumeet Bhargava, p. 147-157.

77. Exception to 10 days rule is

(a) Women who denied recent sexual intercourse
(b) Women who were menstruating at that time
(c) Women who had had an oral contraceptive for no fewer than 3 months and were satisfied
(d) All above

Ans. (d). A Guide to Radiological Procedures, Chapman, 4th ed., p. 2.

78. Exception to 10 days rule is

(a) Women who had sterilized
(b) Women who had had an intrauterine contraceptive for no fewer than 3 months and found it effective
(c) Both (a) and (b)
(d) None of the above

Ans. (c). A Guide to Radiological Procedures, Chapman, 4th ed., p. 2.

79. Argument against 10 days rule is

(a) Orgogenesis occurs during the 4–8 weeks after conception, hence irradiation after 10 days of the menstrual cycle but before next cycle will not result in radiation damage
(b) Irradiation of the unfertilized ovum – no evidence suggest that the irradiation of the concepts is any more dangerous than irradiation of the unfertilized ovum
(c) The risks are small and are greatly outweighed by the likely benefits to the mother or fetus for an early diagnosis
(d) All above

***Ans.* (*d*).** *A Guide to Radiological Procedures, Chapman, 4th ed., p. 3.*

80. The deterministic effect of radiation is

(a) Skin erythema
(b) Leukemia
(c) Skin cancer
(d) Breast cancer

***Ans.* (*a*).** *Textbook of Radiology for Residents & Technicians, 5th ed., S.K. Bhargava & Sumeet Bhargava, p. 149.*

81. Unit for measuring the equivalent doses

(a) Sievert
(b) Gray
(c) Rad
(d) Roentgen

***Ans.* (*a*).** *Textbook of Radiology for Residents & Technicians, 5th ed., S.K. Bhargava & Sumeet Bhargava, p. 98.*

82. Dose to the patient may be increased by using

(a) Collimators
(b) High KV
(c) A grid
(d) Fast screen

***Ans.* (*c*).** *Textbook of Radiology for Residents & Technicians, 5th ed., S.K. Bhargava & Sumeet Bhargava, p. 201.*

83. Following type of wave/particle has maximum radiation weighing factor

(a) Gamma rays
(b) Alpha
(c) Beta rays
(d) X-rays

***Ans.* (*b*).** *Textbook of Radiology for Residents & Technicians, 5th ed., S.K. Bhargava & Sumeet Bhargava, p. 98.*

84. Upper limit of the effective dose for public (in mSv) is

(a) 1
(b) .01
(c) 10
(d) 100

***Ans.* (*a*).** *Textbook of Radiology for Residents & Technicians, 5th ed., S.K. Bhargava & Sumeet Bhargava, p. 150.*

85. The effective dose in CT (in mSv) is

(a) 10
(b) 20
(c) 30
(d) 1

***Ans.* (*a*).** *Textbook of Radiology for Residents & Technicians, 5th ed., S.K. Bhargava & Sumeet Bhargava, p. 145.*

86. Film dose meters

(a) Have two emulsions
(b) Have two screens
(c) Are most expensive dose meters

(d) Single film can be used many times

Ans. (a). *Textbook of Radiology for Residents & Technicians, 5th ed., S.K. Bhargava & Sumeet Bhargava, p. 146.*

87. Upper dose limit for cataract formation based on IRCP is (in mSv)

(a) 1000
(b) 150
(c) 3000
(d) 10

Ans. (b). *Textbook of Radiology for Residents & Technicians, 5th ed., S.K. Bhargava & Sumeet Bhargava, p. 151.*

88. Radiation dose to cause lethal effects/death is (in Gy)

(a) 5
(b) 50
(c) 500
(d) 5000

Ans. (a). *Textbook of Radiology for Residents & Technicians, 5th ed., S.K. Bhargava & Sumeet Bhargava, p. 151.*

89. Which source is the source of maximum natural radiation

(a) Carbon
(b) Phosphorus
(c) Radon
(d) Potassium

Ans. (c). *Textbook of Radiology for Residents & Technicians, 5th ed., S.K. Bhargava & Sumeet Bhargava, p. 150.*

90. Standard thickness of lead used in lead aprons

(a) 0.5 mm
(b) 5 mm
(c) 50 mm
(d) 500 mm

Ans. (a). *Textbook of Radiology for Residents & Technicians, 5th ed., S.K. Bhargava & Sumeet Bhargava, p. 154.*

91. Way to reduce dose to the patient

(a) Using the anti-scatter grid
(b) Decreased filtration
(c) Collimation
(d) Increasing mAs

Ans. (c). *Textbook of Radiology for Residents & Technicians, 5th ed., S.K. Bhargava & Sumeet Bhargava, p. 196.*

92. Example of stochastic effect

(a) Erythema
(b) Cataract
(c) Sterility
(d) Cancer

Ans. (d). *Textbook of Radiology for Residents & Technicians, 5th ed., S.K. Bhargava & Sumeet Bhargava, p. 150.*

93. 10 days rule applies to

(a) Radiation protection in males
(b) Radiation protection in females

(c) Image quality
(d) Spatial resolution

Ans. (b). *Textbook of Radiology for Residents & Technicians, 5th ed., S.K. Bhargava & Sumeet Bhargava, p. 193.*

94. Filtration of the tube is measured in terms of

(a) mm of iron (b) mm of aluminium
(c) mm of lead (d) mm of carbon

Ans. (b). *Textbook of Radiology for Residents & Technicians, 5th ed., S.K. Bhargava & Sumeet Bhargava, p. 120.*

95. The usual dose limit for cataract formation in IRCP is (mSv)

(a) 1000 (b) 150
(c) 3000 (d) 10

Ans. (b). *Textbook of Radiology for Residents & Technicians, 5th ed., S.K. Bhargava & Sumeet Bhargava, p. 150.*

96. 1 gray equals to

a) 100 rads (b) 1000 rads
(c) 10000 rads (d) 10 rads

Ans. (a). *Textbook of Radiology for Residents & Technicians, 5th ed., S.K. Bhargava & Sumeet Bhargava, p. 150.*

97. The largest single source of population radiation exposure from man-made source is

(a) Nuclear power plant (b) Atomic bomb test product
(c) Medical use of X-rays (d) Radio and television

Ans. (c). *Textbook of Radiology for Residents & Technicians, 5th ed., S.K. Bhargava & Sumeet Bhargava, p. 148.*

98. Latest, annual maximum whole body effective dose limit for radiation workers in mSv is

(a) 20 (b) 50
(c) 100 (d) 1

Ans. (a). *Textbook of Radiology for Residents & Technicians, 5th ed., S.K. Bhargava & Sumeet Bhargava, p. 148.*

99. To differentiate between muscle and fat use

(a) 100 kVp to take advantage of both photoelectric effect
(b) Moderate kVp to take advantage of both photoelectric and compton
(c) High kVp to take advantage of compton effect
(d) High kVp to take advantage of photoelectric effect

Ans. (a). *Textbook of Radiology for Residents & Technicians, 5th ed., S.K. Bhargava & Sumeet Bhargava, p. 148.*

100. A full CT scan of the skull delivery a dose to the midline is approximately

(a) 8 (b) 3
(c) 0.3 (d) 30

Ans. (c). Textbook of Radiology for Residents & Technicians, 5th ed., S.K. Bhargava & Sumeet Bhargava, p. 149.

101. In medicolegal cases, which information is not necessary to obtain?

(a) Date of birth (b) Patient identification number
(c) A right or left side marker (d) Date of examination

Ans. (a). Textbook of Radiology for Residents & Technicians, 5th ed., S.K. Bhargava & Sumeet Bhargava, p. 188-195.

102. The usual patient preparation for an upper GI examination is

(a) Upto 8 hr fasting
(b) Light breakfast
(c) Clear fluid on the morning of the examination
(d) Castor oil and enemas until clear

Ans. (a). Textbook of Radiology for Residents & Technicians, 5th ed., S.K. Bhargava & Sumeet Bhargava, p. 188-195.

103. The radiographer must perform which of the following procedures prior to entering a contact isolation room with a mobile X-ray unit?

(a) Put on gown and gloves only
(b) Put on gown, gloves, mask and cap
(c) Clean the mobile X-ray unit
(d) All of the above

Ans. (b). Textbook of Radiology for Residents & Technicians, 5th ed., S.K. Bhargava & Sumeet Bhargava, p. 188-195.

104. What is the normal adult oral temperature?

(a) 36.2°C (b) 36.4°C
(c) 37°C (d) 39°C

Ans. (c). Textbook of Radiology for Residents & Technicians, 5th ed., S.K. Bhargava & Sumeet Bhargava, p. 188-195.

105. Into which position should a patient be moved to avoid vomiting?

(a) Lateral recumbent (b) Sitting
(c) Prone (d) Both (a) and (b)

Ans. (d). Textbook of Radiology for Residents & Technicians, 5th ed., S.K. Bhargava & Sumeet Bhargava, p. 188-195.

106. Which was the first X-ray tube used in India?

(a) Cargo
(b) Heavy duty
(c) Crook
(d) Grid controlled

Ans. (a). *Textbook of Radiology for Residents & Technicians, 5th ed., S.K. Bhargava & Sumeet Bhargava, p. 147-157.*

107. In which year the first X-ray induced skin cancer was reported?

(a) 1902
(b) 1921
(c) 1947
(d) 1949

Ans. (a). *Textbook of Radiology for Residents & Technicians, 5th ed., S.K. Bhargava & Sumeet Bhargava, p. 147-157.*

108. In ___ the ___ made the first radiation protection recommendations.

(a) 1895, Canadian Society
(b) 1921, British Roentgen Society
(c) 1928, ICRP
(d) 1946, NCRP

Ans. (b). *Textbook of Radiology for Residents & Technicians, 5th ed., S.K. Bhargava & Sumeet Bhargava, p. 147-157.*

109. Which of the following is the first standard setting body formed, for the purpose of radiological safety?

(a) NCRP
(b) BEIR
(c) ICRP
(d) UNSCEAR

Ans. (c). *Textbook of Radiology for Residents & Technicians, 5th ed., S.K. Bhargava & Sumeet Bhargava, p. 147-157.*

110. The unit of exposure is

(a) Kerma
(b) Roentgen
(c) Absorbed dose
(d) Effective dose

Ans. (b). *Textbook of Radiology for Residents & Technicians, 5th ed., S.K. Bhargava & Sumeet Bhargava, p. 147-157.*

111. 1 R =

(a) 1000 rads
(b) 100 mREM
(c) 1 C/kg
(d) 2.58×10^{-4} C/kg

Ans. (d). *Textbook of Radiology for Residents & Technicians, 5th ed., S.K. Bhargava & Sumeet Bhargava, p. 147-157.*

112. Absorbed dose is

(a) The amount of energy liberated per unit mass.
(b) The amount of energy absorbed per unit mass.

(c) The amount of energy passed per unit mass.
(d) The amount of energy interacted with mass.

Ans. (b). *Textbook of Radiology for Residents & Technicians, 5th ed., S.K. Bhargava & Sumeet Bhargava, p. 147-157.*

113. The unit of absorbed dose is

(a) Roentgen (b) Rad
(c) Sievert (d) Gray

Ans. (b). *Textbook of Radiology for Residents & Technicians, 5th ed., S.K. Bhargava & Sumeet Bhargava, p. 147-157.*

114. The relation between rad and gray is

(a) 1 Gy = 1 rad (b) 1 Gy = 100 rad
(c) 1 Gy = 1000 rad (d) 1 Gy = 10^4 rad

Ans. (b). *Textbook of Radiology for Residents & Technicians, 5th ed., S.K. Bhargava & Sumeet Bhargava, p. 147-157.*

115. The unit of activity is

(a) Bacquerel (b) Curie
(c) Roentgen (d) Kerma

Ans. (b). *Textbook of Radiology for Residents & Technicians, 5th ed., S.K. Bhargava & Sumeet Bhargava, p. 147-157.*

116. ______ is the SI unit of equivalent dose.

(a) Gray (b) Roentgen
(c) Rad (d) Sievert

Ans. (d). *Textbook of Radiology for Residents & Technicians, 5th ed., S.K. Bhargava & Sumeet Bhargava, p. 147-157.*

117. What is the relation between sievert and rem?

(a) 1 Sv = 1 rem
(b) 1 Sv = 10 rem
(c) 1 Sv = 100 rem
(d) 1 Sv = 1000 rem

Ans. (c). *Textbook of Radiology for Residents & Technicians, 5th ed., S.K. Bhargava & Sumeet Bhargava, p. 147-157.*

118. The difference between equivalent dose and effective dose is

(a) Tissue weighing factor introduced in effective dose.
(b) Tissue weighing factor introduced in equivalent dose.
(c) Equivalent is smaller dose.
(d) Effective is smaller dose.

Ans. (a). *Textbook of Radiology for Residents & Technicians, 5th ed., S.K. Bhargava & Sumeet Bhargava, p. 147-157.*

119. Who introduced ALARA?

(a) NCRP (b) British Committee
(c) BEIR (d) ICRP

Ans. (d). *Textbook of Radiology for Residents & Technicians, 5th ed., S.K. Bhargava & Sumeet Bhargava, p. 147-157.*

120. ALARA

(a) As Low As Radiation Achievable
(b) As Low As Reasonably Achievable
(c) A Lower Radiation Area
(d) None of the above

Ans. (b). *Textbook of Radiology for Residents & Technicians, 5th ed., S.K. Bhargava & Sumeet Bhargava, p. 147-157.*

121. How much percentage of exposure arises from technologic enhancement and artificial radiation source?

(a) 82% (b) 18%
(c) 3% (d) Negligible

Ans. (b). *Textbook of Radiology for Residents & Technicians, 5th ed., S.K. Bhargava & Sumeet Bhargava, p. 147-157.*

122. LET

(a) Low Energy Transmission (b) Linear Energy Transfer
(c) Local Energy Transmission (d) None of the above

Ans. (b). *Textbook of Radiology for Residents & Technicians, 5th ed., S.K. Bhargava & Sumeet Bhargava, p. 147-157.*

123. LET expressed in

(a) keV/μm (b) V/μm
(c) keV/mAs (d) keV/m

Ans. (a). *Textbook of Radiology for Residents & Technicians, 5th ed., S.K. Bhargava & Sumeet Bhargava, p. 147-157.*

124. In which phase of cell division, cells are more radiosensitive?

(a) Meiosis (b) Mitosis
(c) Prophase (d) Anaphase

Ans. (b). *Textbook of Radiology for Residents & Technicians, 5th ed., S.K. Bhargava & Sumeet Bhargava, p. 147-157.*

125. BEIR

(a) Breast Effect of Ionizing Radiation
(b) Biological Effects of Ionizing Radiation
(c) Body Effects of Ionizing Radiation
(d) None of the above

Ans. ***(b).*** *Textbook of Radiology for Residents & Technicians, 5th ed., S.K. Bhargava & Sumeet Bhargava, p. 147-157.*

126. 'Ten day' rule was postulated by

(a) ICRP
(b) AERB
(c) BEIR
(d) UNSCEAR

Ans. ***(a).*** *Textbook of Radiology for Residents & Technicians, 5th ed., S.K. Bhargava & Sumeet Bhargava, p. 147-157.*

127. 'Ten day' rule was postulated for

(a) Pregnant lady
(b) Reproductive age group females
(c) Menopause females
(d) Both male and female reproductive age group

Ans. ***(b).*** *Textbook of Radiology for Residents & Technicians, 5th ed., S.K. Bhargava & Sumeet Bhargava, p. 147-157.*

128. Which of the following are the least radiosensitive cells?

(a) Bone marrow
(b) Nerve cells
(c) Blood cells
(d) Intestinal epithelium

Ans. ***(b).*** *Textbook of Radiology for Residents & Technicians, 5th ed., S.K. Bhargava & Sumeet Bhargava, p. 147-157.*

129. Which of the following concepts deals with keeping exposure to a minimum?

(a) Benefit-risk analysis
(b) Justification
(c) ALARA
(d) Dose limit

Ans. ***(c).*** *Textbook of Radiology for Residents & Technicians, 5th ed., S.K. Bhargava & Sumeet Bhargava, p. 147-157.*

130. The annual dose limit for radiologic worker is

(a) 50 mSv
(b) 30 mSv
(c) 20 mSv
(d) 5 mSv

Ans. ***(c).*** *Textbook of Radiology for Residents & Technicians, 5th ed., S.K. Bhargava & Sumeet Bhargava, p. 147-157.*

131. The annual dose limit for public is

(a) 1 mSv
(b) 5 mSv
(c) 10 mSv
(d) 20 mSv

Ans. ***(a).*** *Textbook of Radiology for Residents & Technicians, 5th ed., S.K. Bhargava & Sumeet Bhargava, p. 147-157.*

132. The inverse square law states that the intesity of radiation

(a) Increases as the distance increases.

(b) Directly proportional to the mass.
(c) Inversely as the square of the distance.
(d) Directly as the square of the distance.

Ans. (c). *Textbook of Radiology for Residents & Technicians, 5th ed., S.K. Bhargava & Sumeet Bhargava, p. 147-157.*

133. In India, which of the following is the most significant in the development of radiation protection standard?

(a) AERB (b) BARC
(c) NCRP (d) ICRP

Ans. (a). *Textbook of Radiology for Residents & Technicians, 5th ed., S.K. Bhargava & Sumeet Bhargava, p. 147-157.*

134. What threshold embryo dose corresponds to a radiation risk smaller than those normally encountered during pregnancy?

(a) 1 Gy (b) 100 mGy
(c) 50 Gy (d) 0.1 mGy

Ans. (b). *Textbook of Radiology for Residents & Technicians, 5th ed., S.K. Bhargava & Sumeet Bhargava, p. 147-157.*

135. By rule, the fetus of an X-ray technologist should receive

(a) No more than 0.5 mSv (b) Less than 50 mSv
(c) Less than 20 mSv (d) All of the above

Ans. (a). *Textbook of Radiology for Residents & Technicians, 5th ed., S.K. Bhargava & Sumeet Bhargava, p. 147-157.*

136. The typical entrance skin exposure in CT is

(a) 5 mGy (b) 30 mGy
(c) 40 mGy (d) 10 mGy

Ans. (b). *Textbook of Radiology for Residents & Technicians, 5th ed., S.K. Bhargava & Sumeet Bhargava, p. 147-157.*

137. The basic methods by which radiation exposures to persons can be minimized by is/are

(a) Time (b) Distance
(c) Shielding (d) All of the above

Ans. (d). *Textbook of Radiology for Residents & Technicians, 5th ed., S.K. Bhargava & Sumeet Bhargava, p. 147-157.*

138. Which of the following materials is/are used as a primary barrier shielding?

(a) Concrete (b) Lead
(c) Steel (d) All of the above

Ans. (d). Textbook of Radiology for Residents & Technicians, 5th ed., S.K. Bhargava & Sumeet Bhargava, p. 147-157.

139. The exposure due to leakage radiation cannot exceed ____ at 1 m from the source.

(a) 100 mR/wk (b) 100 mR/yr
(c) 100 mR/hr (d) 100 mR/day

Ans. (c). Textbook of Radiology for Residents & Technicians, 5th ed., S.K. Bhargava & Sumeet Bhargava, p. 147-157.

140. If the X-ray installation is located in a residential complex, then it shall be ensured that the walls of the X-ray rooms on which primary X-ray beam falls is not less than

(a) 9 inch (b) 14 inch
(c) 20 inch (d) 24 inch

Ans. (b). Textbook of Radiology for Residents & Technicians, 5th ed., S.K. Bhargava & Sumeet Bhargava, p. 147-157.

141. Which of the following is used to measure instant radiation dose?

(a) TLD (b) OSL
(c) Film badge (d) Pocket dosimeter

Ans. (d). Textbook of Radiology for Residents & Technicians, 5th ed., S.K. Bhargava & Sumeet Bhargava, p. 147-157.

142. In India, personnel monitoring services is offered by

(a) NCRP (b) BARC
(c) AERB (d) All of the above

Ans. (b). Textbook of Radiology for Residents & Technicians, 5th ed., S.K. Bhargava & Sumeet Bhargava, p. 147-157.

143. A film badge consist of

(a) Luminesence powder (b) Photographic film
(c) Ionization chamber (d) All of the above

Ans. (b). Textbook of Radiology for Residents & Technicians, 5th ed., S.K. Bhargava & Sumeet Bhargava, p. 147-157.

144. Film badge holder is made-up of

(a) Plastic (b) Paper
(c) Glass (d) Cardboard

Ans. (a). Textbook of Radiology for Residents & Technicians, 5th ed., S.K. Bhargava & Sumeet Bhargava, p. 147-157.

145. At which level film badge should be worn?

(a) Neck (b) Chest

(c) Hip (d) Abdomen

Ans. (b). *Textbook of Radiology for Residents & Technicians, 5th ed., S.K. Bhargava & Sumeet Bhargava, p. 147-157.*

146. If a lead apron is used, then at which level the film badge is worn?

(a) Under the apron (b) Over the apron
(c) Both (a) and (b) (d) No need to wear

Ans. (a). *Textbook of Radiology for Residents & Technicians, 5th ed., S.K. Bhargava & Sumeet Bhargava, p. 147-157.*

147. Why is it necessary to wear film badge at the chest level?

(a) Because it represents the thorax dose equipment.
(b) Because it represents the whole body dose equipment.
(c) Because chest is very sensitive to radiation.
(d) All of the above

Ans. (b). *Textbook of Radiology for Residents & Technicians, 5th ed., S.K. Bhargava & Sumeet Bhargava, p. 147-157.*

148. Which of the following personnel monitoring devices are used currently in India?

(a) Pocket dosimeter (b) TLD
(c) Film badge (d) Sensitometer

Ans. (b). *Textbook of Radiology for Residents & Technicians, 5th ed., S.K. Bhargava & Sumeet Bhargava, p. 147-157.*

149. TLD is based on the phenomenon of

(a) Induction (b) Thermionic emission
(c) Thermoluminescence (d) Photographic effect

Ans. (c). *Textbook of Radiology for Residents & Technicians, 5th ed., S.K. Bhargava & Sumeet Bhargava, p. 147-157.*

150. During fluoroscopy, it is preferable for the radiologist/radio-technologist to wear a TLD badge at the level of

(a) Head (b) Collar
(c) Chest (d) Pelvis

Ans. (b). *Textbook of Radiology for Residents & Technicians, 5th ed., S.K. Bhargava & Sumeet Bhargava, p. 147-157.*

151. Pregnant radiation workers should wear a monitoring badge at the level of

(a) Chest (b) Collar
(c) Waist (d) Upper abdomen

Ans. (c). *Textbook of Radiology for Residents & Technicians, 5th ed., S.K. Bhargava & Sumeet Bhargava, p. 147-157.*

152. The lead apron should have a lead equivalent thickness of

(a) 0.25–0.5 mm (b) 0.5–2 mm
(c) 1–5 mm (d) 5–10 mm

Ans. (a). *Textbook of Radiology for Residents & Technicians, 5th ed., S.K. Bhargava & Sumeet Bhargava, p. 147-157.*

153. 95–99% scattered radiations are attenuated by using

(a) 5 mm lead equivalent (b) 1 mm lead equivalent
(c) 0.5 mm lead equivalent (d) 0.25 mm lead equivalent

Ans. (c). *Textbook of Radiology for Residents & Technicians, 5th ed., S.K. Bhargava & Sumeet Bhargava, p. 147-157.*

154. Disadvantage of lead apron is

(a) It does not cover the arms (b) It has much weight
(c) It does not cover thyroid (d) All of the above

Ans. (d). *Textbook of Radiology for Residents & Technicians, 5th ed., S.K. Bhargava & Sumeet Bhargava, p. 147-157.*

155. The use of gonadal shield can reduce the absorbed dose to the testes by upto

(a) 100% (b) 95%
(c) 70% (d) 50%

Ans. (b). *Textbook of Radiology for Residents & Technicians, 5th ed., S.K. Bhargava & Sumeet Bhargava, p. 147-157.*

156. Ionizing radiation causes

(a) Mutation (b) Point mutation
(c) Chromosomal anomalies (d) Enzyme defects

Ans. (c). *Textbook of Radiology for Residents & Technicians, 5th ed., S.K. Bhargava & Sumeet Bhargava, p. 147-157.*

157. When a technologist is exposed to a chest X-ray during the course of his/her work, then the dose resulting from such exposure is considered as

(a) Medical exposure (b) Occupational exposure
(c) Public exposure (d) None of the above

Ans. (a). *Textbook of Radiology for Residents & Technicians, 5th ed., S.K. Bhargava & Sumeet Bhargava, p. 147-157.*

158. Which of the following shows a relationship between radiation dose and the proportion of cells that remain alive?

(a) Cell life curve (b) Dead cell curve
(c) Cell survival curve (d) GSD

Ans. (c). *Textbook of Radiology for Residents & Technicians, 5th ed., S.K. Bhargava & Sumeet Bhargava, p. 147-157.*

159. Exposure at the stage of major organogenesis of fetal development results in a high incidence of

(a) Prenatal death
(b) Cancer
(c) Neonatal death
(d) Congenital abnormalities

Ans. (d). *Textbook of Radiology for Residents & Technicians, 5th ed., S.K. Bhargava & Sumeet Bhargava, p. 147-157.*

160. The height of protective barriers should be at least

(a) 2.1 m
(b) 5 m
(c) 7 m
(d) 10 m

Ans. (a). *Textbook of Radiology for Residents & Technicians, 5th ed., S.K. Bhargava & Sumeet Bhargava, p. 147-157.*

161. To protect the patient's reproductive organs, which of the following method will be used?

(a) Distance
(b) Inverse square law
(c) Room shielding
(d) Gonadal shielding

Ans. (d). *Textbook of Radiology for Residents & Technicians, 5th ed., S.K. Bhargava & Sumeet Bhargava, p. 147-157.*

162. The lead equivalent thickness of the glass viewing window of the control panel is

(a) 2.0 mm
(b) 1.5 mm
(c) 3.0 mm
(d) 1.0 mm

Ans. (b). *Textbook of Radiology for Residents & Technicians, 5th ed., S.K. Bhargava & Sumeet Bhargava, p. 147-157.*

CHAPTER

7

Radiological Procedures

PART 1

ARTERIAL SYSTEM AND VENOUS SYSTEM

1. Arteries used for catheterisation are

(a) Femoral artery (b) Brachial artery
(c) Axillary artery (d) All of the above

Ans. (d). *A Guide to Radiological Procedures, Chapman, 4th ed., p. 215.*

2. Seldinger technique uses

(a) Double wall needle puncture (b) Guide wire
(c) Both of above (d) None of above

Ans. (c). *A Guide to Radiological Procedures, Chapman, 4th ed., p. 215.*

3. Femoral artery puncture should be preferably done on the

(a) Symptomatic side (b) Asymptomatic side
(c) Right (d) Left

Ans. (b). *A Guide to Radiological Procedures, Chapman, 4th ed., p. 218.*

4. The incidence of complications is lowest on the following puncture site

(a) Femoral (b) Brachial
(c) Axillary (d) Popliteal

Ans. (a). *A Guide to Radiological Procedures, Chapman, 4th ed., p. 217.*

5. To prevent air embolism syringe during injection should be kept on the following position

(a) Vertical (b) Horizontal
(c) Oblique (d) Any of the above

Ans. (a). *A Guide to Radiological Procedures, Chapman, 4th ed., p. 219.*

6. Catheters that can be used for ascending aortography are

(a) Pigtail (b) Gensini
(c) NIH (d) All of the above

Ans. (d). *A Guide to Radiological Procedures, Chapman, 4th ed., p. 224.*

7. Contrast used for arteriography

(a) HOCM (b) LOCM
(c) Barium (d) Oil based contrast media

Ans. (b). *A Guide to Radiological Procedures, Chapman, 4th ed., p. 226.*

8. Catheters used for vascular dilatation are

(a) Gruntzig double lumen dilatation catheter
(b) Van Andel dilatation catheter
(c) Straight Teflon catheter
(d) All of the above

Ans. (d). *A Guide to Radiological Procedures, Chapman, 4th ed., p. 227.*

9. Contrast medium used for peripheral venography is

(a) LOCM 240 (b) LOCM 300
(c) LOCM 360 (d) HOCM

Ans. (a). *A Guide to Radiological Procedures, Chapman, 4th ed., p. 234.*

10. The site for injection in peripheral venography is

(a) Palm (b) Median cubital vein
(c) Popliteal vein (d) Dorsum of foot

Ans. (d). *A Guide to Radiological Procedures, Chapman, 4th ed., p. 234.*

11. Contrast medium used for upper limb venography is

(a) LOCM 300 (b) LOCM 360
(c) LOCM 400 (d) HOCM

Ans. (a). *A Guide to Radiological Procedures, Chapman, 4th ed., p. 235.*

12. In upper limb venography, butterfly needle is inserted in

(a) Median cubital vein (b) Cephalic vein
(c) Basilic vein (d) Axillary vein

Ans. (a). *A Guide to Radiological Procedures, Chapman, 4th ed., p. 236.*

13. Methods for portal venography are

(a) Trans splenic approach
(b) Trans hepatic approach
(c) Paraumbilical vein catheterisation
(d) All of the above

Ans. (d). *A Guide to Radiological Procedures, Chapman, 4th ed., p. 239.*

14. The maximum width of normal portal vein is

(a) 1 cm (b) 3 cm
(c) 2 cm (d) 4 cm

Ans. (c). *A Guide to Radiological Procedures, Chapman, 4th ed., p. 241.*

15. On ultrasonography acute thrombus is

(a) Hyperechoic (b) Hypoechoic
(c) Non-echogenic (d) Any of the above

Ans. (c). *A Guide to Radiological Procedures, Chapman, 4th ed., p. 244.*

BRAIN

1. Frequency used for sonographic examination of infant brain is

(a) 5 MHz (b) 10 MHz
(c) 15 MHz (d) 2 MHz

Ans. (a). *Textbook of Radiology for Residents & Technicians, 5th ed., S.K. Bhargava & Sumeet Bhargava, p. 352.*

2. Contrast media used for ventriculography

(a) Ionic (b) Non-ionic
(c) Oil-based (d) Barium

Ans. (b). *Radiological Procedures, S.K. Bhargava & Sumeet Bhargava, 2nd ed., Pee Pee Publishers, p. 101-103.*

3. For the cure of hypotension following ventriculography, patient should be placed in

(a) Head-up position (b) Supine
(c) Head-down position (d) Prone

Ans. (c). *Radiological Procedures, S.K. Bhargava & Sumeet Bhargava, 2nd ed., Pee Pee Publishers, p. 101-103.*

4. Contraindication for cisternography are

(a) Raised intracranial pressure
(b) Suspected diastematomyelia
(c) Local cellulitis
(d) All of the above

Ans. (d). *Radiological Procedures, S.K. Bhargava & Sumeet Bhargava, 2nd ed., Pee Pee Publishers, p. 101-103.*

5. In lateral cervical punctu:_ for cisternography, level of puncture is

(a) C_1-C_2
(b) C_2-C_3
(c) C_3-C_4
(d) C_4-C_5

Ans. (a). *Radiological Procedures, S.K. Bhargava & Sumeet Bhargava, 2nd ed., Pee Pee Publishers, p. 101-103.*

6. In cisternography contrast is injected in

(a) Epidural space
(b) Subdural space
(c) Subarachnoid space
(d) Subpial space

Ans. (c). *Radiological Procedures, S.K. Bhargava & Sumeet Bhargava, 2nd ed., Pee Pee Publishers, p. 101-103.*

7. Site of cisternal puncture is

(a) Caudal to C_2
(b) Cephalad to C_2
(c) Caudal to C_4
(d) Caudal to C_6

Ans. (b). *Radiological Procedures, S.K. Bhargava & Sumeet Bhargava, 2nd ed., Pee Pee Publishers, p. 101-103.*

8. During cisternal puncture, patient's position is

(a) Standing
(b) Prone
(c) Supine
(d) Lateral decubitus

Ans. (d). *Radiological Procedures, S.K. Bhargava & Sumeet Bhargava, 2nd ed., Pee Pee Publishers, p. 101-103.*

9. In infants, contrast injection for ventriculography is through

(a) Posterior fontanelle
(b) Anterior fontanelle
(c) Lateral fontanelle
(d) Cervical spine

Ans. (b). *Radiological Procedures, S.K. Bhargava & Sumeet Bhargava, 2nd ed., Pee Pee Publishers, p. 101-103.*

10. Needle used for cisternal puncture should be

(a) 26 G
(b) 28 G
(c) 22 G
(d) 18 G

Ans. (c). *Radiological Procedures, S.K. Bhargava & Sumeet Bhargava, 2nd ed., Pee Pee Publishers, p. 101-103.*

MAMMOGRAPHY

1. Projections used in mammography
(a) Mediolateral oblique
(b) Craniocaudal
(c) Both of the above
(d) None of the above

Ans. (b). *Radiological Procedures, S.K. Bhargava & Sumeet Bhargava, 2nd ed., Pee Pee Publishers, p. 210-214.*

2. For a good mediolateral view a small amount of following muscle should be visible
(a) Pectoralis major
(b) Pectoralis minor
(c) Serratus anterior
(d) Teres minor

Ans. (a). *Radiological Procedures, S.K. Bhargava & Sumeet Bhargava, 2nd ed., Pee Pee Publishers, p. 210-214.*

3. Extended craniocaudal view is done to look for abnormalities in
(a) Upper inner quadrant
(b) Lower inner quadrant
(c) Lower outer quadrant
(d) Upper outer quadrant

Ans. (d). *Radiological Procedures, S.K. Bhargava & Sumeet Bhargava, 2nd ed., Pee Pee Publishers, p. 210-214.*

4. Magnification technique is adopted for better visualisation of
(a) Macrocalcification
(b) Microcalcification
(c) Margins
(d) Location

Ans. (b). *Radiological Procedures, S.K. Bhargava & Sumeet Bhargava, 2nd ed., Pee Pee Publishers, p. 210-214.*

5. Magnification view is obtained by
(a) Increasing target object distance
(b) Larger focal spot
(c) Reducing target object distance
(d) Using grid

Ans. (c). *Radiological Procedures, S.K. Bhargava & Sumeet Bhargava, 2nd ed., Pee Pee Publishers, p. 210-214.*

6. Category 0 in Birads classification refers to
(a) Incomplete assessment
(b) Benign
(c) Suspicious
(d) Highly suggestive of malignant

Ans. (a). *Radiological Procedures, S.K. Bhargava & Sumeet Bhargava, 2nd ed., Pee Pee Publishers, p. 210-214.*

7. Xeroradiography is used to see small lesions because of

(a) Edge enhancement (b) Magnification
(c) Blurring (d) Focussed view

Ans. (a). *Radiological Procedures, S.K. Bhargava & Sumeet Bhargava, 2nd ed., Pee Pee Publishers, p. 210-214.*

8. Breast ultrasound is done normally using frequency

(a) 5–10 MHz (b) 15–20 MHz
(c) 10–15 MHz (d) 2–5 MHz

Ans. (a). *Radiological Procedures, S.K. Bhargava & Sumeet Bhargava, 2nd ed., Pee Pee Publishers, p. 210-214.*

9. Technique of choice for evaluation of breast implants are

(a) Mammography (b) MRI
(c) Ultrasonography (d) Scintigraphy

Ans. (b). *Radiological Procedures, S.K. Bhargava & Sumeet Bhargava, 2nd ed., Pee Pee Publishers, p. 210-214.*

10. For breast MRI, patient should be placed in

(a) Prone position (b) Supine position
(c) Lateral (d) Head down

Ans. (a). *Radiological Procedures, S.K. Bhargava & Sumeet Bhargava, 2nd ed., Pee Pee Publishers, p. 210-214.*

GENERAL NOTES – CONTRAST

1. Preliminary film in any examination is taken for

(a) To make adjustment in exposure factors
(b) To check patient position
(c) To demonstrate, identify and localise opacities
(d) All of the above

Ans. (d). *A Guide to Radiological Procedures, Chapman, 4th ed., p. 11.*

2. Stochastic effect follows the following phenomenon

(a) All or none (b) Exponential rate
(c) Inverse relation (d) Dose dependence

Ans. (a). *A Guide to Radiological Procedures, Chapman, 4th ed., p. 1.*

3. Linear no threshold phenomenon is seen with

(a) Skin erythema (b) Cataract
(c) Cancer (d) Mucositis

Ans. ***(c).*** *A Guide to Radiological Procedures, Chapman, 4th ed., p. 1.*

4. The dose of iodinated contrast used in children is

(a) 2 ml/kg (b) 20 ml/kg
(c) 200 ml/kg (d) 100 ml/kg

Ans. ***(a).*** *A Guide to Radiological Procedures, Chapman, 4th ed., p. 17.*

5. The amount of oral contrast medium used in CT abdomen is

(a) 1000 ml (b) 100 ml
(c) 10 ml (d) 5 ml

Ans. ***(a).*** *A Guide to Radiological Procedures, Chapman, 4th ed., p. 18.*

6. Number of hours of fasting required before ultrasound scanning

(a) 6–8 (b) 10–12
(c) 12–14 (d) 2–4

Ans. ***(a).*** *A Guide to Radiological Procedures, Chapman, 4th ed., p. 24.*

7. Iohexol comes in the category of

(a) Non-ionic monomer (b) Non-ionic dimer
(c) Ionic monomer (d) Ionic dimer

Ans. ***(a).*** *A Guide to Radiological Procedures, Chapman, 4th ed., p. 28.*

8. Idiosyncratic contrast medium reactions are

(a) Anaphylactoid (b) Anyphylaxis
(c) Delayed hypersensitivity (d) Immune complex type

Ans. ***(a).*** *A Guide to Radiological Procedures, Chapman, 4th ed., p. 35.*

9. Serum creatinine should be measured how long before the contrast examination

(a) 1 month before (b) 1 year before
(c) 6 months before (d) 1 week before

Ans. ***(d).*** *A Guide to Radiological Procedures, Chapman, 4th ed., p. 17.*

10. In sickle cell anaemia following contrast material should be used

(a) Low osmolality contrast media
(b) High osmolality contrast media
(c) Isosmolar
(d) Hyposmolar

Ans. (a). *A Guide to Radiological Procedures, Chapman, 4th ed., p. 43.*

11. Paramagnetic agents cause alteration in

(a) Decrease T_2 relaxation
(b) IncreaseT_2 relaxation
(c) Increase T_1 relaxation
(d) Decrease T_1 relaxation

Ans. (d). *A Guide to Radiological Procedures, Chapman, 4th ed., p. 44.*

12. Supramagnetic particles cause alteration in

(a) Decrease T_2 relaxation
(b) Increase T_2 relaxation
(c) Increase T_1 relaxation
(d) Decrease T_1 relaxation

Ans. (a). *A Guide to Radiological Procedures, Chapman, 4th ed., p. 46.*

13. Nephrogenic systemic fibrosis is caused by

(a) Gadolinium
(b) Barium
(c) Iodine
(d) Urografin

Ans. (a). *A Guide to Radiological Procedures, Chapman, 4th ed., p. 46.*

14. Positive bowel contrast agent for MRI scan is

(a) Ferrite
(b) Gadolinium
(c) Barium sulphate
(d) Water

Ans. (d). *A Guide to Radiological Procedures, Chapman, 4th ed., p. 16.*

15. Breast feeding after contrast administration should be avoided for

(a) 48 hrs
(b) 24 hrs
(c) 1 week
(d) Not required

Ans. (b). *A Guide to Radiological Procedures, Chapman, 4th ed., p. 33.*

GIT

1. Indication for using water soluble contrast media is

(a) Suspected perforation
(b) Ileocaecal tuberculosis
(c) Constipation
(d) Gastroesophageal reflux disease

Ans. (a). *A Guide to Radiological Procedures, Chapman, 4th ed., p. 51.*

2. **Buscopan is contraindicated in all, except**
   (a) Myasthenia gravis
   (b) Paralytic ileus
   (c) Pyloric stenosis
   (d) Open angle glaucoma

   Ans. (d). *A Guide to Radiological Procedures, Chapman, 4th ed., p. 53.*

3. **Glucagon is contraindicated in all, except**
   (a) Insulinoma
   (b) Glucagonoma
   (c) Phacochromocytoma
   (d) Glaucoma

   Ans. (d). *A Guide to Radiological Procedures, Chapman, 4th ed., p. 54.*

4. **Amount and concentration of barium sulphate used for contrast swallow examination is**
   (a) 200-250% 100 ml
   (b) 100% 300 ml
   (c) 100% 50 ml
   (d) 60% 1500 ml

   Ans. (a). *A Guide to Radiological Procedures, Chapman, 4th ed., p. 56.*

5. **Water insoluble contrast medium is used in all except**
   (a) Barium meal follow through
   (b) Barium swallow
   (c) Sinogram
   (d) Barium enema

   Ans. (c). *A Guide to Radiological Procedures, Chapman, 4th ed., p. 57.*

6. **Following material is used for radionuclide imaging of gastro-intestinal bleeding**
   (a) Tc 99 m labelled red blood cells
   (b) Tc 99 m labelled white blood cells
   (c) FDG
   (d) Tc 99 m labelled parathyroid hormone

   Ans. (a). *A Guide to Radiological Procedures, Chapman, 4th ed., p. 101.*

7. **Contrast enema in neonatal bowel obstruction uses**
   (a) Ionic contrast medium
   (b) Non-ionic contrast medium
   (c) Barium
   (d) Air

   Ans. (a). *A Guide to Radiological Procedures, Chapman, 4th ed., p. 79.*

8. In barium meal sequence antrum and body of stomach are visualised in the position

(a) Supine (b) Left anterior oblique
(c) Right posterior oblique (d) Left lateral

Ans. (a). *A Guide to Radiological Procedures, Chapman, 4th ed., p. 59.*

9. For imaging duodenal loop in a barium examination following position is preferred

(a) Supine (b) Prone
(c) Left lateral (d) Right lateral

Ans. (b). *A Guide to Radiological Procedures, Chapman, 4th ed., p. 59.*

10. The method of choice to demonstrate mucosal pattern in barium studies is

(a) Single contrast (b) Non-contrast
(c) Double contrast (d) Intravenous contrast

Ans. (c). *A Guide to Radiological Procedures, Chapman, 4th ed., p. 57.*

HEART

1. Catheter used for pressure measurements in angiocardiography is

(a) Amplatz catheter (b) Judkins catheter
(c) Cournanad catheter (d) NIH catheter

Ans. (c). *A Guide to Radiological Procedures, Chapman, 4th ed., p. 196.*

2. Catheter used for coronary arteriography are

(a) Judkins coronary artery catheter
(b) Amplatz coronary artery catheter
(c) Both of the above
(d) None of the above

Ans. (c). *A Guide to Radiological Procedures, Chapman, 4th ed., p. 199.*

3. Beta blockers are stopped _______ hrs before the procedure.

(a) 24 (b) 48
(c) 72 (d) 96

Ans. (b). *A Guide to Radiological Procedures, Chapman, 4th ed., p. 199.*

4. In radionuclide ventriculography, stannous pyrophosphate injection is given

(a) Intravenously
(b) Intra-arterial
(c) Intra-cardiac
(d) Subcutaneous

Ans. (a). *A Guide to Radiological Procedures, Chapman, 4th ed., p. 201.*

5. In stress radionuclide ventriculography, agent used is

(a) Beta blocker
(b) Paracetamol
(c) Dipyridamole
(d) Dobutamine

Ans. (d). *A Guide to Radiological Procedures, Chapman, 4th ed., p. 203.*

6. Complications of exercise test are

(a) Induction of angina
(b) Cardiac arrhythmia
(c) Cardiac arrest
(d) All of the above

Ans. (d). *A Guide to Radiological Procedures, Chapman, 4th ed., p. 204.*

7. Agent used for imaging of acute myocardial infarction is

(a) In 111 antimyosin
(b) Tc 99 m pyrophosphate
(c) Both of the above
(d) None of the above

Ans. (c). *A Guide to Radiological Procedures, Chapman, 4th ed., p. 212.*

8. Agent used to reverse dobutamine induced arrhythmias

(a) Dipyridamole
(b) Lignocaine
(c) Adenosine
(d) Paracetamol

Ans. (b). *A Guide to Radiological Procedures, Chapman, 4th ed., p. 210.*

9. Redistribution study in thallium test is performed after the administration of

(a) Glyceryl trinitrate
(b) Adenosine
(c) Dipyridamole
(d) Dobutamine

Ans. (a). *A Guide to Radiological Procedures, Chapman, 4th ed., p. 208.*

10. Gold standard test for myocardial viability test is

(a) Radionuclide ventriculography
(b) Thallium test
(c) Echocardiography
(d) ^{18}FDG + blood flow PET

Ans. (d). A Guide to Radiological Procedures, Chapman, 4th ed., p. 206.

11. **Bronchography is the study performed for**
    (a) Bronchial tree (b) Great vessels
    (c) GIT (d) Renal system

    Ans. (a). Radiological Procedures, S.K. Bhargava & Sumeet Bhargava, 2nd ed., Pee Pee Publishers, p. 141-151.

LACRIMAL GLANDS AND SALIVARY GLANDS

1. **Contrast medium used for dacryocystography**
   (a) Water soluble (b) Lipid soluble
   (c) Barium (d) Any of the above

   Ans. (a). Radiological Procedures, S.K. Bhargava & Sumeet Bhargava, 2nd ed., Pee Pee Publishers, p. 192-196.

2. **During dacryocystography contrast is injected in**
   (a) Upper canaliculus (b) Lower canaliculus
   (c) Common canaliculus (d) Nasolacrimal duct

   Ans. (b). Radiological Procedures, S.K. Bhargava & Sumeet Bhargava, 2nd ed., Pee Pee Publishers, p. 192-196.

3. **Term sialography was coined by**
   (a) Wilhelm Roentgen (b) Ollerenshaw
   (c) Antoneduck (d) Rose

   Ans. (c). Radiological Procedures, S.K. Bhargava & Sumeet Bhargava, 2nd ed., Pee Pee Publishers, p. 192-196.

4. **Contraindication for sialography**
   (a) Acute inflammation
   (b) Chronic inflammation
   (c) Calculus
   (d) Sicca syndrome

   Ans. (a). Radiological Procedures, S.K. Bhargava & Sumeet Bhargava, 2nd ed., Pee Pee Publishers, p. 192-196.

5. **Orifice of parotid duct opens opposite the crown of**
   (a) Third molar (b) Second molar
   (c) First molar (d) Second premolar

   Ans. (b). Radiological Procedures, S.K. Bhargava & Sumeet Bhargava, 2nd ed., Pee Pee Publishers, p. 192-196.

6. On the base of frenulum of tongue orifice of following opens
(a) Parotid gland (b) Sublingual gland
(c) Submandibular gland (d) Lacrimal gland

Ans. (c). *Radiological Procedures, S.K. Bhargava & Sumeet Bhargava, 2nd ed., Pee Pee Publishers, p. 192-196.*

7. Post-secretory film in sialography is taken after a duration of
(a) 15 min (b) 5 min
(c) 10 min (d) 20 min

Ans. (b). *Radiological Procedures, S.K. Bhargava & Sumeet Bhargava, 2nd ed., Pee Pee Publishers, p. 192-196.*

8. Sialoscintigraphy is done for the assessment of
(a) Xerostomia (b) Salivary duct patency
(c) Salivary gland function (d) All of the above

Ans. (d). *Radiological Procedures, S.K. Bhargava & Sumeet Bhargava, 2nd ed., Pee Pee Publishers, p. 192-196.*

9. Radiopharmaceutical used for sialoscintigraphy is
(a) 99 m-Tc pertechnate (b) MIBG
(c) FDG (d) Tc HMPAO

Ans. (a). *Radiological Procedures, S.K. Bhargava & Sumeet Bhargava, 2nd ed., Pee Pee Publishers, p. 192-196.*

10. For visualisation of submandibular gland during sialography, following films are taken
(a) Inferosuperior using an occlusal film
(b) Lateral
(c) Both of above
(d) None of above

Ans. (c). *Radiological Procedures, S.K. Bhargava & Sumeet Bhargava, 2nd ed., Pee Pee Publishers, p. 192-196.*

11. Sialography procedure is done for
(a) Parotid or submandibular gland
(b) Thyroid gland
(c) Spleen
(d) Parathyroid

Ans. (a). *Radiological Procedures, S.K. Bhargava & Sumeet Bhargava, 2nd ed., Pee Pee Publishers, p. 192-196.*

12. 'Lemon/vitamin C' tablet
(a) Stimulates the secretion of saliva.
(b) Inhibits the secretion of saliva.

(c) Does not affect the secretion of saliva
(d) Both (a) and (b)

Ans. (a). *Radiological Procedures, S.K. Bhargava & Sumeet Bhargava, 2nd ed., Pee Pee Publishers, p. 192-196.*

13. In sialography, less than _______ masses may not be detected.

(a) 1 cm (b) 2 cm
(c) 3 cm (d) 4 cm

Ans. (a). *Radiological Procedures, S.K. Bhargava & Sumeet Bhargava, 2nd ed., Pee Pee Publishers, p. 192-196.*

14. Which procedure is done by which nasolacrimal duct system is opacified by injecting contrast media into it?

(a) Bronchography (b) Thermography
(c) Dacryocystography (d) None of the above

Ans. (c). *Radiological Procedures, S.K. Bhargava & Sumeet Bhargava, 2nd ed., Pee Pee Publishers, p. 192-196.*

15. Which one is the indication of dacryocystography?

(a) Chronic dacryocystitis (b) Tumors
(c) Epiphora (d) All of the above

Ans. (d). *Radiological Procedures, S.K. Bhargava & Sumeet Bhargava, 2nd ed., Pee Pee Publishers, p. 192-196.*

LIVER AND BILIARY TRACT

1. 95% of adult spleens measure _______ or less in length.

(a) 12 cm (b) 14 cm
(c) 16 cm (d) 10 cm

Ans. (a). *A Guide to Radiological Procedures, Chapman, 4th ed., p. 123.*

2. Intrahepatic ducts are dilated if their diameter is more than _______ of the accompanying portal vein branch.

(a) 60 (b) 50
(c) 30 (d) 40

Ans. (d). *A Guide to Radiological Procedures, Chapman, 4th ed., p. 124.*

3. Upper limit for pancreatic duct measurement is

(a) 8 mm (b) 3 mm
(c) 6 mm (d) 10 mm

Ans. (b). *A Guide to Radiological Procedures, Chapman, 4th ed., p. 127.*

4. After how much of a bolus injection, arterial phase begins for CT abdomen

(a) 50s (b) 100s
(c) 25s (d) 7s

Ans. (c). *A Guide to Radiological Procedures, Chapman, 4th ed., p. 135.*

5. Following is a cholangiographic agent

(a) Meglumine iotroxate (b) Urografin
(c) Barium (d) Iopamidol

Ans. (a). *A Guide to Radiological Procedures, Chapman, 4th ed., p. 108.*

6. Normal liver shows

(a) Increased T_1 signal (b) Increased T_2 signal
(c) Decreased T_1 signal (d) Decreased T_2 signal

Ans. (a). *A Guide to Radiological Procedures, Chapman, 4th ed., p. 132.*

7. MRCP is a non-invasive technique that uses heavily

(a) T_1 weighted (b) PD weighted
(c) T_2 weighted (d) FIESTA

Ans. (c). *A Guide to Radiological Procedures, Chapman, 4th ed., p. 132.*

8. Biliary contrast media are

(a) Triiodobenzoic acid derivatives
(b) Monoiodobenzoic acid derivatives
(c) Iodic acid derivatives
(d) Barium derivatives

Ans. (a). *A Guide to Radiological Procedures, Chapman, 4th ed., p. 104.*

9. T-Tube cholangiography is performed on _______ postoperative day.

(a) Eighth (b) Six
(c) Tenth (d) Two

Ans. (c). *A Guide to Radiological Procedures, Chapman, 4th ed., p. 110.*

10. Following is the indication for biphasic scanning of liver

(a) Cirrhosis (b) Jaundice
(c) Liver tumors (d) Cholelithiasis

Ans. (c). A Guide to Radiological Procedures, Chapman, 4th ed., p. 136.

11. How many days after operation that T-tube cholangiography done?

(a) 8–10 days
(b) 10–12 days
(c) 12–15 days
(d) 15–18 days

***Ans. (a).** Radiological Procedures, S.K. Bhargava & Sumeet Bhargava, 2nd ed., Pee Pee Publishers, p. 67-79.*

12. In T-tube cholangiography, how much contrast is required?

(a) 25–30 cc (b) 15–20 cc
(c) 20–25 cc (d) 30–35 cc

***Ans. (c).** Radiological Procedures, S.K. Bhargava & Sumeet Bhargava, 2nd ed., Pee Pee Publishers, p. 67-79.*

13. Pitfalls of T-tube cholangiography are

(a) Free drainage of contrast media into the duodenum
(b) Differentiate between air bubble and calculi
(c) Taking the oblique/lateral views
(d) Rapid injection of contrast media resulting in spasm of sphincter of Oddi

***Ans. (b).** Radiological Procedures, S.K. Bhargava & Sumeet Bhargava, 2nd ed., Pee Pee Publishers, p. 67-79.*

14. Chiba needle used in PTC is of

(a) 22/23 G (b) 23/24 G
(c) 21/22 G (d) 20/21 G

***Ans. (a).** Radiological Procedures, S.K. Bhargava & Sumeet Bhargava, 2nd ed., Pee Pee Publishers, p. 296-299.*

15. What is the length of Chiba needle?

(a) 15–20 cm (b) 20–25 cm
(c) 25–30 cm (d) 30–35 cm

***Ans. (a).** Radiological Procedures, S.K. Bhargava & Sumeet Bhargava, 2nd ed., Pee Pee Publishers, p. 296-299.*

16. 1 F =______.

(a) 0.0131 inch (b) 0.254 inch
(c) 0.314 inch (d) 0.894 inch

***Ans. (a).** Radiological Procedures, S.K. Bhargava & Sumeet Bhargava, 2nd ed., Pee Pee Publishers, p. 296-299.*

LYMPHATIC SYSTEM

1. **Sentinel node in lymphoscintigraphy refers to**
   (a) Second node
   (b) First node
   (c) Third node
   (d) Fourth node

   Ans. (b). *A Guide to Radiological Procedures, Chapman, 4th ed., p. 248.*

2. **Site of injection ^{99m}Tc colloid for detection of nodes below diaphragm**
   (a) First and second interdigital web space of foot
   (b) Third and fourth interdigital web space of foot
   (c) Popliteal fossa
   (d) Inguinal region

   Ans. (a). *A Guide to Radiological Procedures, Chapman, 4th ed., p. 249.*

3. **Site of injection ^{99m}Tc colloid for detection of nodes in axillary region**
   (a) Cubital fossa
   (b) First and second interdigital webbed space
   (c) Second and third interdigital webbed space
   (d) Axillary region

   Ans. (c). *A Guide to Radiological Procedures, Chapman, 4th ed., p. 249.*

4. **Site of injection ^{99m}Tc colloid for detection of nodes in intermammary region**
   (a) Periosteum of ribs
   (b) Posterior rectus sheath beside the xiphisternum
   (c) Sub-areolar region
   (d) All of the above

   Ans. (d). *A Guide to Radiological Procedures, Chapman, 4th ed., p. 249.*

5. **Site of injection ^{99m}Tc colloid for detection of nodes in ileopelvic region**
   (a) Bilateral ischiorectal fossae
   (b) Suprapubic
   (c) Perianal
   (d) Bilateral thigh

   Ans. (a). *A Guide to Radiological Procedures, Chapman, 4th ed., p. 249.*

6. **Radiopharmaceutical used for imaging of infection**
   (a) ^{111}In-labelled leucocytes
   (b) ^{99m}Tc-HMPAO labelled leucocytes
   (c) ^{67}Ga gallium citrate
   (d) All of the above

   Ans. (d). *A Guide to Radiological Procedures, Chapman, 4th ed., p. 251.*

7. **The diagnosis of bone infection improved by**
   (a) Two-phase imaging
   (b) Three-phase imaging
   (c) Four-phase imaging
   (d) Single-phase imaging

   Ans. (b). *A Guide to Radiological Procedures, Chapman, 4th ed., p. 253.*

8. **Gallium radionuclide tumor imaging is used for the detection of**
   (a) Carcinoma (b) Sarcoma
   (c) Hodgkin lymphoma (d) Leukaemia

   Ans. (c). *A Guide to Radiological Procedures, Chapman, 4th ed., p. 254.*

9. **Thyroid blockade prior to imaging with ^{123}I-metaiodobenzyl-guanidine (MIBG) is done using**
   (a) Potassium perchlorate (b) Lugol's iodine
   (c) Any of the above (d) None of the above

   Ans. (c). *A Guide to Radiological Procedures, Chapman, 4th ed., p. 256.*

10. **Blood glucose prior to imaging with 18F-Fluorodeoxyglucose (FDG) PET scanning should be**
    (a) Normal to high (b) Normal to low
    (c) Very high (d) Very low

    Ans. (b). *A Guide to Radiological Procedures, Chapman, 4th ed., p. 259.*

THYROID AND PARATHYROIDS

1. **Indications for ultrasound of thyroid**
   (a) Palpable thyroid mass (b) Suspected thyroid tumor
   (c) Guided aspiration (d) All of the above

   Ans. (d). *Radiological Procedures, S.K. Bhargava & Sumeet Bhargava, 2nd ed., Pee Pee Publishers, p. 189-191.*

2. Transducer used for scanning of thyroid gland

(a) 5–10 MHz (b) 10–15 MHz
(c) 15–20 MHz (d) 2–5 MHz

Ans. (a). *Radiological Procedures, S.K. Bhargava & Sumeet Bhargava, 2nd ed., Pee Pee Publishers, p. 189-191.*

3. Indications for radionuclide thyroid imaging

(a) Investigation of thyroid nodule
(b) Assessment of goitre
(c) Assessment of thyroid uptake prior to radioiodine therapy
(d) All of the above

Ans. (d). *Radiological Procedures, S.K. Bhargava & Sumeet Bhargava, 2nd ed., Pee Pee Publishers, p. 189-191.*

4. Preferred radiopharmaceutical for thyroid imaging

(a) I–131 (b) I–123
(c) I–125 (d) I–120

Ans. (b). *Radiological Procedures, S.K. Bhargava & Sumeet Bhargava, 2nd ed., Pee Pee Publishers, p. 189-191.*

5. Radiopharmaceuticals used for parathyroid imaging

(a) ^{99m}Tc-MIBI
(b) ^{99m}Tc-tetroformin
(c) ^{201}Tl-thallous chloride
(d) All of the above

Ans. (d). *Radiological Procedures, S.K. Bhargava & Sumeet Bhargava, 2nd ed., Pee Pee Publishers, p. 189-191.*

PART 2

BONES & JOINTS

1. Regarding plain film before arthrography which of the following is true?

(a) Plain film in AP must be taken before arthrography
(b) Plain film is optional, but ultrasonography should be done
(c) Plain film in different views should be taken

Ans. (c). *A Guide to Radiological Procedures, 4th Edition; Chapman, p. 265.*

After injection of contrast, some important findings may be getting obscured; so, plain film in all necessary views should be done prior to arthrography.

2. In which position, second set of images should be taken during shoulder arthrography?

(a) Adduction & internal rotation
(b) Abduction & internal rotation
(c) Adduction & external rotation
(d) Abduction & external rotation

Ans. (d). *A Guide to Radiological Procedures, 4th edition; Chapman, p. 271.*

Shoulder arthrographic images should be taken in two positions; first at neutral and second at Abduction & External Rotation (ABER).

3. Which of the following is false regarding injection of contrast for elbow arthrography?

(a) Injected in lateral approach
(b) Patient should be in prone position
(c) Elbow should be completely extended
(d) 3–6 ml contrast should be injected

Ans. (c). *A Guide to Radiological Procedures, 4th edition; Chapman, p. 274.*

Elbow should be flexed for 90 degrees for shoulder arthrography.

4. 'Mighty elbow position' is best described as

(a) Prone, arm and elbow fully extended overhead
(b) Prone, arm and elbow fully flexed overhead
(c) Supine, arm and elbow fully extended overhead
(d) Supine, arm and elbow fully flexed overhead

Ans. (a). *A Guide to Radiological Procedures, 4th edition; Chapman, p. 274.*

Mighty elbow position is the best position for an elbow to be examined. It is prone with arm, forearm are fully extended overhead.

5. VATER

(a) Vertebral, Anal, Tracheo-esophageal and Renal anomalies
(b) Vertebral, Anus, Tissue-esophageal and Renal anomalies
(c) Vertebral Activity, Tracheo-esophageal and Retroperitoneal anomalies
(d) Vertebral, Anal, Tissue-esophagus and Uterine anomalies

Ans. (a). *Radiological Procedures, S.K. Bhargava & Sumeet Bhargava, 2nd ed., Pee Pee Publishers, p. 115-126.*

CT – PROTOCOLS & EQUIPMENTS

1. Mr. Goyal, 45 years old gentleman, underwent ultrasound for a suspected renal calculus; on ultrasound there was a 7 mm calculus at upper pole calyx of right kidney, in addition he also had an incidental well defined, homogenously hyperechoic 3 cm lesion noted at right adrenal gland. Left adrenal was normal; chest X-ray was done, and that was also normal. He comes to you with provisional diagnosis of adrenal adenoma. Which of the following is true regarding adrenal adenoma?

(a) Adrenal adenoma can be reliably diagnosed with NCCT
(b) Should proceed with contrast whatever may be the finding in NCCT
(c) MRI should be done to diagnose adrenal adenoma
(d) Delayed scans upto 24 hours may be needed

Ans. (a). *Diagnostic imaging series; Amirsys; 5th ed., P: IV-2-2.*

Adrenal adenoma can be reliably diagnosed with NCCT, if the tumor is having HU density less than 15; if not should proceed with adrenal protocol CT.

2. What is 'adrenal CT protocol'?

(a) Taking delayed images at 5 min after contrast administration
(b) Taking delayed images at 10 min after contrast administration
(c) Taking delayed images at 15 min after contrast administration
(d) Taking delayed images at 30 min after contrast administration

Ans. (b). *Diagnostic imaging series; Amirsys; 5th ed., P: IV-2-2.*

Adrenal CT protocol: *When a patient presented with adrenal mass non-contrast scan is mandatory first;then HU value of the adrenal lesion should be measured, if HU value is less than 15, adenoma can be diagnosed reliably and no need of contrast scans. If it is more than 15, then contrast scan should be done, followed by delayed images at 10 minutes and relative and absolute washout should be measured to differentiate adenoma and other tumors.*

3. Non-contrast CT is used to evaluate all of the followings, except

(a) Adrenal adenoma
(b) Urolithiasis
(c) To detect acute hematoma
(d) To evaluate pelvic ureteric junction (PUJ) obstruction

Ans. (d). *Diagnostic imaging series; Amirsys; 5th ed., p. IV-3-2.*

To evaluate PUJ obstruction IVU is preferred., not NCCT.

4. What is the preferred oral contrast for renal MDCT?

(a) Barium (b) Water
(c) 5% iodine contrast (d) 10% iodine contrast

Ans. (b). *Diagnostic imaging series; Amirsys; 5th ed., P: IV-3-2.*

Using positive oral contrast will impair the renal evaluation due to overlaying. Preferred technique for renal CT is 'no oral contrast' or 'water (negative contrast)'.

5. Which vein is preferred to inject contrast for CT scanning?

(a) Lower limb veins (b) Anti-cubital vein
(c) Cephalic vein (d) Basilic vein

Ans. (b). *A Guide to Radiological Procedures, 4th edition; Chapman, p. 143.*

Anti-cubital vein is the preferred vein to inject contrast in any case for CT scanning.

6. Which is the best phase to look for renal mass?

(a) Cortico-medullary phase (CM)
(b) Nephrographic phase (NG)
(c) Delayed phase
(d) Non-contrast scans

Ans. (b). *Diagnostic imaging series; Amirsys; 5th ed., P: IV-3-2.*

In corticomedullary phase hypovascular lesions can be missed, so best phase is NG phase to look for a renal mass.

7. What is the delay given for nephrographic phase in renal MDCT?

(a) 20–40 seconds (b) 60–90 seconds
(c) 90–120 seconds (d) 3–5 mins

Ans. (c). *Diagnostic imaging series; Amirsys; 5th ed., P: IV-3-2.*

CM phase: 25–80 seconds.
NG phase: 90–120 seconds.
Excretory phase: 3–5 mins.

8. Which of the following is false regarding maximum intensity projection (MIP)?

(a) High density structures demonstrated well
(b) Main disadvantage is area of interest may be obscured by other high density structures
(c) It gives 3-D effect
(d) It gives good depth perception

Ans. (d). *Diagnostic Radiology; Grainger & Allison's; 5th edition, p. 189.*

MIP: In this method maximum voxel intensity along the viewer projection is displayed. In this method high density structures demonstrated nicely. It gives a 3-D effect; but there is no depth perception.

9. What is the use of minimal intensity projection in chest CT?

(a) To evaluate chest wall lesions
(b) To evaluate embolism
(c) To improve conspicuity of subtle differences in lung attenuation
(d) To evaluate nodular lesions

Ans. (c). *Diagnostic Radiology; Grainger & Allison's; 5th edition, p. 190.*

Minimal intensity projection (MiniP) will clearly demonstrate subtle differences in lung attenuation, therefore used to highlight the area of air trapping.

10. Which of the following method will be more useful to evaluate chest wall lesions?

(a) MIP (b) MiniP
(c) SSD (d) Curved MPR

Ans. (c). *Diagnostic Radiology; Grainger & Allison's; 5th edition, p. 190.*

Surface shaded display (SSD) displays interfaces, so it is very useful in evaluating chest wall lesions.

11. Which of the following is true regarding CT scanning of patient with pulmonary embolism?

(a) Should be done from craniocaudal direction
(b) Should be done from caudocranial direction
(c) Should be done with respiration hold at expiration
(d) Should be done in prone position

Ans. (b). *Diagnostic imaging series; Amirsys; 5th ed., P: II-4-52.*

In a suspected case of pulmonary embolism, scanning should be taken in caudocranial direction to avoid respiratory motion.

12. What is the scan delay for a case of pulmonary embolism?

(a) 8 sec (b) 15 sec
(c) 20 sec (d) 60 sec

Ans. (c). *Diagnostic imaging series; Amirsys; 5th ed., P: IV-3-2.*

Even though arm-pulmonary artery time is less than 10 sec, preferably scanning should be done after 20 sec letting the pulmonary vein and left atrium filled with contrast.

13. Which of the following is false regarding CT scanning of abdomen?

(a) Negative oral contrast is preferred for most of the GIT conditions
(b) Arm should be by the side of patient when scanning
(c) 50–60 second delay is given for portovenous phase
(d) Scanning at 25 sec delay (arterial phase) should be done in every case

Ans. (b). *Diagnostic imaging series; Amirsys; 5th edition. P: II-5-2.*

For most of the GIT conditions, negative oral contrast is preferred now. After 30–45 min, patient should be positioned at supine with arm above the head to avoid beam hardening artifacts from bones. Arterial phase is not necessary in every case.

14. Which of the following is false regarding thin reconstruction for HRCT?

(a) For HRCT chest thin reconstructions around 1 mm should be made
(b) Sections thinner than 1 mm doesn't increase the information
(c) Making thinner sections, visualizes structures sharply
(d) Making thinner sections decreases noise

Ans. (d). *Diagnostic Radiology; Grainger & Allison's. 5th edition, p. 190.*

Making thinner sections will increase the resolution, but will increase the noise.

16. What is the recommended thickness of sections for staging of lung cancer?

(a) 1 mm (b) 3 mm
(c) 5 mm (d) 7 mm

Ans. (b). *Diagnostic Radiology; Grainger & Allison's; 5th edition, p. 191.*

REPRODUCTIVE SYSTEM

1. Which of the following is the relative contraindication for hysterosalpingography?

(a) Pregnancy
(b) Pelvic inflammatory disease
(c) Active menstruation
(d) Severe iodine allergy

Ans. (c). *A Guide to Radiological Procedures, 4th edition; Chapman, p. 175.*

Active menstrual bleeding may cause extravasation, which may interfere with interpretation; but it is a relative contraindication only; Rests are the absolute contraindications.

2. What is the advantage of oil based contrasts used in HSG?
(a) No risk of embolization
(b) No risk of peritoneal granulomatous reaction
(c) Increased post-test fertility rate
(d) Less painful

Ans. (c). *A Guide to Radiological Procedures, 4th edition; Chapman, p. 175.*

Oil based contrast agents may clear the impaction in tube and show increased post-test fertility rate.

3. Which is the best modality to look for fallopian tubes?
(a) USG (b) MRI
(c) CECT (d) HSG

Ans. (d). *A Guide to Radiological Procedures, 4th edition; Chapman, p. 175.*

MRI and ultrasound are excellent for demonstrating the uterus, but both studies are poor at showing the normal fallopian tubes. Dilated fallopian tubes can be identified on MRI and ultrasound, but abnormality in non-dilated tubes and patency of it is best seen on a hysterosalpingogram.

4. In which time of menstrual cycle HSG should be done?
(a) 6 to 10 days (b) Just before menstruation
(c) At any time (d) 14 to 20 days of cycle

Ans. (a). *A Guide to Radiological Procedures, 4th edition; Chapman, p. 176.*

Rule of ten in radiology: *Any radiological procedure in radiology should be done in first 10 days of menstrual cycle, because chance of pregnancy after ovulation (14th day). During menstruation risk of intravasation is high. Immediately after menstruation endometrium will be thin so that it will be easy to interpret. So, HSG can be best done during 6th to 10th day of cycle.*

5. All of the followings are the common indications for HSG, except
(a) Infertility
(b) Post-menopausal bleeding
(c) Post-tubal surgery
(d) Recurrent spontaneous abortions

Ans. (b). *A Guide to Radiological Procedures, 4th edition; Chapman, p. 176.*

HSG is not much useful to evaluate endometrial diseases, which are the main reason for post-menopausal bleeding. But, it is mainly used to look for tubal patency in infertility patients and post-tubal surgeries. It also can be used in cases of recurrent abortions, to look for any mullerian anomalies.

6. **True about virtual hysterosalpingography is**
   (a) It is done by using 3D ultrasound
   (b) Can be done at any time in menstrual cycle
   (c) No need to inject contrast
   (d) No radiation exposure to staff

   Ans. (d). *Virtual hysterosalpingography; Radiographics 2010; 30: 643-663.*

   Virtual hysterosalpingography is a new method done by using multi-slice CT, after injecting iodine-based contrast though cervix, and making 3D reconstruction. Advantages over conventional HSG are it provides complete evaluation of pelvis, nearly equal radiation exposure (using low dose protocol) and no radiation exposure to the staff.

7. **What is the advantage of hysterosalpingography over sono-hysterography?**
   (a) Better for endometrial lesions than sonohysterography
   (b) No radiation exposure
   (c) No need of iodine contrast
   (d) Better tubal assessment than sonohysterography

   Ans. (d). *Hysterosalpingography; March 2006 Radiographics, 26, 419-431.*

   Sonohysterography is done by injecting saline, Echovist or air into cervix under ultrasound examination. It gives better assessment of endometrium than conventional HSG, but less effective for tubal assessment.

8. **Non-distensible endometrial cavity with multiple filling defects on HSG is seen in**
   (a) Endometrial carcinoma (b) Endometrial polyps
   (c) Asherman's syndrome (d) Unicornuate uterus

   Ans. (c). *Diagnostic imaging series; Amirsys; 5th edition. P: II-58.*

   Multiple filling defects can be seen in endometrial carcinoma & polyp also; but, ***non-distensible endometrial cavity*** *is diagnostic of Asherman's syndrome.*

9. **Which of the following point favors diagnosis of salpingitis isthmica nodosa (SIN), rather than tuberculosis on HSG?**

(a) Small outpouchings in isthmic portion of fallopian tube
(b) Fimbrial stenosis
(c) Normal tubal diameter
(d) Loculated peritoneal spill

Ans. (c). *Diagnostic imaging series; Amirsys; 5th ed., P: VII-22.*

SIN: *Small outpouchings are seen in isthmic portion of fallopian tube, which also can be seen in tuberculosis. But in SIN tube will be having normal diameter and fimbrial end will be normal unlike tuberculosis.*

10. Which is the best imaging modality for salpingitis isthmica nodosa?

(a) MRI
(b) CECT
(c) HSG
(d) Sonohysterography

Ans. (c). *Diagnostic imaging series; Amirsys; 5th ed., P: VII-22.*

HSG is the best investigation to diagnose salpingitis isthmica nodosa, as it shows outpouchings very clearly and also the tubal caliber can be well assessed.

11. HSG is done for

(a) Uterus
(b) Uterine cavity
(c) Fallopian tubes
(d) All of the above

Ans. (d). *Radiological Procedures, S.K. Bhargava & Sumeet Bhargava, 2nd ed., Pee Pee Publishers, p. 132-140.*

12. Indication of HSG

(a) Infertility
(b) Recurrent abortion
(c) Migrated IUCD and uterine and tubal lesion
(d) All of the above

Ans. (d). *Radiological Procedures, S.K. Bhargava & Sumeet Bhargava, 2nd ed., Pee Pee Publishers, p. 132-140.*

13. Leech Wilkinson cannula used in

(a) Barium swallow
(b) IVU
(c) HSG
(d) MCU

Ans. (c). *Radiological Procedures, S.K. Bhargava & Sumeet Bhargava, 2nd ed., Pee Pee Publishers, p. 132-140.*

14. The ideal period for HSG is

(a) Any time
(b) After ovulation
(c) End of mens
(d) Between 8th and 10th days

Ans. (d). *Radiological Procedures, S.K. Bhargava & Sumeet Bhargava, 2nd ed., Pee Pee Publishers, p. 132-140.*

SPINE

1. Which is the modality of choice to look for CSF leak following myelography?

(a) CECT
(b) MRI
(c) Repeat myelography without further injection
(d) Nucleotide imaging

Ans. (d). *A Guide to Radiological Procedures; Chapman.4th edition, p. 308.*

Radionucleotide imaging is able to pick-up CSF collection in basal cisterns following myelography.

2. Which is the best imaging modality for a suspected case of disc herniation?

(a) Plain radiograph (b) NCCT
(c) MRI (d) Myelography

Ans. (c). *A Guide to Radiological Procedures; Chapman.4th edition, p. 310.*

CT and MRI have rendered invasive techniques such as epidurography and lumbar epidural venography obsolete.They replaced myelography as the first method for investigating suspected disc prolapse. High quality axial imaging by CT is an accurate means of demonstration of disc herniation, but in practice, many studies are less than optimal due to obesity, scoliosis and beam-hardening effects due to dense bone sclerosis. For these reasons, and because of better contrast resolution, MRI is the preferred technique.

3. Which is the time delay given in CT myelography after injection of contrast?

(a) Upto 10 min (b) Upto 30 min
(c) Upto 2 hours (d) Upto 4 hours

Ans. (d). *A Guide to Radiological Procedures; Chapman, 4th edition, p. 319.*

CT myelography should be delayed for upto 4 hr to allow dilution of the contrast medium. A very high concentration may cause difficulty in resolving the cervical nerve roots. Turning the patient a few times prior to CT ensures even distribution and reduces layering effects. In studying the spinal cord a delay is not required, though again good mixing of the CSF with contrast medium is essential.

4. **Which of the following is false regarding lumbar puncture in a case of myelodysraphism?**
   (a) There is increased risk of spinal cord damage due to low lying cord
   (b) Cervical spine should be examined for cerebellar tonsillar herniation before starting puncture
   (c) Thecal sac will be narrow in these conditions
   (d) Needle should be placed laterally in sac

   Ans. (c). *A Guide to Radiological Procedures; Chapman, 4th edition, p. 320.*

   Lumbar puncture in cases of spinal dysraphism carries the risk of damaging a low-lying cord due to teethering.the thecal sac is usually wide in these conditions and the needle should be placed laterally in the thecal sac. In addition, as low a puncture as possible will minimize the risk, though in practice spinal cord injury is very uncommon or masked by the neurologic deficit already present. In dysraphism,the frequent association of cerebellar tonsillar herniation precludes lateral C1/2 puncture.

5. **Most common complication of myelography is**
   (a) Hallucination
   (b) Nausea
   (c) Headache
   (d) Sub-dural injection of contrast medium

   Ans. (c). *A Guide to Radiological Procedures; Chapman, 4th edition, p. 320.*

6. **Which of the following is true regarding guided biopsy from vertebra?**
   (a) Chiba needle is most commonly used
   (b) Preliminary CT is must even when biopsy will be done under fluoroscopy guidance
   (c) Biopsy needles should be used rather than FNA for a highly vascular lesion
   (d) Can be done even coagulation profile is altered because of surrounding bone

   Ans. (b). *A Guide to Radiological Procedures; Chapman.4th edition, p. 325.*

   Vertebral body lesions may be biopsied under either CT or fluoroscopic control. Small lesions, especially those located in the posterior neural arch, are best done under CT control. A preliminary CT scan is helpful, whatever method is finally chosen to control the procedure.

7. Contrast most commonly incorrectly injected into which of the following space?

(a) Spinal canal
(b) Epidural space
(c) Subcutaneous space
(d) Thecal space

Ans. (b). *A Guide to Radiological Procedures; Chapman. 4th edition, p. 320.*

Contrast most commonly injected incorrectly into epidural space. So, examiner should be keen about the space of injection.

8. Which of the following is a contraindication of myelogram?

(a) Local sepsis
(b) Clotting disorder
(c) Iodine sensitivity
(d) All of the above

Ans. (d). *Radiological Procedures, S.K. Bhargava & Sumeet Bhargava, 2nd ed., Pee Pee Publishers, p. 104-114.*

9. Which one of the following contrast media is used in myelogram?

(a) Isohexol
(b) Urografin
(c) ProHance
(d) Gadobutrol

Ans. (a). *Radiological Procedures, S.K. Bhargava & Sumeet Bhargava, 2nd ed., Pee Pee Publishers, p. 104-114.*

10. In myelography, low viscosity of contrast media provides

(a) Excellent filling of nerve root
(b) Less quantity is used
(c) Reaction chances decrease
(d) Easy to fill-up by syringe

Ans. (a). *Radiological Procedures, S.K. Bhargava & Sumeet Bhargava, 2nd ed., Pee Pee Publishers, p. 104-114.*

URINARY TRACT

1. A patient is send to you by a clinician for IVP, but the patient has history of allergic reaction for contrast previously; what will be your action?

(a) IVP could not be done for such patient
(b) No precaution needed
(c) Can be done with low osmolar contrast medium (LOCM)
(d) Can be done under steroid cover and using low osmolar contrast media

Ans. (d). *A Guide to Radiological Procedures, 4th edition; Chapman, p. 142.*

Patient with previous allergic reactions should undergo other modality, if possible. If IVU is mandatory, should be started with methyl prednisolone 32 mg orally, 12 and 2 hours prior to injection of i.v. contrast media in addition to ensuring that LOCM is used.

2. What is the role of preliminary oblique view in IVU?

(a) Should be done routinely
(b) Should be done in suspected cases of renal cell carcinoma
(c) Should be done in cases of hematuria
(d) Should be done in suspected cases of renal calculi but no calculus is seen in preliminary KUB film

Ans. (d). *A Guide to Radiological Procedures, 4th edition; Chapman, p. 142.*

When calculus is suspected strongly on clinical grounds, but no calculus is seen in KUB film a oblique film should be taken; in this view any calculus over sacrum can be picked up, where it is easily missed.

3. Regarding injection of contrast during IVU which of the following is correct?

(a) Should be given slowly
(b) Should be given as rapid bolus
(c) Can be given by either way

Ans. (b). *A Guide to Radiological Procedures, 4th edition; Chapman, p. 143.*

Contrast should be given as rapid bolus to increase the density of nephrogram.

4. Which of the following is true regarding 5 min film of IVU?

(a) Not mandatory
(b) Invaluable in modifying the examination
(c) Compression should be applied prior to 5 min film
(d) Pelvicalyceal system is clearly seen in this film

Ans. (b). *A Guide to Radiological Procedures, 4th edition; Chapman, p. 143.*

5 min film in IVU is mandatory and it is used to look for symmetric excretion of contrast and used to modify the exam e.g. a further injection of contrast medium if there has been poor initial opacification. Compression should be applied after 5 min film.

5. Compression is contraindicated in all of the following conditions except

(a) Following recent surgery
(b) Following recent trauma
(c) In cases with renal calculus
(d) In cases with abdominal masses

Ans. (c). *A Guide to Radiological Procedures, 4th edition; Chapman, p. 143.*

Compression is contraindicated in cases where complete obstruction of urinary tract is seen or suspected, not in every cases of renal calculus.

6. Post-micturition film should be taken with following method

(a) Full-length abdominal film or a coned view of the bladder with the tube angled 30° caudal and centered at the symphysis pubis
(b) Full-length abdominal film or a coned view of the bladder with the tube angled 15° caudal and centered 5 cm above the symphysis pubis
(c) Full-length abdominal film or a coned view of the bladder with the tube directed perpendicularly and centered 5 cm above the symphysis pubis
(d) Full-length abdominal film or a coned view of the bladder with the tube angled 15° cephalad and centered 5 cm above the symphysis pubis

Ans. (b). *A Guide to Radiological Procedures, 4th edition; Chapman, p. 144.*

The principal value of this film is to assess bladder emptying, to demonstrate a return to normal of dilated upper tracts with relief of bladder pressure, to aid the diagnosis of bladder tumors, to confirm ureterovesical junction calculi and, uncommonly, to demonstrate a urethral diverticulum in females.

7. Which is the best view for UV junction calculus?

(a) Plain film
(b) Full film with compression
(c) Post-release film
(d) Post-micturition film

Ans. (d). *A Guide to Radiological Procedures, 4th edition; Chapman, p. 144.*

On post-micturition film with tube directed 15° caudally, UV calculus and retained column of contrast in ureter is best seen.

8. What is the role of prone film in IVU?

(a) To look for residual urine
(b) To look for upper ureter
(c) To look for pelvi-ureteric junction of lower ureter
(d) To look for urinary bladder

Ans. (c). *A Guide to Radiological Procedures, 4th edition; Chapman, p. 144.*

Lower part of ureter is difficult to visualize in some cases. In such cases patient should be asked to lay prone, radiograph should be taken after 1–2 min after letting the lower ureter to fill by gravity.

9. In cases where feces filled transverse colon obscures renal area, how will you visualize the kidney?

(a) By taking delayed films
(b) By taking film with 30° caudal angulation
(c) By taking lateral films
(d) By taking films with 10° caudal angulation

Ans. (b). *A Guide to Radiological Procedures, 4th edition; Chapman, p. 144.*

Taking films with 30° caudal angulation will throw the transverse colon out of kidney, so we can well visualize the kidney.

10. Which of the following is true regarding IVU in infant?

(a) IVU is a preferred modality of imaging in infants
(b) Should be done with compression
(c) Optimum visualization of the upper urinary tract may not occur until 1–3 hrs.
(d) Multiple films should be taken in first hour

Ans. (c). *A Guide to Radiological Procedures, 4th edition; Chapman, p. 144.*

In infants IVU is seldom indicated, rather USG and radio-nucleotide imaging should be done.

But when it is done, optimum visualization will not occur until 1–3 hours, so multiple images on first hour will not help.

11. Which is the best position to demonstrate the ureterocele?

(a) Supine position
(b) Prone position
(c) Dead lateral view
(d) 30° oblique position

Ans. (d). *A Guide to Radiological Procedures, 4th edition; Chapman, p. 144.*

Position of lower ureter and ureterocele is best demonstrated when the child is in 30° oblique position.

12. What is the major indication of retrograde pyelography?

(a) When patient is having urinary tract infection
(b) When ureterocele is suspected
(c) To demonstrate ureteric calculus
(d) To demonstrate lower limit of ureteric obstruction

Ans. (d). *A Guide to Radiological Procedures, 4th edition; Chapman, p. 154.*

Major indication of retrograde ureterography is to demonstrate of the site, length, lower limit and, if possible, the nature of an obstructive lesion.

13. Which of the following is true regarding Conray-400?

(a) It is a non-ionic contrast
(b) It gives better image quality than omnipaque on IVP
(c) It is associated with fewer incidences of contrast reactions
(d) Less cost effective

Ans. (b). *Radiology Sourcebook, A Practical Guide for Reference and Training; Douglas P. Beall, p. 13.*

Conray-400: *It is an ionic contrast; so, it is cheaper, but incidence of contrast reaction is high; but image quality will be always better with ionic contrasts on IVP.*

14. Which of the following is true regarding micturating cysto-urethrography?

(a) Bladder should be full before starting the procedure
(b) It can be done when there is acute urinary tract infection
(c) It must be done with low osmolar contrasts
(d) It should be examined during initial filling phase with fluoroscopy

Ans. (d). *A Guide to Radiological Procedures, 4th edition; Chapman, p. 157.*

Fluoroscopic examination during initial filling phase is must; because if the tip of the catheter is in the lower ureter it may be misinterpreted as reflux.

15. Lower ureter is best seen in which of the following position?

(a) Anterior oblique position of that side
(b) Anterior oblique position of opposite side
(c) Posterior oblique position of that side
(d) Posterior oblique position of that side

Ans. (a). *A Guide to Radiological Procedures, 4th edition; Chapman, p. 143.*

16. In IVU, scout film is taken

(a) To check the exposure factors (b) To check bowel preparation
(c) To see any calculus (d) All of the above

Ans. (d). *Radiological Procedures, S.K. Bhargava & Sumeet Bhargava, 2nd ed., Pee Pee Publishers, p. 80-100.*

17. In IVU, what is the name of radiograph which is taken after 5 minutes of injection of contrast media?

(a) Nephrogram (b) Pyelogram
(c) Ureterogram (d) Full film

Ans. (b). *Radiological Procedures, S.K. Bhargava & Sumeet Bhargava, 2nd ed., Pee Pee Publishers, p. 80-100.*

18. Standard film taking timing in IVU is

(a) 1 min, 5 min, 10 min, 15 min
(b) 1 min, 8 min, 10 min, 25 min
(c) 5 min, 15 min, 25 min, 35 min
(d) 1 min, 3 min, 5 min, 7 min

Ans. (a). *Radiological Procedures, S.K. Bhargava & Sumeet Bhargava, 2nd ed., Pee Pee Publishers, p. 80-100.*

19. In IVU, why compression band is applied on the patient

(a) To provide good contrast between ureter and soft tissue.
(b) To provide better pelvicalyceal distension.
(c) To minimize the dose of contrast media.
(d) All of the above

Ans. (b). *Radiological Procedures, S.K. Bhargava & Sumeet Bhargava, 2nd ed., Pee Pee Publishers, p. 80-100.*

20. In which condition compression band is contraindicated?

(a) Renal trauma
(b) After abdominal surgery
(c) Abdominal mass
(d) All of the above

Ans. (d). *Radiological Procedures, S.K. Bhargava & Sumeet Bhargava, 2nd ed., Pee Pee Publishers, p. 80-100.*

21. In IVU, which one of the following projections will you take to project the ureter away from spine and to separate overlying shadows minicking calculi?

(a) Erect projection
(b) Prone film
(c) Delayed
(d) Oblique projection

Ans. (d). *Radiological Procedures, S.K. Bhargava & Sumeet Bhargava, 2nd ed., Pee Pee Publishers, p. 80-100.*

22. Which one of the following drugs is used in diuretic urogram to induce diuresis which distends the renal pelvis?

(a) Buscopan
(b) Normal saline
(c) Frusemide
(d) Diazepam

Ans. (c). *Radiological Procedures, S.K. Bhargava & Sumeet Bhargava, 2nd ed., Pee Pee Publishers, p. 80-100.*

ULTRASOUND EQUIPMENT & PROTOCOLS

1. Which is the most important factor determining resolution of a ultrasound image?

(a) Mechanical index
(b) Lateral resolution
(c) Axial resolution
(d) Slice thickness

Ans. (d). *Zwiebel; Introduction to Vascular Sonography, 5th edition, p. 35.*

The slice thickness is the thickness of the scanned section of tissue that contributes to the image. It depends on the width of the ultrasound beam perpendicular to the image plane, often called the ***elevational beam width****. Many phased, linear, and curvilinear array transducers still use a one dimensional array along with a mechanical lens to provide focusing in this direction. While the inplane beam width and, hence,the lateral resolution is exquisitely controlled by electronic focusing, the slice thickness for these units is not the elevational focusing. Mechanical lens provides good detail near the focal zone but poor detail at depths proximal and distal to this zone. Not surprising, therefore, slice thickness is the worst aspect of the resolution of array transducers. So, whenever we are operating ultrasound machine these aspects should be set first.*

2. Which of the following is used to avoid reverberation artifacts, thereby to improve the quality of images in tubular structures like common bile duct?

(a) Color doppler (b) Pulsed doppler
(c) Harmonic imaging (d) Elastography

Ans. (c). *Courtesy of: Zwiebel; Introduction to Vascular Sonography, 5th edition.*

Harmonic imaging is supposed to help reduce reverberation noise in images and thus improve image quality.

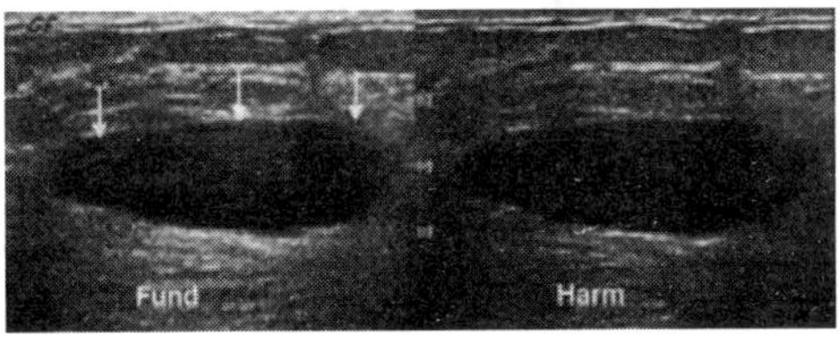

Image of breast cyst with fundamental and harmonic imaging.

3. Which of the following is false regarding instrumentation for harmonic imaging?

(a) Probe with wide frequency range is needed
(b) Waves with high mechanical index are being transmitted
(c) Waves with high frequencies are being transmitted
(d) Waves with frequencies double of the transmitted will be received

Ans. (c). *Zwiebel; Introduction to Vascular Sonography, 5th edition, p. 31.*

During harmonic imaging waves with low frequencies will be transmitted, but only the waves with double the frequencies of the transmitted will be receives. So, the frequency range for probe should be high.

4. Which of the following is true regarding linear array probes?

(a) It has low frame rate
(b) It produces beams that sweep out a rectangular two-dimensional plane
(c) Lens is needed to focus in transverse plane
(d) Beam thickness is constant throughout the depth

Ans. (c).

Linear probes	*Sector probes*
They have good transverse focus throughout the depth of field	*They provide potentially high frame rates*
They have to be mechanically scanned to obtain a two-dimensional image	*A disadvantage is that they must be focused in the transverse direction with physical acoustics using a lens or curved surface.the result is a beam thickness that changes the transverse dimension with depth*

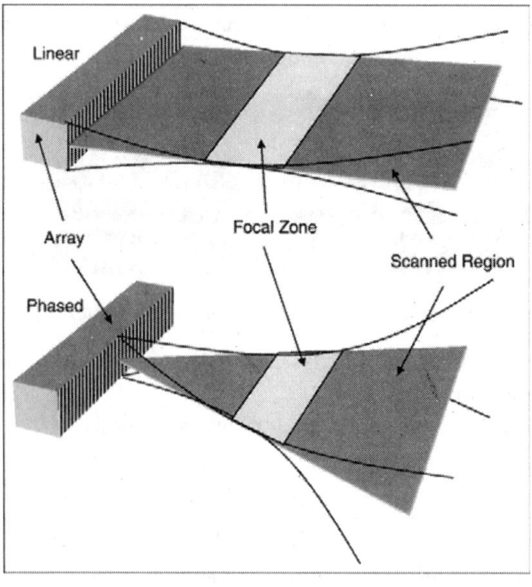

Courtesy: Armin Ernst; Ultrasound-Guided Procedures & Investigations

5. Which of the following needle comes with ultrasound enhancement to increase the visibility of needle under ultrasound?

(a) Chiba needle (b) Westcott needle
(c) Trocar needle (d) Turner needle

Ans. (a). *Radiology Sourcebook: A Practical Guide for Reference and Training; Douglas P. Beall; p. 18.*

Chiba needle comes with ultrasound enhancement to increase the visibility of needle during USG guided procedures.

6. Which of the following is Westcott needle?

(a) 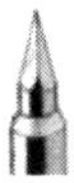 (b) 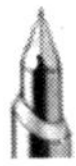

(c) 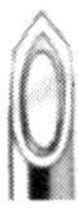 (d) 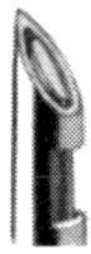

Ans. (d). *These are the different types of needles used in guided procedures; Westcott needle will provide good amount of tissue due to presence of the slot.*

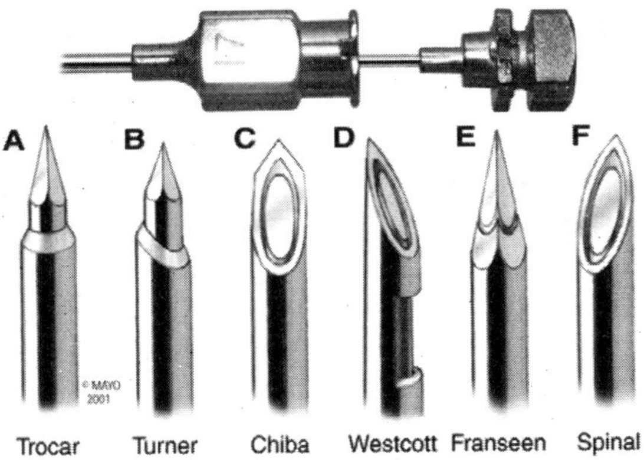

Courtesy: Douglas P. Beall. Radiology Sourcebook; A Practical Guide for Reference and Training.

7. Which of the following is FALSE regarding power mode imaging, when comparing it with color mode?

(a) Energy mode seems to be more sensitive to low- and weak-flow states than color velocity
(b) Angle effects on the Doppler frequency are ignored in power imaging
(c) Power imaging is sensitive to aliasing
(d) Flow direction could not be commented with power imaging

Ans. (c). *Zwiebel; Introduction to Vascular Sonography, 5th edition, p. 54.*

Color flow imaging displays scatterer velocities relative to the interrogating ultrasound beam direction at positions throughout the scanned field. An alternative processing method, power imaging ignores the velocity and simply estimates the strength (power or energy) of the Doppler signal detected from each location.

This power imaging is more sensitive than color imaging, it does not affected by aliasing; but we cannot see the direction of flow in power mode.

8. Which of the following is false regarding positioning patient for ultrasonography for venous incompetence?

(a) In supine position thigh should be externally rotated
(b) In supine position head end should be slightly elevated
(c) In standing position leg should be immobile throughout the examination
(d) In standing position body should be mainly supported by ipsilateral leg

Ans. (d). *Zwiebel; Introduction to Vascular Sonography, 5th edition, p. 435.*

Positioning patient for USG for venous system:
Supine: Mild external rotation of thigh.
Knee should be flexed for few degrees.
Standing position:
Weight should be laid on contralateral leg.
Patient should be immobile throughout the examination to prevent muscle contraction.

9. Which of the following is related to 'mechanical index'?

(a) Related ability to detect flow
(b) Related ability to detect direction
(c) Related to cavitation
(d) Related to heat generation

Ans. (c). *Zwiebel; Introduction to vascular sonography, 5th edition. p. 22.*

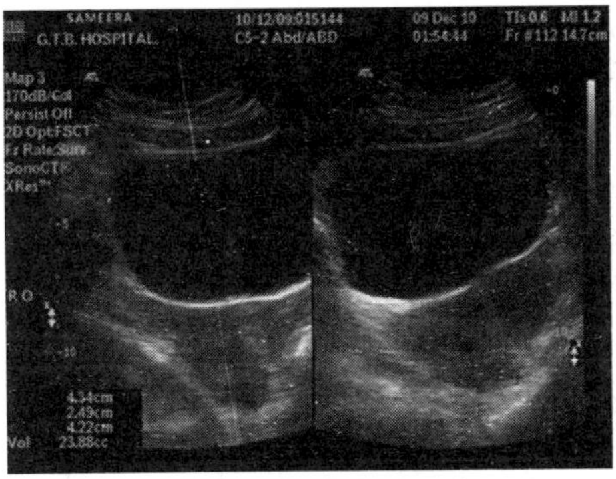

Radiologist should follow 'ALARA' principle during ultrasound examination. Even though biological effect of ultrasound on patients is not clear, there are some adverse effects. They are cavitation and thermal generation. Way of measuring cavitation is 'mechanical index'. Index of thermal generation is 'thermal index'. They will be displayed on the screen.

10. By controlling which of the following we can adjust the receiving signal from the tissue in a particular depth?

(a) Overall gain
(b) Output power control
(c) Frequency of transducer
(d) Time gain compensation

Ans. (d). *Zwiebel; Introduction to Vascular Sonography, 5th edition, p. 37.*

Time gain compensation is used to compensate for attenuation of the ultrasound beam in tissue. With time gain compensation, the receiver amplification increases automatically with the depth of origin of the echoes, so echo signals from deep structures, which have undergone significant attenuation, are amplified more than signals from shallow structures that have undergone less attenuation. Time gain compensation is controlled in most machines using a set of six to eight gain knobs, each adjusting the receiver gain at a different depth.

11. 'Increased through transmission' is seen in

(a) Any hypoechoic lesions
(b) Any cystic lesions
(c) Any necrotic lymph nodes
(d) Bone

Ans. (b). *Diagnostic Radiology; Grainger & Allison's; 5th edition, p. 54.*

Increased through transmission: *When a region of tissue has a lower than average attenuation, the Time Gain Compensation (which is adjusted to compensate for the average attenuation) is inappropriately high for that region so that echoes from deeper tissues are over amplified. The phenomenon is the hallmark of cystic spaces and the 'bright up' is often accentuated by the darker banding lines of the edge shadows typically formed from the cyst wall. Even those fluid cavities that contain echogenic material, such as suspended crystals in the gallbladder, pus, blood or necrotic tissue, usually still produce increased transmission, depending largely on the proportion of fluid present. However, some solid tissues also show increased sound transmission, usually because they have a high proportion of fluid. Many tumors fall into this category,* ***especially fibroadenomas in the breast, while lymphomatous deposits and inflammatory masses may behave in the same way.***

GENITOURINARY SYSTEM

1. Before taking IVU, the patient is taken the history of

(a) Allergy of food
(b) Allergy from drug or contrast media
(c) Bronchial asthma
(d) All above

Ans. (d). *Textbook of Radiology for Residents & Technicians, 5th ed., S.K. Bhargava & Sumeet Bhargava, p. 259-262.*

2. Before doing the IVU, the blood investigation indicated are

(a) Serum sodium and calcium (b) Blood urea and creatinine
(c) Serum potassium (d) Serum bilirubin

Ans. (b). *Textbook of Radiology for Residents & Technicians, 5th ed., S.K. Bhargava & Sumeet Bhargava, p. 259-262.*

3. Which of the following is not film in routine IVU?

(a) Plain X-ray film (b) Nephrogram
(c) Pyelogram (d) Rt. anterior oblique view

Ans. (d). *Textbook of Radiology for Residents & Technicians, 5th ed., S.K. Bhargava & Sumeet Bhargava, p. 259-262.*

4. Pyelogram in IVU is taken

(a) 5 mts. after contrast injection
(b) 15 mts. after contrast injection
(c) 25 mts. after contrast injections
(d) 40 mts. after contrast injections

Ans. (a). *Textbook of Radiology for Residents & Technicians, 5th ed., S.K. Bhargava & Sumeet Bhargava, p. 259-262.*

5. Compression band is applied in IVU for

(a) Better delineation of urinary bladder
(b) Better delineation of post void contrast
(c) Better delineation of PCS and upper ureter
(d) Better delineation of lower ureter

Ans. (c). *Textbook of Radiology for Residents & Technicians, 5th ed., S.K. Bhargava & Sumeet Bhargava, p. 259-262.*

6. Compression band is contraindicated in

(a) Blunt trauma abdomen
(b) Abdominal aortic aneurysm
(c) Children
(d) All of the above

Ans. (d). *Textbook of Radiology for Residents & Technicians, 5th ed., S.K. Bhargava & Sumeet Bhargava, p. 259-262.*

7. If compression band is contraindicated, we do

(a) Head end lower
(b) Feet end lower
(c) Make patient lie right lateral
(d) Make patient lie left lateral

Ans. (a). *Textbook of Radiology for Residents & Technicians, 5th ed., S.K. Bhargava & Sumeet Bhargava, p. 259-262.*

8. Indication of IVU includes

(a) Hematuria
(b) Congenital anomaly of the urinary tract
(c) In donor for renal transplant
(d) All above

Ans. (d). *Textbook of Radiology for Residents & Technicians, 5th ed., S.K. Bhargava & Sumeet Bhargava, p. 259-262.*

9. Plain X-ray KUB is done before IVU for

(a) To see bowel preparation
(b) Abnormal radio-opaque shadows or any other abnormality
(c) B/L psoas shadow or vertebral anomaly
(d) All above

Ans. (d). *Textbook of Radiology for Residents & Technicians, 5th ed., S.K. Bhargava & Sumeet Bhargava, p. 259-262.*

10. Nephrogram in IVU is for

(a) Assessing renal function
(b) To visualize the calculus in the kidney
(c) Assessing the ureter
(d) Assessing the urinary bladder

Ans. ***(a).*** *Textbook of Radiology for Residents & Technicians, 5th ed., S.K. Bhargava & Sumeet Bhargava, p. 259-262.*

11. Full bladder film is taken for

(a) Visualizing any abnormality in urinary bladder
(b) Visualizing any abnormality in PCS
(c) Visualizing any abnormality in kidney
(d) Visualizing any abnormality of the ureter

Ans. ***(a).*** *Textbook of Radiology for Residents & Technicians, 5th ed., S.K. Bhargava & Sumeet Bhargava, p. 259-262.*

12. Compression band is usually applied at

(a) 10–15 mts (b) 2–3 mts
(c) 30–45 mts (d) 1–2 hrs

Ans. ***(a).*** *Textbook of Radiology for Residents & Technicians, 5th ed., S.K. Bhargava & Sumeet Bhargava, p. 259-262.*

13. HSG is indicated for

(a) Patency of the fallopian tubes
(b) Congenital anomalies of the uterus
(c) Check for the recannalization of the tubes
(d) All of the above

Ans. ***(d).*** *Textbook of Radiology for Residents & Technicians, 5th ed., S.K. Bhargava & Sumeet Bhargava, p. 263.*

14. HSG is contraindicated in

(a) Pus discharge from vagina (b) Primary infertility
(c) Secondary infertility

Ans. ***(a).*** *Textbook of Radiology for Residents & Technicians, 5th ed., S.K. Bhargava & Sumeet Bhargava, p. 263.*

15. HSG is done during

(a) 7–10 days of the menstrual cycle
(b) 10–14 days of the menstrual cycle
(c) 14–18 days of the menstrual cycle
(d) 18–22 days of the menstrual cycle

Ans. ***(a).*** *Textbook of Radiology for Residents & Technicians, 5th ed., S.K. Bhargava & Sumeet Bhargava, p. 263.*

16. Normal length of the fallopian tube is

(a) 5 cm (b) 10 cm
(c) 15 cm (d) 20 cm

Ans. ***(b).*** *Textbook of Radiology for Residents & Technicians, 5th ed., S.K. Bhargava & Sumeet Bhargava, p. 263.*

17. Which is not the part of the fallopian tube?

(a) Isthmus
(b) Interstitial
(c) Ampulla
(d) Cornua

Ans. (d). *Textbook of Radiology for Residents & Technicians, 5th ed., S.K. Bhargava & Sumeet Bhargava, p. 263.*

18. MCU is indicated for

(a) Visualization of the posterior urethra
(b) To see for vesico-ureteric reflex
(c) To see the bladder abnormalities
(d) All above

Ans. (d). *Textbook of Radiology for Residents & Technicians, 5th ed., S.K. Bhargava & Sumeet Bhargava, p. 259-262.*

19. RGU is contraindicated in

(a) Pus discharge from urethra
(b) Urine discharge from urethra
(c) Pain during micturation
(d) Injury to urethra

Ans. (a). *Textbook of Radiology for Residents & Technicians, 5th ed., S.K. Bhargava & Sumeet Bhargava, p. 259-262.*

20. Exception to 10 day rule is

(a) Women who denied recent sexual intercourse
(b) Women who were menstruating at that time
(c) Women who had an oral contraceptive for no fewer than 3 months and were satisfied
(d) All above

Ans. (d). *A Guide to Radiological Procedures, Chapman, 4th ed., p. 2.*

21. Exception to 10 day rule is

(a) Women who had sterilized
(b) Women who had had an intrauterine contraceptive for not fewer than 3 months and found it effective
(c) Both (a) and (b)
(d) None of the above

Ans. (c). *A Guide to Radiological Procedures, Chapman, 4th ed., p. 2.*

22. Argument against 10 day rule is

(a) Orgogenesis occurs during the 4–8 weeks after conception. Hence irradiation after 10 days of the menstrual cycle but before next cycle will not result in radiation damage

(b) Irradiation of the unfertilized ovum – no evidence suggest that the irradiation of the concepts is any more dangerous than irradiation of the unfertilized ovum
(c) The risk are small and are greatly outweighted by the likely benefits to the mother or fetus for an early diagnosis
(d) All of the above

Ans. (d). *A Guide to Radiological Procedures, Chapman, 4th ed., p. 3.*

23. The LOCM has following advantages

(a) Less tissue toxicity
(b) Less adverse reactions
(c) More comfortable in I.V. injection and arteriography
(d) All of the above

Ans. (d). *A Guide to Radiological Procedures, Chapman, 4th ed., p. 40.*

24. The main advantage of barium contrast over water soluble contrast in GIT examinations are

(a) Excellent coating
(b) Cost
(c) Both (a) and (b)
(d) None

Ans. (c). *A Guide to Radiological Procedures, Chapman, 4th ed., p. 51.*

25. The main disadvantages of barium in GIT examination are

(a) High morbidity associated with barium in the paritoneal cavity
(b) Clearance of the barium takes long time so patient has to wait long time for ultrasound/examination
(c) Both (a) and (b)
(d) None

Ans. (c). *A Guide to Radiological Procedures, Chapman, 4th ed., p. 51.*

26. Gastrograffin contains

(a) Meglumine diatrizoate 66% w/v, sodium diatrizoate 10% and 370 mg iodine concentration/ml
(b) Meglumine diatrizoate 10% w/v, sodium diatrizoate 67% and 370 mg iodine concentration/ml
(c) Meglumine diatrizoate 66% w/v, sodium diatrizoate 10% and 270 mg iodine concentration/ml
(d) Meglumine diatrizoate 10% w/v, sodium diatrizoate 67% and 270 mg iodine concentration/ml

Ans. (a). *A Guide to Radiological Procedures, Chapman, 4th ed., p. 52.*

27. Indication of water-soluble contrast media in GIT are

(a) Suspected perforation
(b) Meconium ileus
(c) To distinguish bowel from other structures during CT examination
(d) All above

Ans. (d). *A Guide to Radiological Procedures, Chapman, 4th ed., p. 52.*

28. During peroral pneumocolon, the air is injected/given

(a) Orally
(b) Via anus
(c) Via nasogastric tube
(d) None of the above

Ans. (b). *A Guide to Radiological Procedures, Chapman, 4th ed., p. 89.*

29. Common complications with water soluble contrast media during GIT examination are

(a) Pulmonary edema if aspirated
(b) Hypovolemia in children due to hyperosmolarity of the contrast media
(c) Allergic reaction
(d) All above

Ans. (d). *A Guide to Radiological Procedures, Chapman, 4th ed., p. 52.*

30. Buscopan used as antimuscarinic agent to inhibit intestinal motility is contraindicated in

(a) Closed angle glaucoma
(b) Myasthenia gravis
(c) Paralytic ileus
(d) All above

Ans. (d). *A Guide to Radiological Procedures, Chapman, 4th ed., p. 54.*

31. The adult dose of the buscopan used in GIT is

(a) 20 mgm/IV
(b) 40 mgm/IV
(c) 20 mgm/S/C
(d) None above

Ans. (a). *A Guide to Radiological Procedures, Chapman, 4th ed., p. 53.*

32. In GIT double contrast effect is produced due to

(a) CO_2
(b) Air
(c) Both
(d) None

Ans. (c). *A Guide to Radiological Procedures, Chapman, 4th ed., p. 52–53.*

33. The action of metacloramide (Mexolon) are

(a) Stimulate gastric emptying
(b) Enhanced transit of barium during follow-through
(c) Antiemetic
(d) All above

Ans. (d). *A Guide to Radiological Procedures, Chapman, 4th ed., p. 55.*

34. The best position for barium swallow is

(a) Erect RAO view
(b) Lateral view
(c) P.A. view
(d) None above

Ans. (a). *A Guide to Radiological Procedures, Chapman, 4th ed., p. 56.*

35. Oesophageal varices are best seen in

(a) Prone RPO position (Right Postero-Oblique position)
(b) Supine RPO position
(c) Prone lateral view
(d) None above

Ans. (a). *A Guide to Radiological Procedures, Chapman, 4th ed., p. 56.*

36. To see mucosal pattern of stomach, the investigation of the choice is

(a) Barium full of stomach
(b) Single contrast
(c) Double contrast
(d) None above

Ans. (c). *A Guide to Radiological Procedures, Chapman, 4th ed., p. 57.*

37. For visualization of the duodenal cap, the best position is

(a) ROA position
(a) LOA position
(c) Supine
(d) Prone

Ans. (a). *A Guide to Radiological Procedures, Chapman, 4th ed., p. 60.*

38. Enteroclysis of the small bowel is superior to barium follow through as

(a) Continuous column of the contrast medium
(b) No segmentation
(c) No flocculation
(d) All above

Ans. (d). *A Guide to Radiological Procedures, Chapman, 4th ed., p. 64.*

39. In enteroclysis, the tip of the tube (Bilbao-Dotter tube) is placed
- (a) Beyond duodeno-jejunal flexure
- (b) 1st part of duodenum
- (c) 2nd part of duodenum
- (d) At pylorus

Ans. (a). *A Guide to Radiological Procedures, Chapman, 4th ed., p. 73.*

40. The "instant enema" is advised in
- (a) To identify the level of suspected large bowel obstruction
- (b) To show the extent and severity of mucosal lesion in active ulcerative colitis
- (c) Both (a) and (b)
- (d) None of the above

Ans. (c). *A Guide to Radiological Procedures, Chapman, 4th ed., p. 73.*

41. Balloon dilatation of the esophageal stricture is contraindicated in
- (a) Achalasia cardia
- (b) Esophageal tumours
- (c) Anastomotic strictures
- (d) Tracheo-oesophageal fistula

Ans. (d). *A Guide to Radiological Procedures, Chapman, 4th ed., p. 74.*

42. Reduction of the intussusception should not attempted in patient of
- (a) Peritonitis
- (b) Perforation
- (c) Advanced (more than 24 hrs) intestinal obstruction
- (d) All above

Ans. (d). *A Guide to Radiological Procedures, Chapman, 4th ed., p. 75.*

43. Which of the following are not the colonic causes of the neonatal low intestinal obstruction requiring contrast enema
- (a) Hirschsprung's disease
- (b) Functional immaturity of the colon
- (c) Colonic atresia
- (d) Meconium ileus

Ans. (d). *A Guide to Radiological Procedures, Chapman, 4th ed., p. 79.*

44. The indication of the oral cholecystography in era of the ultrasound

(a) Ultrasound not available
(b) Ultrasound failed to demonstrate the gall bladder
(c) Both above
(d) None

Ans. (c). *A Guide to Radiological Procedures, Chapman, 4th ed., p. 105.*

45. Post-operative T-tube cholangiogram is done

(a) Immediately or next post-operative day
(b) 7th post-operative day
(c) 10th post-operative day
(d) 15th post-operative day

Ans. (c). *A Guide to Radiological Procedures, Chapman, 4th ed., p. 110.*

46. Which of the following condition, percutaneous extraction of the retained biliary calculi (Burhenne technique) is contraindicated

(a) Small/tortous T-tube
(b) Acute pancreatitis
(c) Drain in situ
(d) All above

Ans. (d). *A Guide to Radiological Procedures, Chapman, 4th ed., p. 111.*

47. Which are advantages of the ERCP over PTC?

(a) Ability to visualize and biopsy ampullary lesions
(b) Demonstrate biliary tree and pancreatic duct
(c) Therapeutic potential
(d) All above

Ans. (d). *A Guide to Radiological Procedures, Chapman, 4th ed., p. 113.*

48. MCU

(a) Micturating Cystoureterography
(b) Modified Cystourethrogram
(c) Micturating Cystourethrography
(d) Micturating Cystourography

Ans. (c). *Radiological Procedures, S.K. Bhargava & Sumeet Bhargava, 2nd ed., Pee Pee Publishers, p. 132-140.*

49. Spot film is taken in MCU

(a) After the micturation
(b) Before the micturation
(c) During the micturation
(d) Before filling the bladder

Ans. (c). *Radiological Procedures, S.K. Bhargava & Sumeet Bhargava, 2nd ed., Pee Pee Publishers, p. 132-140.*

50. In RGU, which of the following contrast media is used?

(a) Urografin 60% (b) Urografin 76%
(c) Barium sulphate (d) Air

Ans. (a). *Radiological Procedures, S.K. Bhargava & Sumeet Bhargava, 2nd ed., Pee Pee Publishers, p. 132-140.*

51. In which position patient is adjusted, so that the bladder neck and urethra can be radiographed free of body superimposition?

(a) Prone (b) Supine
(c) Oblique (d) Erect

Ans. (c). *Radiological Procedures, S.K. Bhargava & Sumeet Bhargava, 2nd ed., Pee Pee Publishers, p. 132-140.*

52. Arthrography is done for

(a) Spine study (b) Lung cavity
(c) Joints (d) Bone study

Ans. (c). *Radiological Procedures, S.K. Bhargava & Sumeet Bhargava, 2nd ed., Pee Pee Publishers, p. 115-126.*

RADIOLOGICAL PROCEDURES (SPECIAL INVESTIGATION)

1. To visualize the urinary system, the method used are

(a) Intravenous urography/pyelography
(b) Retrograde pyelography
(c) Antegrade pyelography
(d) All above

Ans. (d). *Textbook of Radiology for Residents & Technicians, 5th ed., S.K. Bhargava & Sumeet Bhargava, p. 259-262.*

2. Intravenous pyelography is indicated in

(a) Obstructive uropathy like stone etc.
(b) Congenital anomalies involving kidneys
(c) In investigating hypertension
(d) All above

Ans. (d). *Textbook of Radiology for Residents & Technicians, 5th ed., S.K. Bhargava & Sumeet Bhargava, p. 259-262.*

3. Intravenous pyelography is advised in

(a) To know the function of the kidney
(b) Hematuria with or without blunt injury of the abdomen
(c) Abdominal mass suspected to arise from urinary system
(d) All above

Ans. ***(d).*** *Textbook of Radiology for Residents & Technicians, 5th ed., S.K. Bhargava & Sumeet Bhargava, p. 259-262.*

4. IVP not recommended, if

(a) Sensitive to iodine or previous reaction to contrast media
(b) Intractable cardiac or renal failure
(c) Patient is pregnant or suffering from multiple myeloma
(d) All above

Ans. ***(d).*** *Textbook of Radiology for Residents & Technicians, 5th ed., S.K. Bhargava & Sumeet Bhargava, p. 259-262.*

5. In renal failure the requirement is

(a) High dose of contrast with delayed radiographs
(b) Low dose contrast with delayed radiographs
(c) High dose contrast with normal 30 mts. film (no delayed radiograph)
(d) Low dose contrast with normal 30 mts. film (no delayed radiograph)

Ans. ***(d).*** *Textbook of Radiology for Residents & Technicians, 5th ed., S.K. Bhargava & Sumeet Bhargava, p. 259-262.*

6. In hypertension, to compare the rate of excretion from each kidney during IVP, the requirement is

(a) Normal sequence exposure
(b) Rapid sequence exposure in 1st 5–6 mts
(c) None
(d) Both

Ans. ***(b).*** *Textbook of Radiology for Residents & Technicians, 5th ed., S.K. Bhargava & Sumeet Bhargava, p. 259-262.*

7. To assess better intraluminal growth in urinary bladder and bladder diverticulae during IVP, the views required are

(a) AP view
(b) PA view
(c) Oblique view
(d) None

Ans. ***(c).*** *Textbook of Radiology for Residents & Technicians, 5th ed., S.K. Bhargava & Sumeet Bhargava, p. 259-262.*

8. To assess the delayed excretion from the kidneys, views to be taken upto

(a) 25–30 mts (b) 45–50 mts
(c) 12 hrs (d) 24 hrs

Ans. ***(d).*** *Textbook of Radiology for Residents & Technicians, 5th ed., S.K. Bhargava & Sumeet Bhargava, p. 259-262.*

9. Nephrotomography is a technique to get the detailed information about

(a) Renal outline (b) Renal parenchyma
(c) Renal medulla (d) None

Ans. (a). *Textbook of Radiology for Residents & Technicians, 5th ed., S.K. Bhargava & Sumeet Bhargava, p. 259-262.*

10. Antegrade pyelography is done for

(a) The combination of inadequate information from IV pyelography with failed retrograde pyelogram
(b) To demonstrate the pelvi-ureteric obstruction
(c) Not able to conduct retrograde pyelography due to ureteric implantation
(d) All above

Ans. (d). *Textbook of Radiology for Residents & Technicians, 5th ed., S.K. Bhargava & Sumeet Bhargava, p. 259-262.*

11. The sequence of the film during I.V.P. are

(a) 1 mt, 5 mts, 15 mts, prone, 30–45 mts
(b) 5 mts, 20 mts, and 60 mts
(c) 1 mts, 10 mts, 20 mts, 60 mts
(d) None of the above

Ans. (a). *Textbook of Radiology for Residents & Technicians, 5th ed., S.K. Bhargava & Sumeet Bhargava, p. 259-262.*

12. MCU (micturating cystogram) is indicated to

(a) Assess the urethrae for any abnormality/ outflow obstruction
(b) Stress incontinence
(c) To demonstrate vesico-ureteric reflux
(d) All above

Ans. (d). *Textbook of Radiology for Residents & Technicians, 5th ed., S.K. Bhargava & Sumeet Bhargava, p. 259-262.*

13. Contrast medium used in MCUIs

(a) Sodium iodide in concentration of 12% w/v
(b) Sodium chloride in concentration of 12% w/v
(c) Sodium iodide in concentration of 20% w/v
(d) Sodium iodide in concentration of 50% w/v

Ans. (a). *Textbook of Radiology for Residents & Technicians, 5th ed., S.K. Bhargava & Sumeet Bhargava, p. 259-262.*

14. The main indication of hysterosalpingography in present imaging era is

(a) Infertility (b) Dysmenorrhoea

(c) Endometrial polyp (d) Fibroid uterus

Ans. (a). *Textbook of Radiology for Residents & Technicians, 5th ed., S.K. Bhargava & Sumeet Bhargava, p. 263.*

15. Best time to do hysterosalpingogram is

(a) 7–10 days from menstruation
(b) Any time in cycle
(c) 10–15 days from menstruation
(d) None of the above

Ans. (a). *Textbook of Radiology for Residents & Technicians, 5th ed., S.K. Bhargava & Sumeet Bhargava, p. 263.*

16. Barium swallow is the technique to visualize the

(a) Esophagus (b) Stomach
(c) Small Intestine (d) Large Intestine

Ans. (a). *Textbook of Radiology for Residents & Technicians, 5th ed., S.K. Bhargava & Sumeet Bhargava, p. 263-266.*

17. For single contrast barium swallow, barium mixture used is

(a) 100% w/v (b) 250 % w/v
(c) 350% w/v (d) None above

Ans. (a). *Textbook of Radiology for Residents & Technicians, 5th ed., S.K. Bhargava & Sumeet Bhargava, p. 263-266.*

18. For double contrast barium swallow, barium mixture used is

(a) 100% w/v (b) 250% w/v
(c) 350% w/v (d) None above

Ans. (b). *Textbook of Radiology for Residents & Technicians, 5th ed., S.K. Bhargava & Sumeet Bhargava, p. 263-266.*

19. Examination of small bowel by giving barium by mouth is known as

(a) Barium meal follow-through (b) Enteroclysis
(c) Barium enema (d) None

Ans. (a). *Textbook of Radiology for Residents & Technicians, 5th ed., S.K. Bhargava & Sumeet Bhargava, p. 263-266.*

20. For conventional barium enema, the concentration of barium required is

(a) 15% w/v (b) 30% w/v
(c) 60% w/v (d) 100% w/v

Ans. (b). *Textbook of Radiology for Residents & Technicians, 5th ed., S.K. Bhargava & Sumeet Bhargava, p. 263-266.*

21. For double contrast barium enema, the concentration of barium required is

(a) 15% w/v (b) 30% w/v
(c) 60% w/v (d) 100% w/v

Ans. (d). *Textbook of Radiology for Residents & Technicians, 5th ed., S.K. Bhargava & Sumeet Bhargava, p. 263-266.*

22. Comparing the male and female bony pelvis, it is noted that male pelvis has the following features

(a) Greater or false pelvis is deep
(b) Pubic angle is less than 90%
(c) Ileum more vertical
(d) All above

Ans. (d). *Tortera & Derickson, p. 244.*

23. Investigation of the barium enema is contraindicated in which of the following conditions

(a) Suspected perforation of the hollow viscous
(b) Suspected large bowel obstruction
(c) Presurgical patients
(d) All above

Ans. (d). *Ballinger & Frank, Vol. 2, p. 94.*

24. The usual patient for an upper GI series examination

(a) Clear fluids 8 hrs. before examination
(b) Nil orally after 8 p.m. proceeding the night before examination
(c) Enema until clear fluid before examination
(d) Light breakfast the day of the examination

Ans. (b). *Textbook of Radiology for Residents & Technicians, 5th ed., S.K. Bhargava & Sumeet Bhargava, p. 263-266.*

25. During myelography, contrast medium is introduced into the

(a) Subarachnoid space
(b) Subdural space
(c) Epidural space
(d) Epidermal space

Ans. (a). *Textbook of Radiology for Residents & Technicians, 5th ed., S.K. Bhargava & Sumeet Bhargava, p. 271.*

26. Myelography can be done

(a) Spinal cisternal route (b) Spinal lumbar route
(c) Both (d) None

Ans. (c). *Textbook of Radiology for Residents & Technicians, 5th ed., S.K. Bhargava & Sumeet Bhargava, p. 271.*

27. These days the contrast media used in myelography is

(a) Water soluble contrast media
(b) Oil based contrast media
(c) Both
(d) None

Ans. (a). *Textbook of Radiology for Residents & Technicians, 5th ed., S.K. Bhargava & Sumeet Bhargava, p. 271.*

28. Which of the following examination involves the introduction of radio opaque contrast media using lumbar puncture needle?

(a) Retrograde pyelogram
(b) Hysterosalpingogram
(c) Voiding cystourethrogram
(d) Myelogram

Ans. (d). *Textbook of Radiology for Residents & Technicians, 5th ed., S.K. Bhargava & Sumeet Bhargava, p. 271.*

29. Which of the following examination involves the introduction of the contrast media using uterine cannula?

(a) Retrograde pyelogram
(b) Hysterosalpingogram
(c) Myelogram
(d) Voiding cystourethrogram

Ans. (b). *Textbook of Radiology for Residents & Technicians, 5th ed., S.K. Bhargava & Sumeet Bhargava, p. 263.*

30. Patients are instructed to remove all prosthesis, coins, credit cards etc. before entering the room for an examination in

(a) Ultrasound examination
(b) CT (Computed Tomography)
(c) Magnetic resonance imaging
(d) Nuclear medicine

Ans. (c). *Textbook of Radiology for Residents & Technicians, 5th ed., S.K. Bhargava & Sumeet Bhargava, p. 408.*

31. The investigation of the choice to visualize the gall bladder

(a) Ultrasonography (b) Oral cholecystography
(c) CT (d) None

Ans. (a). *Textbook of Radiology for Residents & Technicians, 5th ed., S.K. Bhargava & Sumeet Bhargava, p. 266-268.*

32. Intravenous choledochography is done to

(a) Visualize the ducts for any stone
(b) When oral cholecystography fails

(c) Both
(d) None

Ans. (c). Textbook of Radiology for Residents & Technicians, 5th ed., S.K. Bhargava & Sumeet Bhargava, p. 267.

33. Endoscopic Retrograde Choledochopancreatography (ERCP) usually involves

(a) Intubation of the papilla of the vater and injection of the contrast medium
(b) By intravenous injection of the contrast medium
(c) Introduction of the barium directly into the duodenum.
(d) None of the above

Ans. (a). Textbook of Radiology for Residents & Technicians, 5th ed., S.K. Bhargava & Sumeet Bhargava, p. 267.

34. ERCP is not advised when

(a) Patient has positive serological test and Australian antigen
(b) Patient with acute pancreatitis
(c) When not able to negotiate the endoscope
(d) All above

Ans. (d). Textbook of Radiology for Residents & Technicians, 5th ed., S.K. Bhargava & Sumeet Bhargava, p. 267.

35. ERCP is advised in

(a) Investigation of the jaundice of the obscure origin
(b) When other techniques fails for pancreatic disease
(c) For collection of biliary and pancreatic sample and biopsy
(d) All above

Ans. (d). Textbook of Radiology for Residents & Technicians, 5th ed., S.K. Bhargava & Sumeet Bhargava, p. 267.

36. During upper GE examination, trendelenburg position is used to demonstrate

(a) Hiatus hernia
(b) Gastric ulcer
(c) Duodenal diverticulae
(d) Duodenal bulb and C-loop

Ans. (a). Textbook of Radiology for Residents & Technicians, 5th ed., S.K. Bhargava & Sumeet Bhargava, p. 264.

37. In which of the following procedure, a catheter is placed within the ureter and contrast media is injected in renal pelvis

(a) Intravenous pyelography
(b) Antegrade pyelography
(c) Micturating cystography
(d) Retrograde urography

Ans. (d). Textbook of Radiology for Residents & Technicians, 5th ed., S.K. Bhargava & Sumeet Bhargava, p. 259-262.

38. To safest and convenient site of the injection of the contrast media in myelography is
(a) Cervical route
(b) Epidural space
(c) Subarachnoid space between 1st and 2nd lumbar vertebrae
(d) Subarachnoid space between 3rd & 4th lumbar vertebrae

Ans. (d). Textbook of Radiology for Residents & Technicians, 5th ed., S.K. Bhargava & Sumeet Bhargava, p. 271.

39. The best method to demonstrate vesico-ureteric reflux in a child is
(a) Color Doppler
(b) Micturating cystourethrogram
(c) Retrograde pyelogram
(d) None of the above

Ans. (a). Textbook of Radiology for Residents & Technicians, 5th ed., S.K. Bhargava & Sumeet Bhargava, p. 259-262.

40. The choice of the contrast media in myelography is
(a) Oily contrast media
(b) Gas
(c) Ionic contrast media
(d) Non-ionic water soluble contrast media

Ans. (d). Textbook of Radiology for Residents & Technicians, 5th ed., S.K. Bhargava & Sumeet Bhargava, p. 271.

41. Patient undergoing IVU should be instructed to
(a) Avoid the meal immediately prior to the examination
(b) Avoid the meal after the examination
(c) Avoid fluid intake
(d) All

Ans. (a). Textbook of Radiology for Residents & Technicians, 5th ed., S.K. Bhargava & Sumeet Bhargava, p. 259-262.

42. Preparation of the IVU study is required to
(a) Avoid overhydration
(b) Avoid dehydration
(c) Avoid abdominal gas
(d) All above

Ans. (d). Textbook of Radiology for Residents & Technicians, 5th ed., S.K. Bhargava & Sumeet Bhargava, p. 259-262.

43. Which of the following statement is false regarding IVU study?
(a) Patient should micturate immediately prior to study
(b) Control radiograph are obtained at a relatively low kV_p
(c) Enema is required to clear the bowel
(d) IVU is contraindicated in pregnancy

Ans. (c). *Textbook of Radiology for Residents & Technicians, 5th ed., S.K. Bhargava & Sumeet Bhargava, p. 259-262.*

44. IVU should be avoided in patient with
(a) Diabetes with renal insufficiency
(b) Hematuria
(c) Persistent pyuria
(d) Renal trauma

Ans. (a). *Textbook of Radiology for Residents & Technicians, 5th ed., S.K. Bhargava & Sumeet Bhargava, p. 259-262.*

45. About bowel preparation for IVU study, following is false
(a) Laxatives are given
(b) Liquid diet advised day before study
(c) Bowel preparation is not required
(d) All of the above

Ans. (c). *Textbook of Radiology for Residents & Technicians, 5th ed., S.K. Bhargava & Sumeet Bhargava, p. 259-262.*

46. Which blood investigation required prior to IVU study
(a) KFT (b) RFT
(c) Uric acid level (d) Iodine level

Ans. (a). *Textbook of Radiology for Residents & Technicians, 5th ed., S.K. Bhargava & Sumeet Bhargava, p. 259-262.*

47. Compression is contraindicated in all except
(a) Urinary tract obstruction (b) Renal failure
(c) Ureteric calculi (d) Renal calculi

Ans. (d). *Textbook of Radiology for Residents & Technicians, 5th ed., S.K. Bhargava & Sumeet Bhargava, p. 259-262.*

48. Charcoal given for bowel preparation acts as
(a) Laxative (b) Gas absorbent
(c) Anti emetic (d) None

Ans. (b). *Textbook of Radiology for Residents & Technicians, 5th ed., S.K. Bhargava & Sumeet Bhargava, p. 259-262.*

49. Fasting is indicated in all except
(a) USG (b) Renal Doppler
(c) FAST (d) Portal vein doppler

Ans. (c). *Textbook of Radiology for Residents & Technicians, 5th ed., S.K. Bhargava & Sumeet Bhargava, p. 344.*

50. Fasting is important in USG abdomen

(a) For visualization of distended gall bladder
(b) To decrease bowel gases
(c) Both
(d) None

Ans. (c). *Textbook of Radiology for Residents & Technicians, 5th ed., S.K. Bhargava & Sumeet Bhargava, p. 344.*

51. Preparation of the TVS include

(a) Fasting
(b) Empty bladder
(c) Must be performed by the female doctor
(d) All of the above

Ans. (b). *Textbook of Radiology for Residents & Technicians, 5th ed., S.K. Bhargava & Sumeet Bhargava, p. 345.*

52. For evaluation of prostate by transabdominal USG

(a) Urinary bladder should be empty
(b) Urinary bladder should be full
(c) Prostate can not be visualized by transabdominal USG
(d) Transrectal USG is indicated in all cases

Ans. (b). *Textbook of Radiology for Residents & Technicians, 5th ed., S.K. Bhargava & Sumeet Bhargava, p. 345.*

53. What is the name of the flexure that lies between transverse colon and the ascending colon?

(a) Splenic (b) Ileocecal
(c) Hepatic (d) Sigmoid

Ans. (c). *Radiological Procedures, S.K. Bhargava & Sumeet Bhargava, 2nd ed., Pee Pee Publishers, p. 43-66.*

54. Fluoroscopic imaging of the ileocecal valve is generally part of an

(a) Esophagogram (b) Upper GI series
(c) Small bowel series (d) Barium enema

Ans. (c). *Radiological Procedures, S.K. Bhargava & Sumeet Bhargava, 2nd ed., Pee Pee Publishers, p. 43-66.*

55. Which is recommended to demonstrate small amounts of air within the peritoneal cavity?

(a) Lateral decubitus, affected side-up

(b) Lateral decubitus, affected side-down
(c) AP Trendelenburg
(d) AP supine

Ans. (a). *Radiological Procedures, S.K. Bhargava & Sumeet Bhargava, 2nd ed., Pee Pee Publishers, p. 43-66.*

56. Which radiographic projection of the large intestine best demonstrate the rectum?

(a) Oblique (b) Upright
(c) Lateral (d) PA

Ans. (c). *Radiological Procedures, S.K. Bhargava & Sumeet Bhargava, 2nd ed., Pee Pee Publishers, p. 43-66.*

57. To demonstrate the large bowel, which view separates the overlying loops of sigmoid colon?

(a) Right lateral decubitus
(b) Supine, with the tube angled 45° caudally
(c) Oblique, with the tube angled 45° caudally
(d) Prone

Ans. (b). *Radiological Procedures, S.K. Bhargava & Sumeet Bhargava, 2nd ed., Pee Pee Publishers, p. 43-66.*

58. Where is the vermiform appendix attached to?

(a) Rectum (b) Sigmoid
(c) Caecum (d) Hepatic flexure

Ans. (c). *Radiological Procedures, S.K. Bhargava & Sumeet Bhargava, 2nd ed., Pee Pee Publishers, p. 43-66.*

59. What is part of the preferred preparation for small intestine?

(a) A soft or low residue diet 2 days before
(b) Nothing to eat 24 hr before exam
(c) By cleansing enema only
(d) All of the above

Ans. (a). *Radiological Procedures, S.K. Bhargava & Sumeet Bhargava, 2nd ed., Pee Pee Publishers, p. 43-66.*

60. For the esophagus RAO, how much is the patient obliqued?

(a) 35– 40 (b) 45
(c) 25 –30 (d) 10–15

Ans. (a). *Radiological Procedures, S.K. Bhargava & Sumeet Bhargava, 2nd ed., Pee Pee Publishers, p. 43-66.*

61. In high kV_p technique, barium sulphate suspension used is of

(a) 30% (b) 80%

(c) 100% (d) 200–250%

Ans. (a). *Radiological Procedures, S.K. Bhargava & Sumeet Bhargava, 2nd ed., Pee Pee Publishers, p. 43-66.*

62. For double contrast study, contrast media should have

(a) High density, high viscosity 200–250%
(b) High density, low viscosity 100–200%
(c) Low density, high viscosity 200–250%
(d) High density, low viscosity 200–250%

Ans. (d). *Radiological Procedures, S.K. Bhargava & Sumeet Bhargava, 2nd ed., Pee Pee Publishers, p. 43-66.*

63. Effervescent powder is given for

(a) Single contrast study (b) Double contrast study
(c) Triple phase study (d) All of the above

Ans. (b). *Radiological Procedures, S.K. Bhargava & Sumeet Bhargava, 2nd ed., Pee Pee Publishers, p. 43-66.*

64. When mecholyl is administered there will be hyperperistalsis, pain and streaks of contrast entering the stomach confirming the diagnosis of

(a) Carcinoma (b) Pharyngeal web
(c) Achalasia (d) Perforation

Ans. (c). *Radiological Procedures, S.K. Bhargava & Sumeet Bhargava, 2nd ed., Pee Pee Publishers, p. 43-66.*

65. Double contrast barium meal is generally done for

(a) Well-distended stomach
(b) Increased opacity in abdomen
(c) Mucosal pattern/coating
(d) Duodenal cap

Ans. (c). *Radiological Procedures, S.K. Bhargava & Sumeet Bhargava, 2nd ed., Pee Pee Publishers, p. 43-66.*

66. D1 and C loop of duodenum will be seen in the standard view

(a) Prone right side down (b) Supine right side up
(c) Supine left side up (d) All of the above

Ans. (b). *Radiological Procedures, S.K. Bhargava & Sumeet Bhargava, 2nd ed., Pee Pee Publishers, p. 43-66.*

67. Which tube is usually used in barium meal?

(a) Ryle's tube (b) Oesophageal tube
(c) Leach Willkinson tube (d) All of the above

Ans. (a). Radiological Procedures, S.K. Bhargava & Sumeet Bhargava, 2nd ed., Pee Pee Publishers, p. 43-66.

68. Buscopan is given via

(a) IV (b) Orally
(c) Rectally (d) All of the above

Ans. (a). Radiological Procedures, S.K. Bhargava & Sumeet Bhargava, 2nd ed., Pee Pee Publishers, p. 43-66.

69. Buscopan is given

(a) Prior to barium study (b) After barium study
(c) During barium study (d) Can be given any time

Ans. (a). Radiological Procedures, S.K. Bhargava & Sumeet Bhargava, 2nd ed., Pee Pee Publishers, p. 43-66.

70. Generally, ____amount of high density low viscosity barium is given in barium meal procedure.

(a) 100–150 ml (b) 200 ml
(c) 50 ml (d) 50–100 ml

Ans. (a). Radiological Procedures, S.K. Bhargava & Sumeet Bhargava, 2nd ed., Pee Pee Publishers, p. 43-66.

71. Which investigation will be done in case of Crohn's disease?

(a) BMFT (b) Barium meal
(c) Barium swallow (d) Barium enema

Ans. (a). Radiological Procedures, S.K. Bhargava & Sumeet Bhargava, 2nd ed., Pee Pee Publishers, p. 43-66.

72. Which one is a indication of BMFT?

(a) Unexplained hematuria (b) Heart burn
(c) Malabsorption (d) Colonic obstruction

Ans. (c). Radiological Procedures, S.K. Bhargava & Sumeet Bhargava, 2nd ed., Pee Pee Publishers, p. 43-66.

73. Paralytic ileus is the contraindication of

(a) Barium swallow (b) Barium meal
(c) BMFT (d) Barium enema

Ans. (c). Radiological Procedures, S.K. Bhargava & Sumeet Bhargava, 2nd ed., Pee Pee Publishers, p. 43-66.

74. Which barium suspension is used in BMFT?

(a) 100% w/v (b) 150% w/v
(c) 50–60% w/v (d) 220% w/v

Ans. (c). Radiological Procedures, S.K. Bhargava & Sumeet Bhargava, 2nd ed., Pee Pee Publishers, p. 43-66.

75. Prior to GIT study, colon should be cleaned by

(a) Castor oil (b) Buscopan
(c) Purgative (d) Barium suspension

Ans. (c). *Radiological Procedures, S.K. Bhargava & Sumeet Bhargava, 2nd ed., Pee Pee Publishers, p. 43-66.*

76. Peroral pneumocolon is done

(a) Before the BMFT (b) During the BMFT
(c) At the end of BMFT (d) None of the above

Ans. (c). *Radiological Procedures, S.K. Bhargava & Sumeet Bhargava, 2nd ed., Pee Pee Publishers, p. 43-66.*

77. In which condition Ryle's tube is used?

(a) In perforated patient (b) Hypersensitive to contrast
(c) Asthamatic patient (d) Old age patient

Ans. (a). *Radiological Procedures, S.K. Bhargava & Sumeet Bhargava, 2nd ed., Pee Pee Publishers, p. 43-66.*

78. Feathery appearance is shown in

(a) Duodenum (b) Ileum
(c) Jejunum (d) Colon

Ans. (c). *Radiological Procedures, S.K. Bhargava & Sumeet Bhargava, 2nd ed., Pee Pee Publishers, p. 43-66.*

79. Length of small intestine is approximately

(a) 5–6 metres (b) 1–4 metres
(c) 6–7 metres (d) 10–12 metres

Ans. (c). *Radiological Procedures, S.K. Bhargava & Sumeet Bhargava, 2nd ed., Pee Pee Publishers, p. 43-66.*

80. Which one is not an indication of enteroclysis?

(a) Crohn's disease (b) Meckel's diverticulum
(c) Malabsorption (d) Paralytic ileus

Ans. (d). *Radiological Procedures, S.K. Bhargava & Sumeet Bhargava, 2nd ed., Pee Pee Publishers, p. 43-66.*

81. In enteroclysis, which tube is used?

(a) Ryle's tube (b) Bilbao-Dotter tube
(c) Catheter (d) None of the above

Ans. (b). *Radiological Procedures, S.K. Bhargava & Sumeet Bhargava, 2nd ed., Pee Pee Publishers, p. 43-66.*

82. Bilbao Dotter tube is

(a) 22 F and 150 cm long (b) 18 F and 150 cm long

(c) 20 F and 130 cm long (d) 18 F and 130 cm long

Ans. (a). *Radiological Procedures, S.K. Bhargava & Sumeet Bhargava, 2nd ed., Pee Pee Publishers, p. 43-66.*

83. The first modern double contrast medium enema with air insufflation was performed by

(a) Fischer in 1923 (b) Luelin in 1938
(c) Pauter in 1901 (d) Hodd in 1995

Ans. (a). *Radiological Procedures, S.K. Bhargava & Sumeet Bhargava, 2nd ed., Pee Pee Publishers, p. 43-66.*

84. We give 30° cranial angulation to the tube with the patient supine so that pubic symphysis and sacral promentary overlap for the

(a) Pelvic outlet view for rectum.
(b) Pelvic inlet view for rectum.
(c) This view is not done in barium enema.
(d) Both (a) and (b)

Ans. (a). *Radiological Procedures, S.K. Bhargava & Sumeet Bhargava, 2nd ed., Pee Pee Publishers, p. 43-66.*

85. In which modality 'no radiations' are involved?

(a) Virtual colonoscopy (b) CT colonography
(c) MR colonography (d) Barium enema

Ans. (c). *Radiological Procedures, S.K. Bhargava & Sumeet Bhargava, 2nd ed., Pee Pee Publishers, p. 43-66.*

EMERGENCY DRUGS

1. Which of the following is not the emergency drug?

(a) Adrenaline (b) Atropine
(c) Buscopan (d) Amphetamine

Ans. (d). *Textbook of Radiology for Residents & Technicians, 5th ed., S.K. Bhargava & Sumeet Bhargava, p. 302-303.*

2. Adrenaline is used in all of the following conditions, except

(a) Cardiac arrest (b) Anaphylactic reaction
(c) Hypertension (d) Cardiac asystole

Ans. (c). *Textbook of Radiology for Residents & Technicians, 5th ed., S.K. Bhargava & Sumeet Bhargava, p. 302-303.*

3. Adrenaline is given by which route

(a) IV only (b) SC only
(c) Orally (d) SC, IM, IV

***Ans. (d).** Textbook of Radiology for Residents & Technicians, 5th ed., S.K. Bhargava & Sumeet Bhargava, p. 302-303.*

4. During CPR, following drugs may be considered except

(a) VT or VF-Lignocaine
(b) Severe bradycardia-atropine
(c) Hypertension-adrenaline
(d) All of the above

***Ans. (c).** Textbook of Radiology for Residents & Technicians, 5th ed., S.K. Bhargava & Sumeet Bhargava, p. 302-303.*

5. Atropine causes

(a) Bradycardia
(b) Tachycardia
(c) Hypertension
(d) None

***Ans. (b).** Textbook of Radiology for Residents & Technicians, 5th ed., S.K. Bhargava & Sumeet Bhargava, p. 302-304.*

6. Atenolol is indicated in

(a) Bradycardia
(b) Post acute MI
(c) Hypotension
(d) All of the above

***Ans. (b).** Textbook of Radiology for Residents & Technicians, 5th ed., S.K. Bhargava & Sumeet Bhargava, p. 302-304.*

7. All of the following are true about atropine except

(a) Pre-anaesthetic medicine
(b) Lessen the degree of A-V block
(c) Overcome the severe carotid sinus reflex
(d) Decrease the heart rate

***Ans. (d).** Textbook of Radiology for Residents & Technicians, 5th ed., S.K. Bhargava & Sumeet Bhargava, p. 302-304.*

8. True statement is

(a) Nitroglycerine is indicated in angina pectoris
(b) Nitroglycerine increases the myocardial consumption
(c) It is vasoconstrictor
(d) Side effect of nitroglycerine is hypertension

***Ans. (a).** Textbook of Radiology for Residents & Technicians, 5th ed., S.K. Bhargava & Sumeet Bhargava, p. 302-304.*

9. Lignocaine is used as

(a) Antiarrhythmics
(b) Anaesthetics
(c) Both
(d) None

***Ans. (b).** Textbook of Radiology for Residents & Technicians, 5th ed., S.K. Bhargava & Sumeet Bhargava, p. 302-304.*

10. Dopamine is used for

(a) To treat anaphylaxis
(b) To treat shock
(c) To treat hypertension
(d) To treat asthma

Ans. (b). *Textbook of Radiology for Residents & Technicians, 5th ed., S.K. Bhargava & Sumeet Bhargava, p. 302-304.*

11. Drugs used in anaphylactic reaction are all except

(a) Adrenaline
(b) Hydrocortisone
(c) Antihistaminic
(d) Atenolol

Ans. (d). *Textbook of Radiology for Residents & Technicians, 5th ed., S.K. Bhargava & Sumeet Bhargava, p. 302-304.*

12. True about diphenhydramine

(a) It is antihistaminic drug
(b) Used in the treatment of allergic reaction
(c) Used in cardiac block
(d) Both (a) and (b)

Ans. (d). *Textbook of Radiology for Residents & Technicians, 5th ed., S.K. Bhargava & Sumeet Bhargava, p. 302-304.*

13. 1st step in CPR is

(a) Circulation maintenance
(b) Airways clearance
(c) Breathing management
(d) BP monitoring

Ans. (b). *Textbook of Radiology for Residents & Technicians, 5th ed., S.K. Bhargava & Sumeet Bhargava, p. 327-333.*

14. Salbutamol is used in

(a) Bronchial asthma
(b) Hypotension
(c) Cardiac arrest
(d) Shock

Ans. (a). *Textbook of Radiology for Residents & Technicians, 5th ed., S.K. Bhargava & Sumeet Bhargava, p. 302-304.*

CONTRAST MEDIA

HOCM (High Osmolar Contrast Media); LOCM (Low Osmolar Contrast Media)

1. Iohexol is

(a) Ionic monomer
(b) Non-ionic monomer
(c) Ionic dimer
(d) Non-ionic dimer

Ans. (b). *Textbook of Radiology for Residents & Technicians, 5th ed., S.K. Bhargava & Sumeet Bhargava, p. 298-326.*

2. Monomer of the iodinated contrast media contains how many atoms of iodine

(a) 1 atom (b) 2 atoms
(c) 3 atoms (d) 4 atoms

Ans. (c). *Textbook of Radiology for Residents & Technicians, 5th ed., S.K. Bhargava & Sumeet Bhargava, p. 298-326.*

3. Characteristic of the iodinated contrast media are

(a) Very hydrophilic (b) Low lipid solubility
(c) Low binding affinity to protein (d) All of the above

Ans. (d). *Textbook of Radiology for Residents & Technicians, 5th ed., S.K. Bhargava & Sumeet Bhargava, p. 298-326.*

4. Which of the following is HOCM?

(a) Diatrizoate (b) Iohexol
(c) Iopamidol (d) All

Ans. (a). *Textbook of Radiology for Residents & Technicians, 5th ed., S.K. Bhargava & Sumeet Bhargava, p. 298-326.*

5. IV contrast media are predominantly excreted by

(a) Glomerular filtration by kidney
(b) Tubular secretion by kidney
(c) Intestine
(d) Liver

Ans. (a). *Textbook of Radiology for Residents & Technicians, 5th ed., S.K. Bhargava & Sumeet Bhargava, p. 298-326.*

6. Atomic weight of iodine used for contrast media is

(a) 125 (b) 127
(c) 53 (d) 55

Ans. (b). *Textbook of Radiology for Residents & Technicians, 5th ed., S.K. Bhargava & Sumeet Bhargava, p. 298-326.*

7. These are the salts consisting of a sodium or meglumine cation

(a) Ionic monomers (b) Ionic dimers
(c) Non-ionic monomers (d) Non-ionic dimers

Ans. (a). *Textbook of Radiology for Residents & Technicians, 5th ed., S.K. Bhargava & Sumeet Bhargava, p. 298-326.*

8. Iodine in contrast media is attached to benzoic acid at

(a) 1, 2, 3 positions (b) 2, 4, 6 positions
(c) 1, 3, 5 positions (d) 1, 4, 6 positions

Ans. (b). *Textbook of Radiology for Residents & Technicians, 5th ed., S.K. Bhargava & Sumeet Bhargava, p. 298-326.*

9. Ionic particle ratio of ionic monomers (i.e. conventional contrast media) is

(a) 3:1 (b) 3:2
(c) 6:1 (d) 6:2

Ans. (b). *Textbook of Radiology for Residents & Technicians, 5th ed., S.K. Bhargava & Sumeet Bhargava, p. 298-326.*

10. In ionic contrast media, the iodine acts as

(a) Cation (b) Anion
(c) Both (d) None

Ans. (b). *Textbook of Radiology for Residents & Technicians, 5th ed., S.K. Bhargava & Sumeet Bhargava, p. 298-326.*

11. Urografin which is commonly used for IVU study is

(a) Ionic monomers (b) Nonionic monomers
(c) Ionic dimers (d) None

Ans. (a). *Textbook of Radiology for Residents & Technicians, 5th ed., S.K. Bhargava & Sumeet Bhargava, p. 298-326.*

12. Radio-opacity is dependant on the

(a) Iodine concentration
(b) Number of the particles in solute
(c) Both
(d) None

Ans. (a). *Textbook of Radiology for Residents & Technicians, 5th ed., S.K. Bhargava & Sumeet Bhargava, p. 298-326.*

13. Which of the following is ionic dimer?

(a) Urografin (b) Hexabrix
(c) Omnipaque (d) Angiografin

Ans. (b). *Textbook of Radiology for Residents & Technicians, 5th ed., S.K. Bhargava & Sumeet Bhargava, p. 298-326.*

14. Contrast media used for myelography are

(a) Ionic (b) Non-ionic
(c) Water soluble (d) None

Ans. (b). *Textbook of Radiology for Residents & Technicians, 5th ed., S.K. Bhargava & Sumeet Bhargava, p. 298-326.*

15. Contrast media used in cerebral angiography contains

(a) Sodium cation (b) Meglumine cation
(c) Both (d) None

Ans. (b). *Textbook of Radiology for Residents & Technicians, 5th ed., S.K. Bhargava & Sumeet Bhargava, p. 298-326.*

16. Idiosyncratic anaphylactic reactions to the iodinated contrast media usually begins

(a) During or immediately after injection of contrast media
(b) 30 mts. after injection
(c) Next morning
(d) After 5 days

Ans. (a). *Textbook of Radiology for Residents & Technicians, 5th ed., S.K. Bhargava & Sumeet Bhargava, p. 298-326.*

17. Idiosyncratic anaphylactoid reactions to iodinated contrast media is

(a) Dose dependent
(b) Dose independent
(c) Sometimes dependant and sometimes not
(d) None

Ans. (b). *Textbook of Radiology for Residents & Technicians, 5th ed., S.K. Bhargava & Sumeet Bhargava, p. 298-326.*

18. Adverse drug reaction to IV injection of iodinated contrast media is more common for

(a) HOCM
(b) LOCM
(c) Does not depend upon osmolality
(d) None

Ans. (a). *Textbook of Radiology for Residents & Technicians, 5th ed., S.K. Bhargava & Sumeet Bhargava, p. 298-326.*

19. Safest contrast media from the following is

(a) Hexabrix (b) Urografin
(c) Omnipaque (Iohexol) (d) Angiografin

Ans. (c). *Textbook of Radiology for Residents & Technicians, 5th ed., S.K. Bhargava & Sumeet Bhargava, p. 298-326.*

20. Contrast media of the choice for Myelography is

(a) Urografin (b) Conray
(c) Iohexol (d) Biligrafin

Ans. (c). *Textbook of Radiology for Residents & Technicians, 5th ed., S.K. Bhargava & Sumeet Bhargava, p. 298-326.*

21. Which of the following is MOST prone to causing contrast reactions?

(a) Non-ionic monomers (b) Non-ionic dimers
(c) Ionic monomers (d) Ionic dimer

Ans. (c). *Textbook of Radiology for Residents & Technicians, 5th ed., S.K. Bhargava & Sumeet Bhargava, p. 298-326.*

22. Which of the following statement is false?
- (a) Non-ionic contrast media are safer than ionic contrast media
- (b) Reaction rates are proportional to the amount of iodine administered
- (c) The adverse drug reaction from HOCM and LOCM is about the same
- (d) Osmolality does not depend upon on iodine concentration

Ans. (c). *Textbook of Radiology for Residents & Technicians, 5th ed., S.K. Bhargava & Sumeet Bhargava, p. 298-326.*

23. Regarding non-anaphylactoid reactions, which is true?
- (a) Chemotoxic reactions are more common with non-ionic contrast media
- (b) Chemotoxic reactions can cause cardiac arrhythmias
- (c) Vasovagal reactions cause tachycardia and hypotension
- (d) Reaction always present in either anaphylactoid or non-anaphylactoid forms

Ans. (b). *Textbook of Radiology for Residents & Technicians, 5th ed., S.K. Bhargava & Sumeet Bhargava, p. 298-326.*

24. Which of the following is not associated with risk of contrast reactions?
- (a) Renal failure
- (b) LRTI (Low Respiratory Tract Infection)
- (c) Heart failure
- (d) Use of metformin in diabetic patients

Ans. (b). *Textbook of Radiology for Residents & Technicians, 5th ed., S.K. Bhargava & Sumeet Bhargava, p. 298-326.*

25. A patient experiences convulsions after receiving contrast. What would you do?
- (a) Call the emergency medical team
- (b) Check the pulse, start an intravenous line and call the emergency medical team
- (c) Maintain a patent airway, monitor the vital signs, call the emergency medical team, start an intravenous route
- (d) Panic

Ans. (c). *Textbook of Radiology for Residents & Technicians, 5th ed., S.K. Bhargava & Sumeet Bhargava, p. 298-326.*

26. A patient has a decreased heart rate and low blood pressure. Which is wrong?

(a) The effect is caused by vagal stimulation
(b) Treatment options include β-blockers
(c) Treatment option includes atropine
(d) Treatment option include the head low positions

Ans. (b). *Textbook of Radiology for Residents & Technicians, 5th ed., S.K. Bhargava & Sumeet Bhargava, p. 298-326.*

27. Which of the following statement is false?

(a) Most reactions occur about 20 mts. after contrast administration
(b) The mortality rate from HOCM and LOCM is about the same
(c) Patients with various metabolic and hematological disorders is a risk factor for ADR
(d) None

Ans. (a). *Textbook of Radiology for Residents & Technicians, 5th ed., S.K. Bhargava & Sumeet Bhargava, p. 298-326.*

28. Which of the following is true regarding contrast media in pregnancy and breast feeding?

(a) Contrast agents do not cross the placenta and are safe in pregnancy
(b) Breast feeding should be withheld for 5 days after contrast examination
(c) Iodinated contrast agents can cause thyroid disorders in the fetus and newborn
(d) Iodinated contrast agents are absolutely contraindicated in pregnancy

Ans. (c). *Textbook of Radiology for Residents & Technicians, 5th ed., S.K. Bhargava & Sumeet Bhargava, p. 298-326.*

29. Which of the following statement about delayed reaction is true?

(a) More frequent with the LOCM than HOCM
(b) More frequent with dimers than monomers
(c) Both (a) and (b)
(d) None of these

Ans. (c). *Textbook of Radiology for Residents & Technicians, 5th ed., S.K. Bhargava & Sumeet Bhargava, p. 298-326.*

30. Which of the following statement about prevention of contrast reaction is/are true?

(a) Avoid contrast study in old age
(b) Avoid study in patient with coronary artery disease
(c) Diazepam should be used to sedate the patient
(d) All of the above

Ans. (d). *Textbook of Radiology for Residents & Technicians, 5th ed., S.K. Bhargava & Sumeet Bhargava, p. 298-326.*

31. Which of the following is true about treatment of anaphylactic reaction?

(a) Dose of adrenaline is 0.5 ml (1 : 100) SC
(b) Dose of adrenaline is 0.5 ml (1 : 1000) IM
(c) Tracheotomy may be required
(d) All of the above

Ans. (d). *Textbook of Radiology for Residents & Technicians, 5th ed., S.K. Bhargava & Sumeet Bhargava, p. 298-326.*

32. False statement about treatment of cardiac arrest is

(a) CPR should be done
(b) Clear the airways constantly
(c) Continuous cardiac monitoring
(d) Intubation is not required

Ans. (d). *Textbook of Radiology for Residents & Technicians, 5th ed., S.K. Bhargava & Sumeet Bhargava, p. 298-326.*

33. Peak nephrogram in IVU is delayed with

(a) HOCM
(b) LOCM
(c) Not effected by osmolality
(d) Both HOCM and LOCM

Ans. (b). *Textbook of Radiology for Residents & Technicians, 5th ed., S.K. Bhargava & Sumeet Bhargava, p. 298-326.*

34. Which of the following statement is false?

(a) Distension of pelvicalyceal system is less with LOCM than with HOCM
(b) Abdominal compression is more important when non-ionic agents are used
(c) Urinary Iodine content is higher with LOCM than HOCM
(d) LOCM produces a larger osmotic dieresis than HOC

Ans. (d). *Textbook of Radiology for Residents & Technicians, 5th ed., S.K. Bhargava & Sumeet Bhargava, p. 298-326.*

35. Which contrast media are more expensive?

(a) Ionic
(b) Non-ionic
(c) No difference in cost
(d) Gastrografin

Ans. (b). *Textbook of Radiology for Residents & Technicians, 5th ed., S.K. Bhargava & Sumeet Bhargava, p. 298-326.*

36. All of the following procedures demonstrate renal function, except

(a) I.V.P.
(b) Infusion pyelography
(c) Renal scintigraphy
(d) Retrograde pyelography

Ans. (d). *Textbook of Radiology for Residents & Technicians, 5th ed., S.K. Bhargava & Sumeet Bhargava, p. 260.*

37. K-shell binding energy of iodine is _______.

(a) 37.3 (b) 33.7
(c) 19.1 (d) 23.9

Ans. (b). Radiological Procedures, S.K. Bhargava & Sumeet Bhargava, 2nd ed., Pee Pee Publishers, p. 25-42.

38. What is the reason for the outstanding contrast obtained by iodinated contrast agents?

(a) Maximizing the coherent scattering interaction
(b) Non-toxic
(c) Very high K-shell binding energy (73.9)
(d) Maximizing the photoelectric interaction

Ans. (d). Radiological Procedures, S.K. Bhargava & Sumeet Bhargava, 2nd ed., Pee Pee Publishers, p. 25-42.

39. The side chain in non-ionic contrast agents are

(a) Short
(b) Long
(c) Shorter than ionic contrast agent
(d) Equal to ionic contrast agent

Ans. (b). Radiological Procedures, S.K. Bhargava & Sumeet Bhargava, 2nd ed., Pee Pee Publishers, p. 25-42.

40. Iodine has an atomic number of

(a) 37 (b) 53
(c) 74 (d) 24

Ans. (b). Radiological Procedures, S.K. Bhargava & Sumeet Bhargava, 2nd ed., Pee Pee Publishers, p. 25-42.

41. Sodium or meglumine acts as a

(a) Cation
(b) Electrolytes
(c) Anion
(d) Both (b) and (c)

Ans. (a). Radiological Procedures, S.K. Bhargava & Sumeet Bhargava, 2nd ed., Pee Pee Publishers, p. 25-42.

42. Urografin 76% contains

(a) Meglumine diatrizoate 52% + sodium diatrizoate 24%
(b) Meglumine diatrizoate 66% + sodium diatrizoate 10%
(c) Meglumine diatrizoate 70 % + sodium diatrizoate 6%
(d) Meglumine diatrizoate 76% + sodium diatrizoate 0%

Ans. (b). Radiological Procedures, S.K. Bhargava & Sumeet Bhargava, 2nd ed., Pee Pee Publishers, p. 25-42.

43. Urografin 60% contains

(a) Meglumine diatrizoate 30% + sodium diatrizoate 30%
(b) Meglumine diatrizoate 40% + sodium diatrizoate 20%
(c) Meglumine diatrizoate 52% + sodium diatrizoate 8%
(d) Meglumine diatrizoate 60% + sodium diatrizoate 0%

Ans. (c). *Radiological Procedures, S.K. Bhargava & Sumeet Bhargava, 2nd ed., Pee Pee Publishers, p. 25-42.*

44. Currently commercially available ionic monomers include

(a) Iotrolan (b) Iohexol
(c) Iopamidol (d) Urografin

Ans. (d). *Radiological Procedures, S.K. Bhargava & Sumeet Bhargava, 2nd ed., Pee Pee Publishers, p. 25-42.*

45. Gadodiamide is a contrast media which is used in

(a) X-rays (b) CT
(c) MRI (d) USG

Ans. (c). *Radiological Procedures, S.K. Bhargava & Sumeet Bhargava, 2nd ed., Pee Pee Publishers, p. 25-42.*

46. What is the diameter of microbubbles in current generation of US?

(a) 1–5 micrometre (b) 3–9 nanometre
(c) 12–16 picometre (d) 2–3 centimetre

Ans. (a). *Radiological Procedures, S.K. Bhargava & Sumeet Bhargava, 2nd ed., Pee Pee Publishers, p. 25-42.*

47. Levovist, sonovist are the examples of

(a) X-ray contrast agent (b) MRI contrast agent
(c) CT contrast agent (d) USG contrast agent

Ans. (d). *Radiological Procedures, S.K. Bhargava & Sumeet Bhargava, 2nd ed., Pee Pee Publishers, p. 25-42.*

48. Levovist has been developed by

(a) Schering AG (b) Mallincnodt Inc
(c) Raymond (d) Petre Pedigrue

Ans. (b). *Radiological Procedures, S.K. Bhargava & Sumeet Bhargava, 2nd ed., Pee Pee Publishers, p. 25-42.*

49. Shell stabilizers and gases used in levovist are respectively

(a) Galactose and O_2 (b) Galactose and CO_2
(c) Galactose and air (d) Air and galactose

Ans. (c). *Radiological Procedures, S.K. Bhargava & Sumeet Bhargava, 2nd ed., Pee Pee Publishers, p. 25-42.*

50. Shell stabilizer used in sonovist is

(a) Galactose
(b) Palmitic acid
(c) Cyanoacrylate
(d) No need of stabilizer

Ans. (c). *Radiological Procedures, S.K. Bhargava & Sumeet Bhargava, 2nd ed., Pee Pee Publishers, p. 25-42.*

51. Which one is a T1 relaxation agent?

(a) GD-HP-DO3A
(b) SPIO
(c) GD-DTPA
(d) (a) and (c)

Ans. (d). *Radiological Procedures, S.K. Bhargava & Sumeet Bhargava, 2nd ed., Pee Pee Publishers, p. 25-42.*

52. Which of the following was the first US contrast agents?

(a) Echovist
(b) Levovist
(c) Cavisomes
(d) PFOB

Ans. (a). *Radiological Procedures, S.K. Bhargava & Sumeet Bhargava, 2nd ed., Pee Pee Publishers, p. 25-42.*

53. Gadolinium chelates produce

(a) T1 shortening effects
(b) T2 shortening effects
(c) Both (a) and (b)
(d) None of the above

Ans. (c). *Radiological Procedures, S.K. Bhargava & Sumeet Bhargava, 2nd ed., Pee Pee Publishers, p. 25-42.*

CHAPTER

8

Nuclear Medicine and Radiotherapy

1. **Nuclear medicine**
   (a) The field involving the clinical use of sealed radionuclides.
   (b) The field involving the clinical use of non-sealed radionuclides.
   (c) The field involving the non-ionizing radiations.
   (d) A branch in which ionizing radiation is used to treat malignant diseases.

   Ans. (b). *Textbook of Radiology for Residents & Technicians, 5th ed., S.K. Bhargava & Sumeet Bhargava, p. 486-515.*

2. **How many artificial radionuclides are as on date?**
   (a) 114 (b) 3900
   (c) 18000 (d) 2500

   Ans. (d). *Textbook of Radiology for Residents & Technicians, 5th ed., S.K. Bhargava & Sumeet Bhargava, p. 486-515.*

3. **^{99m}Tc is obtained from**
   (a) ^{99}Mo (b) ^{67}Ga
   (c) ^{111}In (d) ^{125}I

   Ans. (a). *Textbook of Radiology for Residents & Technicians, 5th ed., S.K. Bhargava & Sumeet Bhargava, p. 486-515.*

4. **Which radionuclide is an ideal radionuclide and accounts for over 70% in nuclear imaging?**
   (a) ^{131}I (b) ^{99}Mo
   (c) ^{99m}Tc (d) ^{201}Ti

   Ans. (c). *Textbook of Radiology for Residents & Technicians, 5th ed., S.K. Bhargava & Sumeet Bhargava, p. 486-515.*

5. ^{99m}Tc has a half-life of

(a) 128 days (b) 2.5 hr
(c) 6 hr (d) 2 days

Ans. (c). *Textbook of Radiology for Residents & Technicians, 5th ed., S.K. Bhargava & Sumeet Bhargava, p. 486-515.*

6. ^{99m}Tc release _____ gamma rays.

(a) 50% (b) 88%
(c) 95% (d) 99%

Ans. (b). *Textbook of Radiology for Residents & Technicians, 5th ed., S.K. Bhargava & Sumeet Bhargava, p. 486-515.*

7. Iodine has a half life of

(a) 6 hr (b) 8.06 days
(c) 128 days (d) 23 hr

Ans. (b). *Textbook of Radiology for Residents & Technicians, 5th ed., S.K. Bhargava & Sumeet Bhargava, p. 486-515.*

8. Iodine decays by

(a) Electron capture (b) Isomeric transition
(c) Beta emission (d) Alpha emission

Ans. (c). *Textbook of Radiology for Residents & Technicians, 5th ed., S.K. Bhargava & Sumeet Bhargava, p. 486-515.*

9. Iodine gives a whole body dose of

(a) 0.2 to 0.6 mrad/mCi (b) 0.5 to 3.5 rad/mCi
(c) 2 to 4.8 rad/mCi (d) 7 to 12 rad/mCi

Ans. (b). *Textbook of Radiology for Residents & Technicians, 5th ed., S.K. Bhargava & Sumeet Bhargava, p. 486-515.*

10. The time required for a radionuclide to decay to half of its original activity is known as

(a) Decay constant (b) Half life
(c) Curie (d) Activity

Ans. (b). *Textbook of Radiology for Residents & Technicians, 5th ed., S.K. Bhargava & Sumeet Bhargava, p. 486-515.*

11. The relation between the effective biological and physical half life is

(a) $T_e = T_b + T_{1/2}$ (b) $T_e = T^2_b + T^2_{1/2}$
(c) $1/T_e = 1/T_b + 1/T_{1/2}$ (d) $T_e^2 = T_b + T_{1/2}$

Ans. (c). *Textbook of Radiology for Residents & Technicians, 5th ed., S.K. Bhargava & Sumeet Bhargava, p. 486-515.*

12. The detector efficiency is expressed in

(a) Efficiency = number of photons detected × number of photons emitted
(b) Efficiency = number of photons detected / number of photons emitted
(c) Efficiency = √ number of photons detected / √ number of photons emitted
(d) Efficiency = number of photons emitted / number of photons detected

***Ans.* (*b*).** *Textbook of Radiology for Residents & Technicians, 5th ed., S.K. Bhargava & Sumeet Bhargava, p. 486-515.*

13. In technetium generator ________ is passed through the column to remove (elute) Tc^{99m}.

(a) weak HCl (0.2%)
(b) strong NaOH (0.2%)
(c) isotonic saline (0.9%)
(d) distilled water

***Ans.* (*c*).** *Textbook of Radiology for Residents & Technicians, 5th ed., S.K. Bhargava & Sumeet Bhargava, p. 486-515.*

14. Which of the following is used in PET?

(a) NaI:Tl
(b) $Bi_4Ge_3O_{12}$
(c) $CaWO_4$
(d) Xenon

***Ans.* (*b*).** *Textbook of Radiology for Residents & Technicians, 5th ed., S.K. Bhargava & Sumeet Bhargava, p. 486-515.*

15. The atomic number of bismuth is

(a) 83
(b) 4
(c) 74
(d) 131

***Ans.* (*a*).** *Textbook of Radiology for Residents & Technicians, 5th ed., S.K. Bhargava & Sumeet Bhargava, p. 486-515.*

16. PMT supply

(a) 150–250 volts power
(b) 350–800 volts power
(c) 800–1200 volts power
(d) 1200–1800 volts power

***Ans.* (*c*).** *Textbook of Radiology for Residents & Technicians, 5th ed., S.K. Bhargava & Sumeet Bhargava, p. 486-515.*

17. In MCA, when the acquisition of a spectrum begins, the entire channel is set to

(a) Zero
(b) Negative
(c) Positive
(d) None of the above

***Ans.* (*a*).** *Textbook of Radiology for Residents & Technicians, 5th ed., S.K. Bhargava & Sumeet Bhargava, p. 486-515.*

18. DTPA

(a) Di Triamine Penta Amine acid
(b) Diethylene Triamine Penta Acetic acid
(c) Dicyclo Tetraamine Penta Acetic acid
(d) None of the above

Ans. (b). *Textbook of Radiology for Residents & Technicians, 5th ed., S.K. Bhargava & Sumeet Bhargava, p. 486-515.*

19. Radioiodine is used for

(a) Liver scanning
(b) Bone scanning
(c) Thyroid scanning
(d) Lung scanning

Ans. (c). *Textbook of Radiology for Residents & Technicians, 5th ed., S.K. Bhargava & Sumeet Bhargava, p. 486-515.*

20. Radioiodine-labelled hippuran is used to evaluate

(a) Thyroid function
(b) Kidney function
(c) Heart function
(d) Liver function

Ans. (b). *Textbook of Radiology for Residents & Technicians, 5th ed., S.K. Bhargava & Sumeet Bhargava, p. 486-515.*

21. For lung perfusion imaging, which of the following is used?

(a) Cr-51
(b) In-111
(c) Ga-67
(d) Xe-133

Ans. (d). *Textbook of Radiology for Residents & Technicians, 5th ed., S.K. Bhargava & Sumeet Bhargava, p. 486-515.*

22. Gamma scintillation camera was developed by

(a) Macovski
(b) Hookes
(c) Dandy Walker
(d) Haloanger

Ans. (d). *Textbook of Radiology for Residents & Technicians, 5th ed., S.K. Bhargava & Sumeet Bhargava, p. 486-515.*

23. Which of the following is not a radiopharmaceutical localization mechanism?

(a) Diffusion
(b) Phagocytosis
(c) Capillary blockage
(d) Elution

Ans. (d). *Textbook of Radiology for Residents & Technicians, 5th ed., S.K. Bhargava & Sumeet Bhargava, p. 486-515.*

24. PET scanners detect

(a) Positron of the same energy in coincidence.
(b) Positrons and electrons in coincidence.
(c) Photons of different energies in coincidence.
(d) Annihilation photons in coincidence.

Ans. (d). *Textbook of Radiology for Residents & Technicians, 5th ed., S.K. Bhargava & Sumeet Bhargava, p. 626-631.*

25. The best radionuclide spatial resolution is normally achieved by using

(a) SPECT (b) High resolution collimator
(c) PET (d) High sensitivity collimator

Ans. (c). *Textbook of Radiology for Residents & Technicians, 5th ed., S.K. Bhargava & Sumeet Bhargava, p. 626-631.*

26. In which year gamma camera was developed?

(a) 1914 (b) 1950
(c) 1976 (d) 1984

Ans. (b). *Textbook of Radiology for Residents & Technicians, 5th ed., S.K. Bhargava & Sumeet Bhargava, p. 486-515.*

27. NaI crystals are coupled with

(a) PHA (b) SCA
(c) ADC (d) PMT

Ans. (d). *Textbook of Radiology for Residents & Technicians, 5th ed., S.K. Bhargava & Sumeet Bhargava, p. 486-515.*

28. Why crystals and PMT are coupled together?

(a) To reduce patient dose.
(b) To reduce geometric unsharpness.
(c) To decrease artifact.
(d) To improve light transmittance.

Ans. (d). *Textbook of Radiology for Residents & Technicians, 5th ed., S.K. Bhargava & Sumeet Bhargava, p. 486-515.*

29. In SPECT, which of the following collimators is used?

(a) Converging collimator (b) Diverging collimator
(c) Parallel collimator (d) Fan beam collimator

Ans. (d). *Textbook of Radiology for Residents & Technicians, 5th ed., S.K. Bhargava & Sumeet Bhargava, p. 486-515.*

30. Positron annihilation produces two photons of energy

(a) 104 keV (b) 232 keV
(c) 511 keV (d) 1022 keV

Ans. (c). *Textbook of Radiology for Residents & Technicians, 5th ed., S.K. Bhargava & Sumeet Bhargava, p. 486-515.*

31. ACD

(a) Analog to Digital Converter
(b) Annihilation Coincidence Detection

(c) Automatic Converter Device
(d) Direct Amplitude Converter

Ans. ***(b).*** *Textbook of Radiology for Residents & Technicians, 5th ed., S.K. Bhargava & Sumeet Bhargava, p. 486-515.*

32. Which of the following radiopharmaceuticals is used in PET for metabolism study?

(a) ^{13}N
(b) ^{18}F
(c) ^{15}O
(d) ^{11}C

Ans. ***(b).*** *Textbook of Radiology for Residents & Technicians, 5th ed., S.K. Bhargava & Sumeet Bhargava, p. 626-631.*

33. The major limitation of PET is

(a) More radiation to patient
(b) More sensitive to humidity
(c) The large cost of building
(d) All of the above

Ans. ***(c).*** *Textbook of Radiology for Residents & Technicians, 5th ed., S.K. Bhargava & Sumeet Bhargava, p. 626-631.*

RADIOTHERAPY

34. Radiation therapy is a branch of medicine in which

(a) Non-ionizing radiations are used to treat malignant diseases.
(b) Ionizing radiations are used to treat malignant diseases.
(c) Non-sealed radionuclides are used.
(d) None of the above

Ans. ***(b).*** *Textbook of Radiology for Residents & Technicians, 5th ed., S.K. Bhargava & Sumeet Bhargava, p. 537-577.*

35. Grenz-ray therapy is mainly used for

(a) Deep therapy
(b) Internal therapy
(c) Extremities conditions
(d) Dermatological conditions

Ans. ***(d).*** *Textbook of Radiology for Residents & Technicians, 5th ed., S.K. Bhargava & Sumeet Bhargava, p. 537-577.*

36. Grenz-ray therapy provides

(a) Soft X-rays
(b) Hard X-rays
(c) Very hard X-rays
(d) All of the above

Ans. ***(a).*** *Textbook of Radiology for Residents & Technicians, 5th ed., S.K. Bhargava & Sumeet Bhargava, p. 537-577.*

37. Superficial therapy unit is operated at _____ potential.

(a) 50–150 kV_p
(b) 20–30 kV_p
(c) 150–250 kV_p
(d) 250–500 kV_p

Ans. *(a). Textbook of Radiology for Residents & Technicians, 5th ed., S.K. Bhargava & Sumeet Bhargava, p. 537-577.*

38. X-ray machines, which are operated at a potential of 150–500 kV_p are known as

(a) Simulator (b) Telecobalt
(c) Orthovoltage unit (d) Kilovoltage unit

Ans. *(c). Textbook of Radiology for Residents & Technicians, 5th ed., S.K. Bhargava & Sumeet Bhargava, p. 537-577.*

39. Orthovoltage unit is also known as

(a) Simulator (b) Deep therapy units
(c) Kilovoltage unit (d) Telecobalt unit

Ans. *(b). Textbook of Radiology for Residents & Technicians, 5th ed., S.K. Bhargava & Sumeet Bhargava, p. 537-577.*

40. In deep therapy X-ray tube, when the filament is heated, _______ are emitted.

(a) Positron (b) Electron
(c) Neutron (d) All of the above

Ans. *(b). Textbook of Radiology for Residents & Technicians, 5th ed., S.K. Bhargava & Sumeet Bhargava, p. 537-577.*

41. To achieve proper cooling the entire X-ray tube should be

(a) Used at low potential (b) Placed in coal place
(c) Used one day in a week (d) Immersed in oil

Ans. *(d). Textbook of Radiology for Residents & Technicians, 5th ed., S.K. Bhargava & Sumeet Bhargava, p. 537-577.*

42. The leakage radiation at 1 metre from the centre of the source must be less than

(a) 0.0013 mR/hr (b) 0.5 mR/hr
(c) 0.89 mR/hr (d) 2 mR/hr

Ans. *(d). Textbook of Radiology for Residents & Technicians, 5th ed., S.K. Bhargava & Sumeet Bhargava, p. 537-577.*

43. The shielding materials should have

(a) Low atomic number
(b) High atomic number
(c) Maximum unpaired number of electrons
(d) Maximum thickness

Ans. *(b). Textbook of Radiology for Residents & Technicians, 5th ed., S.K. Bhargava & Sumeet Bhargava, p. 537-577.*

44. Collimators is a device, which

(a) Brings the source in the front of an opening.
(b) Is used to control size and shape of the beam.
(c) Is used to absorb scatter and secondary radiation.
(d) All of the above

***Ans. (b).** Textbook of Radiology for Residents & Technicians, 5th ed., S.K. Bhargava & Sumeet Bhargava, p. 537-577.*

45. Collimator is made-up of

(a) Aluminium (b) Lead
(c) Tungsten (d) Nickle

***Ans. (c).** Textbook of Radiology for Residents & Technicians, 5th ed., S.K. Bhargava & Sumeet Bhargava, p. 537-577.*

46. The first LINAC was designed in

(a) 1930 (b) 1928
(c) 1989 (d) 1978

***Ans. (b).** Textbook of Radiology for Residents & Technicians, 5th ed., S.K. Bhargava & Sumeet Bhargava, p. 537-577.*

47. A set of isodose curve is known as

(a) Scatter air ratio (b) Tissue phantom ratio
(c) Isodose chart (d) Isodose family

***Ans. (c).** Textbook of Radiology for Residents & Technicians, 5th ed., S.K. Bhargava & Sumeet Bhargava, p. 537-577.*

48. The aim of treatment planning is

(a) To deliver optimum uniform dose to the target volume.
(b) To deliver optimum uniform dose to the treated volume.
(c) To deliver optimum uniform dose to the normal volume.
(d) All of the above

***Ans. (a).** Textbook of Radiology for Residents & Technicians, 5th ed., S.K. Bhargava & Sumeet Bhargava, p. 537-577.*

49. Low melting alloy is also known as

(a) Weak metal (b) Phantom
(c) Lipowitz metal (d) None of the above

***Ans. (c).** Textbook of Radiology for Residents & Technicians, 5th ed., S.K. Bhargava & Sumeet Bhargava, p. 537-577.*

50. Lipowitz material consists of

1. Bismuth 2. Lead
3. Tin 4. Cadmium

(a) 1, 2 (b) 1, 3
(c) 1, 4 (d) 1, 2, 3, 4

Ans. (d). *Textbook of Radiology for Residents & Technicians, 5th ed., S.K. Bhargava & Sumeet Bhargava, p. 537-577.*

51. Cesium-137 has a half-life of

(a) 5.6 years (b) 30 years
(c) 73.8 days (d) 2.7 days

Ans. (b). *Textbook of Radiology for Residents & Technicians, 5th ed., S.K. Bhargava & Sumeet Bhargava, p. 537-577.*

52. LDR

(a) Local Distance Ratio (b) Low Dose Rate
(c) Less Dose Recorder (d) None of the above

Ans. (b). *Textbook of Radiology for Residents & Technicians, 5th ed., S.K. Bhargava & Sumeet Bhargava, p. 537-577.*

53. Telecobalt therapy units are performed in

(a) A half shielded room (b) A full shielded room
(c) A partial shielded room (d) No need for shielded room

Ans. (b). *Textbook of Radiology for Residents & Technicians, 5th ed., S.K. Bhargava & Sumeet Bhargava, p. 537-577.*

54. Which of the following methods is usually used to calculate treatment time?

(a) Percentage depth dose (b) Tissue air ratio
(c) Back scatter factor (d) Scatter air ratio

Ans. (a). *Textbook of Radiology for Residents & Technicians, 5th ed., S.K. Bhargava & Sumeet Bhargava, p. 537-577.*

CHAPTER

9

Dental Radiology

1. Intraoral radiography is

(a) Bitewing radiography (b) Periapical radiography
(c) Occlusal radiography (d) All of the above

Ans. (d). *Clark's Positioning in Radiography, 12th Edition, p. 279-331.*

2. Periapical radiography view demonstrates

(a) Crowns of the teeth of the premolar and molar region.
(b) Root of the tooth and the surrounding bone.
(c) Occlusal plane.
(d) All of the above

Ans. (b). *Clark's Positioning in Radiography, 12th Edition, p. 279-331.*

3. The deciduous dentition comprises

(a) 18 teeth (b) 20 teeth
(c) 28 teeth (d) 32 teeth

Ans. (b). *Clark's Positioning in Radiography, 12th Edition, p. 279-331.*

4. The part of the tooth that projects above the gingiva (gum) are

(a) Root (b) Apex
(c) Crown (d) Canal

Ans. (c). *Clark's Positioning in Radiography, 12th Edition, p. 279-331.*

5. The part of the tooth that is embedded within the jaw is known as

(a) Root (b) Apex

(c) Crown (d) Canal

Ans. (a). Clark's Positioning in Radiography, 12th Edition, p. 279-331.

6. **The outer surface of the crown of the tooth is**
(a) Gum (b) Enamel
(c) Calcium-coated layer (d) None of the above

Ans. (b). Clark's Positioning in Radiography, 12th Edition, p. 279-331.

7. **_______ covers the dentine of the root.**
(a) Enamel (b) Connective tissue
(c) Cementum (d) Hydroxyapatite

Ans. (c). Clark's Positioning in Radiography, 12th Edition, p. 279-331.

8. **Which teeth are single-rooted?**
(a) Canine (b) Pre-molar
(c) Molar (d) All of the above

Ans. (a). Clark's Positioning in Radiography, 12th Edition, p. 279-331.

9. **Dental formulas for permanent teeth are**
(a) 2122 / 2122 (b) 2103 / 2123
(c) 2123 / 2123 (d) 2023 / 2023

Ans. (c). Clark's Positioning in Radiography, 12th Edition, p. 279-331.

10. **Dental formulas for deciduous teeth are**
(a) 2123 / 2123 (b) 2102 / 2102
(c) 2120 / 2120 (d) 2122 / 2122

Ans. (b). Clark's Positioning in Radiography, 12th Edition, p. 279-331.

11. **Intraoral films are**
(a) Single emulsion (b) Double emulsion
(c) Both can be used (d) None of the above

Ans. (b). Clark's Positioning in Radiography, 12th Edition, p. 279-331.

12. **IOPA**
(a) Intraoral Para Apex (b) Intraoral Peri Apical
(c) Interoral Para Align (d) Interoral Peri Apical

Ans. (b). Clark's Positioning in Radiography, 12th Edition, p. 279-331.

13. The paralleling technique using the extension cone, compared with the bisecting angle technique, involves
(a) Greater vertical angulation.
(b) Greater object to the film distance.
(c) Shorter developing time.
(d) Shorter anode to the film distance.

Ans. (b). *Clark's Positioning in Radiography, 12th Edition, p. 279-331.*

14. Image magnifications may be mineralized by
(a) Using a long cone.
(b) Using a short cone.
(c) Placing the film as far away from the tooth as possible.
(d) Shortening the exposure time.

Ans. (a). *Clark's Positioning in Radiography, 12th Edition, p. 279-331.*

15. Which tooth has the longest root?
(a) Mandibular canine
(b) Maxillary first premolar
(c) Maxillary canine
(d) Maxillary central

Ans. (c). *Clark's Positioning in Radiography, 12th Edition, p. 279-331.*

CHAPTER

10

Peadiatric Radiography

1. The first textbook of pediatric radiology is an/a

(a) American textbook (b) Indian textbook
(c) British textbook (d) Canadian textbook

Ans. (a). *Textbook of Radiology for Residents & Technicians, 5th ed., S.K. Bhargava & Sumeet Bhargava, p. 516-529.*

2. The first textbook of pediatric radiology was published in

(a) 1935 (b) 1918
(c) 1910 (d) 1896

Ans. (c). *Textbook of Radiology for Residents & Technicians, 5th ed., S.K. Bhargava & Sumeet Bhargava, p. 516-529.*

3. The name of first textbook of pediatric radiology is

(a) The Roentgen method in pediatrics
(b) The positioning of pediatrics
(c) The pediatrics method of Roentgen
(d) The procedure of pediatric

Ans. (a). *Textbook of Radiology for Residents & Technicians, 5th ed., S.K. Bhargava & Sumeet Bhargava, p. 516-529.*

4. Pediatric X-ray diagnosis was published by

(a) John Cattey (b) Thomas M. Rotch
(c) W.C. Roentgen (d) None of these

Ans. (a). *Textbook of Radiology for Residents & Technicians, 5th ed., S.K. Bhargava & Sumeet Bhargava, p. 516-529.*

5. Correct exposure factors should be set on the X-ray machine

(a) After positioning of child (b) Before positioning of child

(c) During positioning of child (d) None of the above

Ans. (b). *Textbook of Radiology for Residents & Technicians, 5th ed., S.K. Bhargava & Sumeet Bhargava, p. 516-529.*

6. **Generators used in pediatric radiography should be**
   (a) High milliampere (800–1000 mA)
   (b) Low milliampere (50 mA)
   (c) Medium milliampere (300–500 mA)
   (d) In any ampere we can use

   Ans. (a). *Textbook of Radiology for Residents & Technicians, 5th ed., S.K. Bhargava & Sumeet Bhargava, p. 516-529.*

7. **In neonates and young infants (< 2 years) radiography should be done**
   (a) With grid
   (b) Without grid
   (c) Grid used only in abdoman and pelvis examination
   (d) Grid used only in chest radiography

   Ans. (b). *Textbook of Radiology for Residents & Technicians, 5th ed., S.K. Bhargava & Sumeet Bhargava, p. 516-529.*

8. **What is the grid ratio for general pediatric radiology?**
   (a) 16 : 1 (b) 12 : 1
   (c) 8 : 1 (d) 4 : 1

   Ans. (c). *Textbook of Radiology for Residents & Technicians, 5th ed., S.K. Bhargava & Sumeet Bhargava, p. 516-529.*

9. **Plastic cassettes are used in pediatric radiography because**
   (a) These are light, so easy to handle.
   (b) These are colourful, so looking attractive.
   (c) Warmer to the touch than metal cassette.
   (d) Cheap and easily available.

   Ans. (c). *Textbook of Radiology for Residents & Technicians, 5th ed., S.K. Bhargava & Sumeet Bhargava, p. 516-529.*

10. **Which type of film screen combination is used in pediatric radiography?**
    (a) Rare earth fast screen film combination.
    (b) Rare earth slow screen film combination.
    (c) Conventional (calcium tungstate) fast screen film combination.
    (d) Conventional (calcium tungstate) slow screen film combination.

    Ans. (a). *Textbook of Radiology for Residents & Technicians, 5th ed., S.K. Bhargava & Sumeet Bhargava, p. 516-529.*

11. Pigg-O-Stat device is used when

(a) Child is in supine position.
(b) Child is in lateral or prone position.
(c) Child is in upright erect position.
(d) Child is in any position.

Ans. (c). *Textbook of Radiology for Residents & Technicians, 5th ed., S.K. Bhargava & Sumeet Bhargava, p. 516-529.*

12. What should be worn by technologist when entering the neonatal intensive care unit?

(a) Should wear lead apron.
(b) Should wear gown.
(c) Should wear white apron.
(d) Should wear formal dress.

Ans. (b). *Textbook of Radiology for Residents & Technicians, 5th ed., S.K. Bhargava & Sumeet Bhargava, p. 516-529.*

CHAPTER

11

Interventional Radiology

1. Who described a method of arterial access that uses a catheter and makes surgery of vessels unnecessary?

(a) Judkin
(b) Sven Ivar Seldinger
(c) Robert Richard
(d) Elbert Seldinger

Ans. (b). *Textbook of Radiology for Residents & Technicians, 5th ed., S.K. Bhargava & Sumeet Bhargava, p. 481-485.*

2. In which year interventional technology was introduced?

(a) 1901
(b) 1953
(c) 1988
(d) 1935

Ans. (b). *Textbook of Radiology for Residents & Technicians, 5th ed., S.K. Bhargava & Sumeet Bhargava, p. 481-485.*

3. Catheters can be classified depending on

(a) Side holes
(b) Sizes
(c) Shapes
(d) All of the above

Ans. (d). *Textbook of Radiology for Residents & Technicians, 5th ed., S.K. Bhargava & Sumeet Bhargava, p. 296-299.*

4. Advantage of having side holes is that

(a) They increase the rate at which the contrast medium can be injected.
(b) They minimize the dissection of the artery.
(c) They maximize the jet effect of the injection.
(d) All of the above

Ans. (a). *Textbook of Radiology for Residents & Technicians, 5th ed., S.K. Bhargava & Sumeet Bhargava, p. 296-299.*

5. Why modern catheters are made-up of polyethylene plastic?

(a) Cheaper
(b) Easily available
(c) Obtain better torque
(d) Available in wide sizes

Ans. (c). *Textbook of Radiology for Residents & Technicians, 5th ed., S.K. Bhargava & Sumeet Bhargava, p. 296-299.*

6. Catheters intended principally for abdominal use are usually ______ in length.

(a) 60–80 cm
(b) 100–140 cm
(c) 150–180 cm
(d) 15–30 cm

Ans. (a). *Textbook of Radiology for Residents & Technicians, 5th ed., S.K. Bhargava & Sumeet Bhargava, p. 296-299.*

7. The catheter's size is numbered in

(a) French
(b) Inchs
(c) Millimetres
(d) Feet

Ans. (a). *Textbook of Radiology for Residents & Technicians, 5th ed., S.K. Bhargava & Sumeet Bhargava, p. 296-299.*

8. In ventricles and arch of aorta only _______ catheter should be used.

(a) Straight catheters
(b) Cobra catheters
(c) Pigtail catheters
(d) Side winder catheters

Ans. (c). *Textbook of Radiology for Residents & Technicians, 5th ed., S.K. Bhargava & Sumeet Bhargava, p. 296-299.*

9. ______________ is mainly used for coronary angiogram.

(a) Judkin's catheter
(b) Simmon's catheter
(c) Stepherd hook stick catheter
(d) Caged balloon catheter

Ans. (a). *Textbook of Radiology for Residents & Technicians, 5th ed., S.K. Bhargava & Sumeet Bhargava, p. 296-299.*

10. Guide wires are made-up of

(a) Polyethylene
(b) Stainless steel
(c) Polymer
(d) Plastic

Ans. (b). *Textbook of Radiology for Residents & Technicians, 5th ed., S.K. Bhargava & Sumeet Bhargava, p. 296-299.*

11. The coating on guide wires is usually done by which material?

(a) Nylon
(b) Teflon
(c) Polyethylene
(d) None of the above

Ans. (b). *Textbook of Radiology for Residents & Technicians, 5th ed., S.K. Bhargava & Sumeet Bhargava, p. 296-299.*

12. ________ catheters are used in angioplasty.

(a) Straight
(b) Judkin
(c) Balloon
(d) J-shaped

Ans. (c). *Textbook of Radiology for Residents & Technicians, 5th ed., S.K. Bhargava & Sumeet Bhargava, p. 296-299.*

13. Guide wire allows

(a) Safe introduction of catheter into vessel.
(b) Safe introduction of catheter into muscular region.
(c) Safe introduction of catheter into oral cavity.
(d) All of the above

Ans. (a). *Textbook of Radiology for Residents & Technicians, 5th ed., S.K. Bhargava & Sumeet Bhargava, p. 296-299.*

CHAPTER

12

Quality Assurance

1. The general criteria of standard of quality are set by the ________.

(a) AERB
(b) ACR
(c) AAPM
(d) All of the above

Ans. (d). *Textbook of Radiological Safety, 1st Edition, p. 119-134.*

2. Which of the following parameters affects the image quality?

(a) kV_p
(b) mA and sec
(c) Focal spot size
(d) All of the above

Ans. (d). *Textbook of Radiological Safety, 1st Edition, p. 119-134.*

3. FFD

(a) Filter to Focal Distance
(b) Focus to Film Distance
(c) Filter to Film Distance
(d) Focus to Floor Distance

Ans. (b). *Textbook of Radiological Safety, 1st Edition, p. 119-134.*

4. Which of the following test tools is used for testing the "congruence of optical and radiation fields"?

(a) kV_p meter
(b) Beam alignment test tool
(c) Focal spot test tool
(d) Collimator test tool

Ans. (d). *Textbook of Radiological Safety, 1st Edition, p. 119-134.*

5. Collimator test tools are made of

(a) Plastic
(b) Fibre glass
(c) Tungsten plate
(d) Molybdenum

Ans. (b). *Textbook of Radiological Safety, 1st Edition, p. 119-134.*

6. **In "congruence of optical and radiation fields" focus to film distance (FFD) is kept at**
   (a) 75 cm (b) 100 cm
   (c) 120 cm (d) 180 cm

   Ans. ***(b).*** *Textbook of Radiological Safety, 1st Edition, p. 119-134.*

7. **What is the suitable kV_p and mAs factor for congruence of radiation and optical field practical?**
   (a) 40 kV_p, 0–4 mAs
   (b) 40–50 kV_p, 50 mAs
   (c) 50–55 kV_p, 10–12 mAs
   (d) 70–80 kV_p, 90–110 mAs

   Ans. ***(c).*** *Textbook of Radiological Safety, 1st Edition, p. 119-134.*

8. **The beam alignment can be tested by using a**
   (a) Collimator test tool
   (b) Spinning top test tool
   (c) Measuring meter test tool
   (d) Beam alignment test tool

   Ans. ***(d).*** *Textbook of Radiological Safety, 1st Edition, p. 119-134.*

9. **The ability for resolving the smallest size of the image in a radiograph depends on the**
   (a) Focal spot size (b) Beam alignment
   (c) Screen (d) All of the above

   Ans. ***(a).*** *Textbook of Radiological Safety, 1st Edition, p. 119-134.*

10. **In focal spot test tool the spacing between two lines is**
    (a) 0.84 LP/mm to 5.6 LP/mm (b) 5 LP/mm to 7 LP/mm
    (c) 7 LP/mm to 10 LP/mm (d) 10 LP/mm to 14 LP/mm

    Ans. ***(a).*** *Textbook of Radiological Safety, 1st Edition, p. 119-134.*

11. **Which one of the following test tools is used for testing the tube voltage?**
    (a) Pocket dosimeter (b) kV_p meter
    (c) Voltmeter (d) Spinning top test tool

    Ans. ***(b).*** *Textbook of Radiological Safety, 1st Edition, p. 119-134.*

12. **ADC**
    (a) Auto Digital Counter
    (b) Analog Digital Circuit
    (c) Auto Direct Converter
    (d) None of the above

    Ans. ***(b).*** *Textbook of Radiological Safety, 1st Edition, p. 119-134.*

13. Which of the following test tools is used to test the timer of the X-ray unit?

(a) Spinning top test tool (b) Collimator test tool

(c) Filter (d) kV_p meter

Ans. (a). *Textbook of Radiological Safety, 1st Edition, p. 119-134.*

14. The coefficient of linearity should not exceed_____.

(a) 0.1 (b) 0.001

(c) 0.1×10^{-8} (d) $0.10 \times 10^{+8}$

Ans. (a). *Textbook of Radiological Safety, 1st Edition, p. 119-134.*